Eat Like a Girl

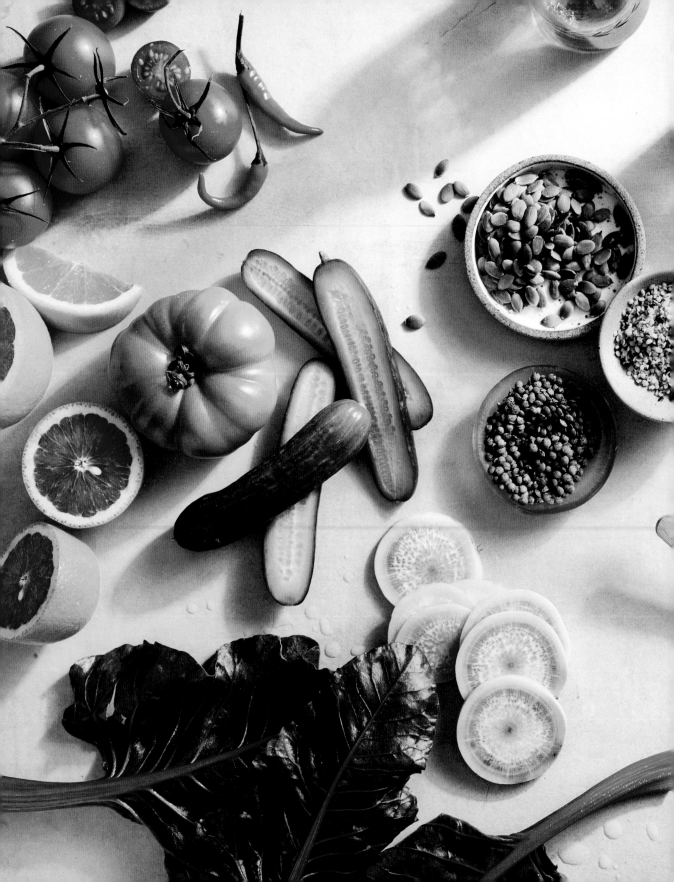

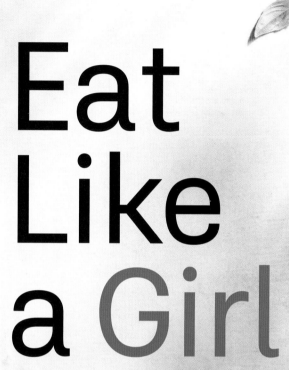
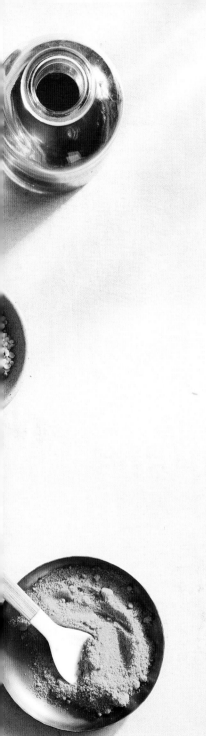

Eat
Like
a Girl

100+ DELICIOUS RECIPES TO BALANCE HORMONES, BOOST ENERGY, AND BURN FAT

Dr. Mindy Pelz

HAY HOUSE LLC

CARLSBAD, CALIFORNIA • NEW YORK CITY
LONDON • SYDNEY • NEW DELHI

Copyright © 2024 by Mindy Pelz

Published in the United States by: Hay House LLC:
www.hayhouse.com®
Published in Australia by: Hay House Australia
Publishing Pty Ltd: www.hayhouse.com.au
Published in the United Kingdom by: Hay House
UK Ltd: www.hayhouse.co.uk
Published in India by: Hay House Publishers (India)
Pvt Ltd: www.hayhouse.co.in

Composition: David Van Ness
Interior/cover photos: Erin Kunkel
Additional photography: Laura Grier (page 101),
Michelle Magdalena Maddox (page 102)
Illustrations: Mark Oehlschlager, Marisol Godinez
Indexer: Kay Banning

Produced by One+One Books

Cataloging-in-Publication Data is on file at the Library of Congress

Hardcover ISBN: 978-1-4019-7944-7
E-book ISBN: 978-1-4019-7945-4
Audiobook ISBN: 978-1-4019-7946-1

10 9 8 7 6 5 4 3 2 1

1st edition, October 2024

Printed in Canada

This product uses responsibly sourced papers and/or recycled materials. For more information see www.hayhouse.com.

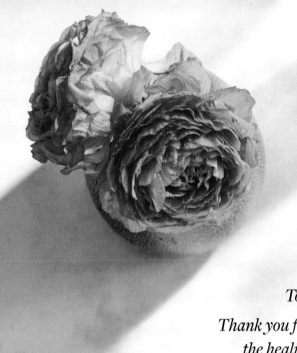

To my mom:

*Thank you for teaching me about
the healing power of food.*

Forever grateful.

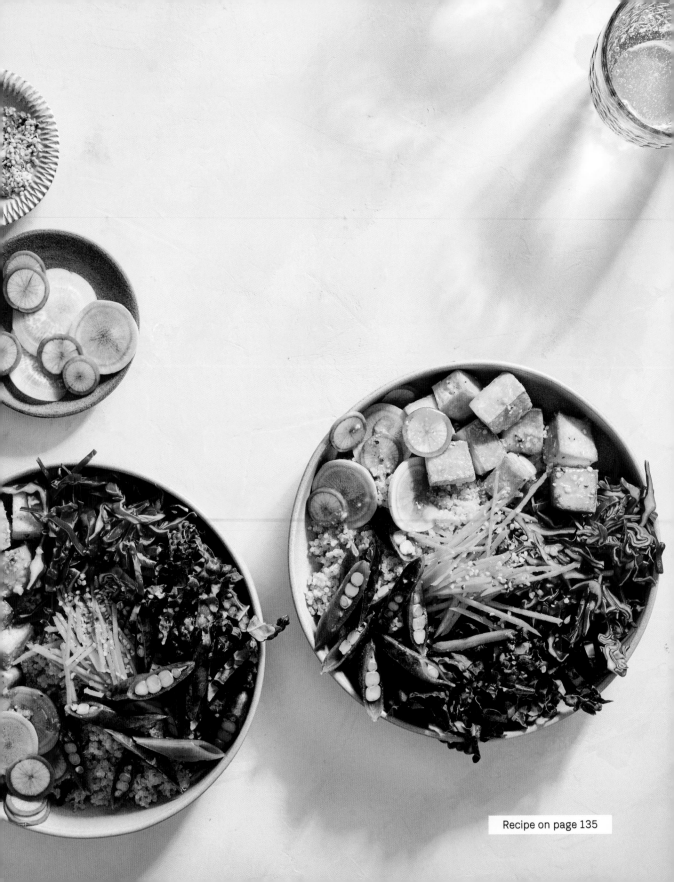

Recipe on page 135

CONTENTS

LETTER FROM DR. MINDY

DEAR READER, When you start to understand the natural rhythms of the feminine body, you will see all aspects of your life differently. Much like you, I spent most of my years building lifestyle tools like a man. I never stopped to ask myself *What does my feminine body need?* When I hit my perimenopause years and my hormones went on a wild ride, I changed that. I started building a lifestyle toolbox that ebbed and flowed with my hormones. A huge part of this new lifestyle was honoring rest. I dramatically changed my perception of grit. Pushing through the tough times in life is no doubt an important skill to have, but for the female body, when stress becomes constant and overwhelming, we need to pause to recover and recalibrate.

This book has been a collaboration of many powerful, successful women and one powerhouse man who is incredibly skilled at supporting women. These are women who know grit very well—women who have trained themselves to push through the tough times and used fierce passion and persistence to reach epic heights in their careers. As strong as these women are, unusual life circumstances can still bring them to their knees. Life moments that tug so deeply on the heart that it's impossible to push through. While writing this book, with deadlines staring us in the face, several of us were reminded of our feminine humanity. Life got turbulent—extremely turbulent. Long-term relationships abruptly ended, dear family members died, and aging parents needed to be immediately tended to. Painful moments that required a drop-everything approach to handle what stood in front of us.

In a patriarchal world that often forces us to persevere through these very human moments, I chose to handle them differently. I wanted to make sure that this book was written with the heart of a girl. That meant allowing these life moments to unfold at a rhythm that gave space for healing. As several members of my team, including me, dealt with these immediate life traumas, my patriarchally conditioned brain kept screaming at me to suck it up and push through. Yet I knew that was incongruent with our feminine bodies. Bodies that would say *Pause the pain, so the compounding stress doesn't destroy us.* So that's what we did. It caused deadlines to be pushed back, even at the possible sacrifice of getting this book out to you. But ultimately, it offered an incredible opportunity to create a new paradigm of performance. Perhaps a softer, more nurturing, matriarchal approach to a project—an approach our world so desperately needs.

As I was describing the life obstacles that kept unfolding for my book team to my husband, he pointed out, "Well, I guess you are writing this book in true *like a girl* fashion." His comment pierced me. He was exactly right. Production at any cost is incredibly expensive for the female body.

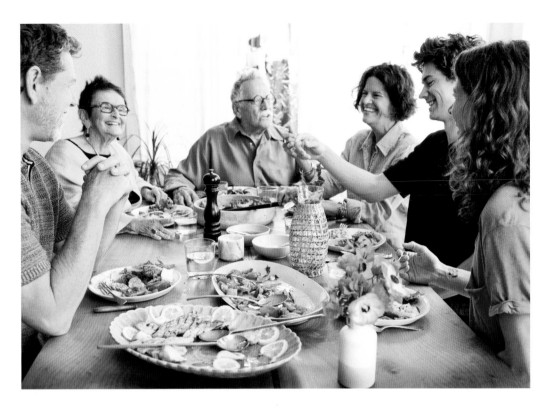

As we all learn to co-regulate our hormones together in this incredibly dysregulated world, I hope this story and what you learn in this book give you the permission to pause when life comes crashing down. As women, we sit in a unique moment in time. As our bodies are screaming *Rest!* at us, we have an opportunity to slow down and listen. In doing so, every food and fasting principle you discover in this book will work more effortlessly for you.

It's with great honor I bring you *Eat Like a Girl*. A heartfelt book brought to you by a group of women and one man who stayed true to living like a girl. I hope that, in these pages, you too find your natural female rhythm. That you learn how to live like a girl, giving yourself permission to courageously rest when life demands it. You deserve to live in a body you love—a healthy, happy, vibrant body that lives congruently with your hormonal wisdom.

Much love,

Dr. Mindy

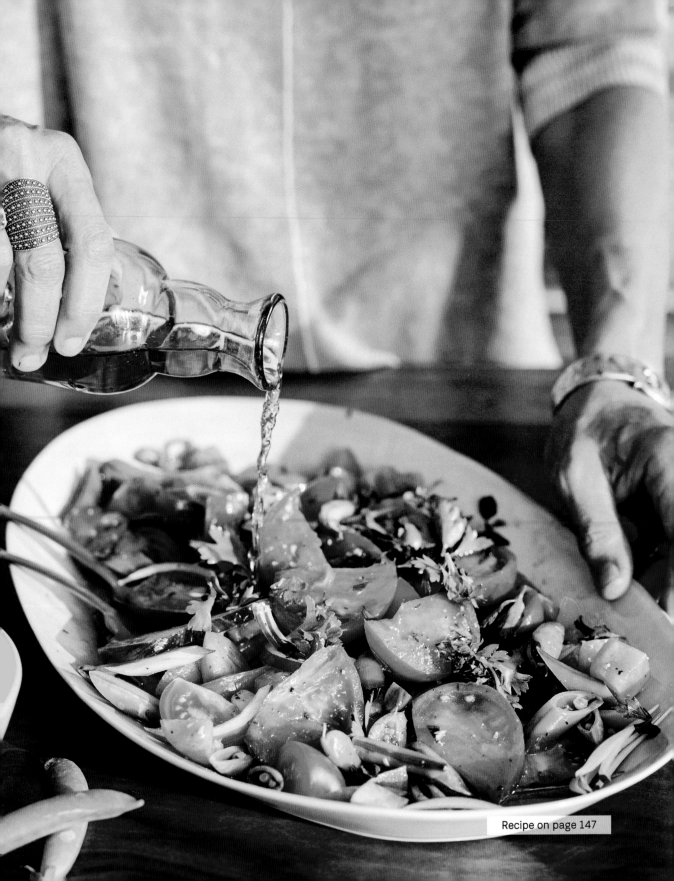

Recipe on page 147

INTRODUCTION

WHEN *FAST LIKE A GIRL* launched into the world at the end of 2022, never in my wildest dreams did I imagine the impact it would make on women all over the world. I knew that fasting held the key to unlocking profound health benefits. I had spent years immersed in the research and interpreting how it applied to women. I had witnessed firsthand the transformative results fasting provided. In my heart, I knew that if women truly understood how the body heals in the fasted state, we would not only end the massive metabolic mess that plagues so many, but women would finally have a free tool they could use to heal themselves.

Women became fired up after reading the book. A movement of empowered women began to emerge. Although my original intention was to give women a fasting manual that was unique to their bodies, I quickly discovered that they were deeply longing to understand their bodies. Women have also been desperately searching for simple, easy-to-apply, no-cost lifestyle tools that finally give them results for their growing hormonal challenges.

It's interesting because when you talk to many doctors, they will tell you that their patients won't make lifestyle changes to help pull them out of a health crisis. That's not been my experience. In both my practice and from the millions of comments we've received on my socials over the years, women want lifestyle answers. They are exhausted from being gaslighted in their doctor's office. They don't want another pill to cure their symptoms. They don't want to be told there is nothing they can do about their health situation. They are fed up with the roller-coaster ride of hopping on and off trendy diets. They want to be heard. They are ready to do the work. And they are looking for clear science-backed lifestyle solutions to put them back in control of their health.

I am so honored to be on the frontlines, witnessing these newly empowered women emerging from the ashes of a healthcare system that has not listened to their cries. Women all over the world are standing up and asking what does health look like for their unique bodies. These newly empowered women want to do health a woman's way. We are amid an epic moment in history where these inspiring women are cracking open a new health paradigm, one that will benefit many generations to come. I am so proud to be a part of this beautiful unfolding.

Yet, as full as my heart has been watching the world embrace *Fast Like a Girl*, we still have so much more work to do. Women's healthcare is at a crossroads. On one side of the equation, women are opening their eyes to the fact that our traditional healthcare system has been offering a one-size-fits-all formula—a formula that doesn't honor the hormonal rhythm of our female bodies. In this awakening, women are boldly standing up and demanding better solutions from their doctors—healthcare answers that are unique to the feminine body. The old-school health paradigm begins to break apart when we ask the simple question "How does this apply to a woman's body?" Whether it's a new health trend, a diet fad, a promising biohack, or a prescription handed to us by our doctor, the more we demand unique answers, the more we shake the dust off the old healthcare system and create a new one.

On the other side of the healthcare conversation live millions of women who can't find the door out of poor health. Women across the globe are feeling helpless, confused, and out of answers. The path toward health has become needlessly complicated, expensive, and time-consuming. Lifestyle solutions are looked at as mildly effective and rarely offered. Medications are still the primary go-to solution when a woman's health goes awry—a solution that has not even been specifically researched for a woman's body. This ignorance is leaving too many women hating the bodies they are living in. Here's the rub—when a woman feels her body is working against her, she often turns on herself by shaming and guilting herself for doing something wrong. Witnessing the outcry of these women has perhaps tugged on my heart the most. If you are one of them, please know you are not alone. Too many of us feel like we must be doing something wrong that has caused us to suffer within our own skin. We feel inadequate, not enough, and disconnected from our bodies. This mentality is killing us and it needs to stop.

Why do we have to complicate health so much? Health is simple. Our female bodies are always doing the right thing at the right time. Why haven't we been taught how to understand its rhythms? Who is profiting from our disempowerment? Too many of us accept the "There's nothing you can do" answers our healthcare system is providing. We need to bring lifestyle back into the health conversation. It's time to go back to the basics and talk about how our hormones respond to our daily activities, especially those we do repetitively like eating, drinking, sleeping, breathing, and moving.

Every woman deserves an elevated conversation around what exactly is happening with her hormones every month and how we can build a lifestyle that honors those natural rhythms. And when our hormonal cycle changes in our menopausal years, instead of being handed an antidepressant to help us cope, we deserve a conversation about what lifestyle changes we ourselves need to make to smooth the ride. We need to bring *every* woman on this journey back to health with us; no woman should be left behind when it comes to health.

Changing the Course of Women's Health

Empowerment begins with education—we deserve and desperately need in-depth information on how our brilliant bodies work. In *Fast Like a Girl*, I taught you how to create a fasting lifestyle that honors your hormonal rhythms to help you thrive; *Eat Like a Girl* will teach you how to use food to support your body's cyclical nature so that you feel nourished, aligned, and vibrant. For those of you who are familiar with *Fast Like a Girl*, there is so much new and exciting information here for you. And for those of you who are new, welcome! You will easily be able to benefit from what's in this book even if you've never been introduced to my work before. I have summarized many of the principles from *Fast Like a Girl* throughout this book, so you haven't missed out.

We need to stop looking at health as a destination you hopefully will arrive at one day. Health is a continual action. It shouldn't be hard or time-consuming, or cost enormous amounts of money. *Eat Like a Girl* is my attempt to give you a user's manual for your body that will guide you through making smart lifestyle choices around food that support your age-appropriate hormones. Whether you just started your period or your menstrual cycle ended years ago, this book will give you the information you need to use food to love your body again. I often wonder what would be possible if we taught women how to build a lifestyle that matches their hormonal rhythms. Would we see a decline in hormonal cancers, Alzheimer's disease, autoimmune diseases, thyroid challenges, and even the growing menopausal struggles women are facing today? Would we see changes in our collective mental health? Our politics? Our communities? How far could we go if we harness our hormonal superpowers?

FIRING UP YOUR METABOLISM

Before I move into the mechanics of what it looks like to eat like a girl, it's pivotal that you keep in mind that you have two types of metabolism: one that kicks in when you eat food and the other that your body switches over to when you fast. We call the metabolism your body uses when you eat food your *sugar burner system*. I lovingly name your fasting metabolism your *fat burner system*, because the body has to burn fat to create a different fuel source. One reason so many of us have failed at dieting is that we have been trying to control just our sugar burner systems. No one taught us about the fat burner system. The amazing results so many got from *Fast Like a Girl* were largely because women were finally taught how to tap into the fat burner system. Now, keep in mind that the goal of great metabolic health is not to spend most of your time in the fat-burning system; rather, it's to learn the art of switching back and forth between these two systems. This book is going to show you how you can clean up your sugar burner metabolism so that you can metabolically switch effortlessly.

How to Use This Book

This is as much a food book as it is a cookbook. It is a go-to resource to help you navigate your food choices and give your body the nutrients it needs to keep your hormones happy. You are going to learn how each of your sex hormones has slightly different food requirements. Whether you are cycling, have an erratic, unpredictable cycle, or are no longer cycling, I want to take you on a journey of understanding the impact food has on your hormonal health. I also want to highlight what foods are disrupting your hormonal system. The foods you eat are powerful—they can either balance or destroy your hormonal health. Unfortunately, our food system is now filled with convenience items that are laden with hormone-disrupting chemicals. It's time to call these chemicals out.

Once you understand what is destroying your hormones, I want to walk you through all the wonderful ways what you make in your kitchen can balance your hormones. I will introduce you to categories of foods that nourish your hormonal systems. Foods like carbohydrates that our earth has provided us (like fruits and vegetables), plant and animal-based proteins, healthy fats and oils, prebiotic spices, bitter liver-loving vegetables, and fibrous foods that feed the microbes in your gut that break down hormones.

This book is laid out in a unique way—there is nothing traditional about it. When you are shifting paradigms, a different way needs to appear. First, I want to show why so many of the health challenges you are facing are caused by the modern world you live in—a rushing world that is full of fake food, nonstop dopamine hits, and quick-fix promises. Food has become complicated. Ingredients have become toxic. And your taste buds have been hijacked by a food industry that is more interested in profits than health. I want you to understand how to navigate the food world we all find ourselves in now. Then I will dive into the principles of what it means to eat like a girl. Whether you just went through puberty or are entering your menopausal years, you will get to know your glorious hormones and the foods they thrive on. Then I will address many of the questions that arose around food and fasting from readers of *Fast Like a Girl*. Questions like "What can I eat or drink in my fasting window?" or "What breaks a fast?" or "What food is best to break a fast with?" With the help of my celebrity chefs, I have provided you with incredible recipes for fasted snacks and drinks you can have in your fasting window, along with some truly delicious meals to break your fast with that will build muscle and repair your microbiome.

I then move you into the different phases of the fasting cycle, a concept I created that breaks down your menstrual cycle into three phases and teaches you how to eat or fast during each one. Through the lens of this fasting cycle, I will show you what hormones you are building in each phase and what foods best support them.

For my menopausal friends and those of you in your childbearing years who have a missing cycle, don't worry—I didn't leave you out! While you should be sure to read through each phase chapter so you understand your three sex hormones—because you are still producing them even if you do not menstruate!—I wrote an entire chapter that will help you use the principles of the three phases to bring you back into a natural rhythm with your hormones.

I am also excited to include a detailed and expanded layout of the 30-Day Fasting Reset I first shared in *Fast Like a Girl*. This is a 30-day plan that guides you in putting all these principles into place, including menus and resources to help simplify your hormonal journey.

Finally, you'll notice something really special about the recipes in this book: I included both a plant-based and omnivore track. From all the research I have seen, I strongly feel there are benefits to both plant- and animal-based eating. The only diet that I am strongly opposed to is the Standard Western Diet. The one that our food system dishes out. The one that is killing us. With both a plant-based and omnivore track, I am bringing everyone into the food conversation around hormones. You have options based on your personal preferences. I have no doubt you will fall in love with the recipes my chefs have created and understand why I chose them. With each recipe, I include notes about my reasons for picking them.

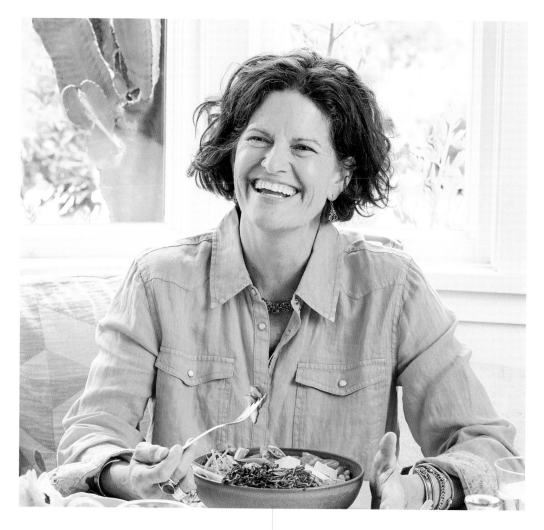

I'm excited to be on this journey with you! Get ready to delve into the nourishing power of food. Within these pages, we celebrate the beautiful feminine body, help you continue on the journey to heal your body through a fasting lifestyle, and dive into the hormone-healing power of food.

Bon appétit, and here's to fueling your journey to hormonal bliss!

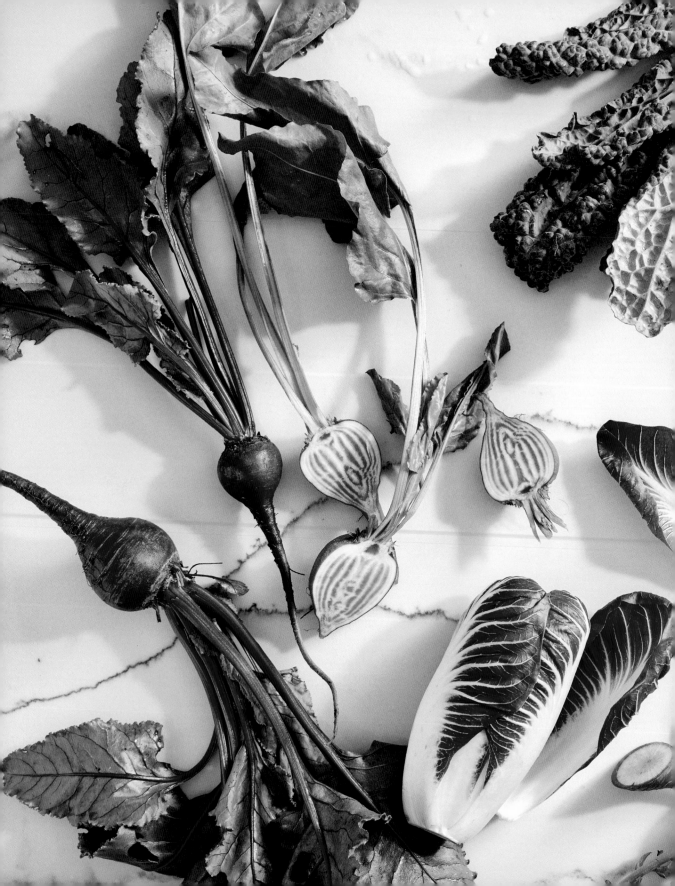

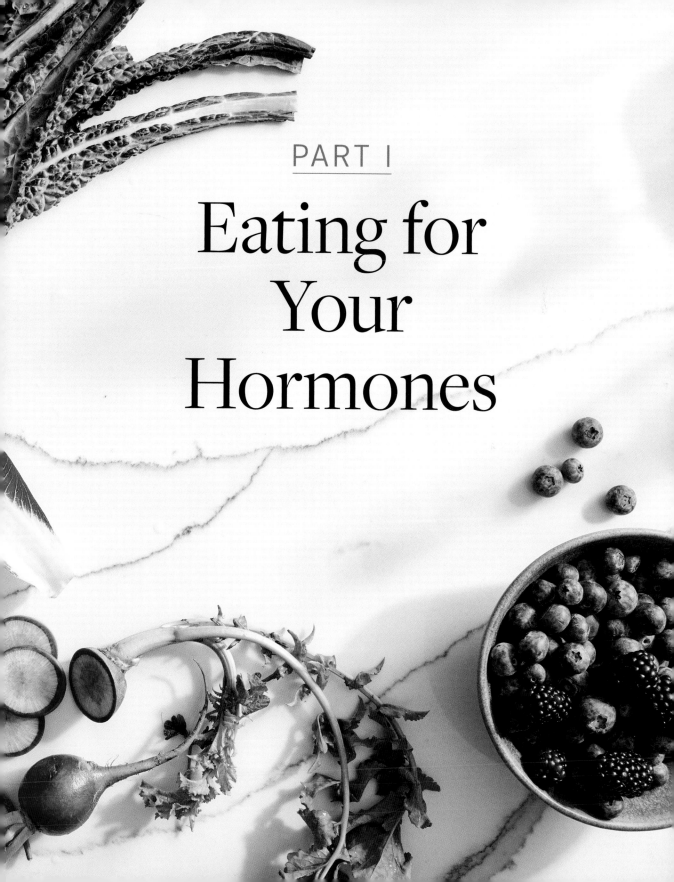

PART I

Eating for Your Hormones

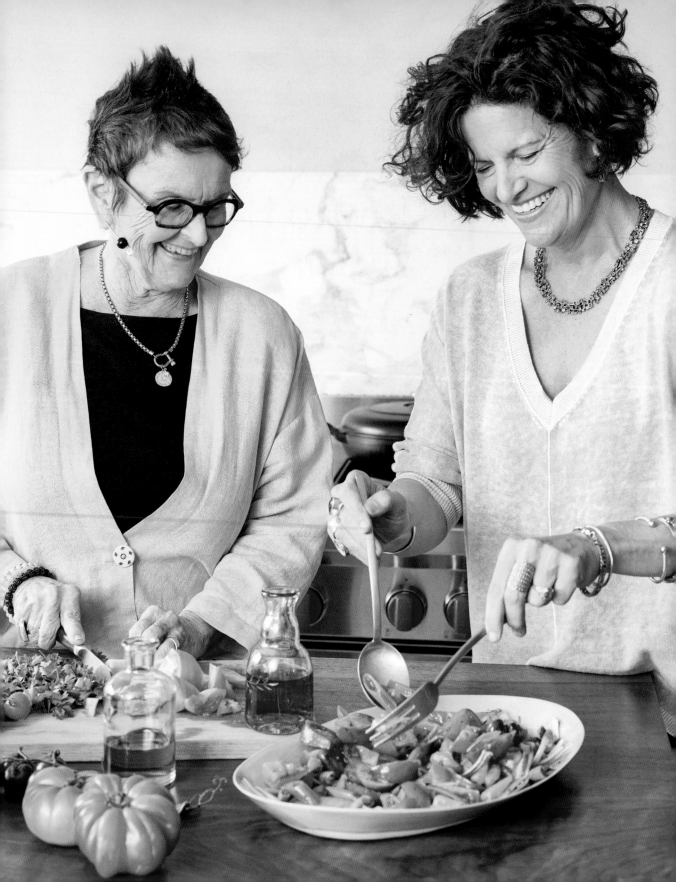

1

How to Eat for Your Hormones

I WAS RAISED BY A MOM who was a health freak. At a time when white bread, TV dinners, Twinkies, sugary cereals, and sodas were the cultural norm, my mom filled our home with healthy, fresh foods that had a short shelf life, didn't require a microwave to heat up, and weren't filled with a long list of ingredients. As grateful as I am now for her approach to food, I remember pleading with her to just make me a "normal" sandwich for my lunch. In the 1970s, that meant a sandwich made with white bread, Skippy peanut butter, and Smucker's grape jam. But she knew better than to succumb to my pleas. She knew how important healthy food is to our growing bodies and brains. A health-food pioneer, she was committed to teaching us the importance of eating chemical-free foods. This meant my lunches were filled with oranges, rice cake sandwiches with natural peanut butter and honey, and string cheese—a far cry from the Twinkies my classmates were getting. As much as I hated my mom's approach, she sent a strong message to my developing brain: The quality of the ingredients in our food matters.

Fast-forward to today's modern world, where food labels and ingredient lists are far beyond what she could have imagined in the 1970s. You practically need a science degree to understand the complexity of the ingredients listed on our nutrition labels. Our food system has become unnecessarily complicated. Ingredient lists are ridiculously long, dangerous chemicals are hidden in misleading buzzwords like *natural flavors*, and ingredients that are scientifically proven hormone disruptors, obesogens, and known carcinogens are allowed to permeate what we eat. The quality of our food has degraded into a package full of toxins, and the metabolic health of our world is collapsing because of it. Obesity rates have skyrocketed, and hormone challenges like polycystic ovary syndrome, infertility, autoimmune conditions, and troubling menopause symptoms have become the norm for women, not the exception. You don't have to look far to see that the female body is struggling amid this massive influx of toxins. Whether you are 15 and just starting your hormonal journey, or 65 and your menstruating years are long behind you, it's time

3

we all learn how to avoid the foods that are destroying our health.

Food and Dysregulation

In so many ways, our female bodies carry the burden of a stressful and toxic world. The patriarchal pace of our culture tells us we're successful only if we're producing, performing, and earning. Our brains are trying to keep up with and absorb an excessive amount of information daily, and during all hours of the day and night, we consume toxic, nutritionally depleted foods that disrupt our natural cycles and cause our health to suffer. Your brilliant body will adapt itself to whatever environment you put yourself in, and unfortunately for the female body, the modern world has offered an unprecedented amount of physical, emotional, and chemical stress.

Much of this chemical stress comes from the food industry and diet culture. The chemicals allowed in our foods have not only hijacked our taste buds but also flipped our metabolic switches for the worse. We are amid a massive food crisis—one that is killing us.

Why are harmful chemicals allowed in our foods? Unfortunately, here in the United States, the joke within the Food and Drug Administration (FDA) is that "the *F* in FDA is silent."[1] This means governmental agencies don't strictly regulate food. The mysterious category of food known as GRAS—generally recognized as safe—is a good example of this. Ingredients are categorized this way when research hasn't been done on their safety. The FDA has an innocent-until-proven-guilty philosophy with ingredients. Unfortunately, it takes years and lots of money to prove an ingredient is damaging to the human body.

Partially hydrogenated oils are the poster child for this. In 2006, this artificial trans fat in food was estimated to cause one in five (up to 250,000) heart attacks and 50,000 deaths a year. Yet it wasn't until 2018, after more than 25 years of advocacy, that the FDA's ban on the use of partially hydrogenated oil (PHO) as a food ingredient went into effect.[2] Why did it take so long to remove this incredibly harmful ingredient? How many people died not knowing that our government was allowing this life-ending ingredient to permeate our everyday foods?

I think of this toxic food stress as a form of dysregulation in our bodies. Toxic foods dysregulate and disrupt your metabolic system, causing you to be insulin-resistant, a state wherein your body produces more glucose that it can use, so it stores it as fat on your belly and in your organs. Your metabolic system is intimately tied to your nervous system; dysregulation there means you are producing too much cortisol, which is a stress hormone. Cortisol signals to your body to become even more insulin-resistant, which then releases extra glucose into your bloodstream. These high levels of glucose and cortisol then dramatically shift your sex hormones into a state of dysregulation. Imbalances in your hormonal system often put you on an emotional roller-coaster that further amplifies your stressed state. Welcome to what I call the dysregulation loop. One system in your body went off course and caused several other systems to follow.

Is it any wonder that so many of us have an internal state of chaos brewing? Our nervous systems are so amped up and frazzled that we can't relax; we've muscled our way through so many trendy diets and workout plans that have destroyed our metabolisms to the point where

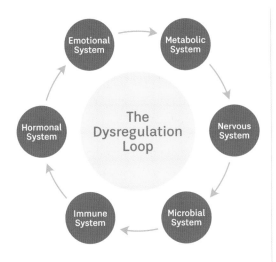

we need drugs to help us lose weight; and we struggle with brain fog, missed periods, tumultuous menopausal symptoms, digestive issues, and so much more. We're battling one hell of a modern-day, humanmade storm.

At the root of this barrage of stressors and the symptoms that accompany them is that our female bodies are out of coherence. We need to build a lifestyle that puts us back in harmony with them. We need to regulate our metabolism so we can also regulate our nervous systems and our sex hormones.

Let's make the interconnectedness of our nervous, metabolic, and hormonal systems work to our advantage. Your body craves balance. It has a homeostatic instinct that wants to bring you back into it. Whether you are trying to heal your metabolic system, calm your fried nervous system, or support the healthy, cyclical nature of your sex hormones, the intelligence inside you will do everything it can to bring you back to a state of health. We just need to help it do so. You can start anywhere, but here's the good news: Just as toxic food is one of the primary sources of dysregulation, healthy food is one of the quickest

(and yummiest) ways to heal. The right foods timed to your hormonal needs create a beautiful state of coherence for your body. Let's start with the Foundational Five—five food principles that regulate many of the systems of your body, not just your metabolic system.

The Foundational Five

Food is complicated. Let's simplify it! The Foundational Five are your guiding lights back to a regulated body. If you ever lose your way with your health, come back and revisit the Five. They will always help you find harmony with your body. If you are getting lost trying to navigate new weight-loss trends or conflicting nutrition opinions, come home to these Five. They are a beautiful lens through which to see food. Plus, they fit both plant-based and omnivore diets. They even work with trendy diets like keto and carnivore. Struggling to get off one of the new weight-loss drugs? These Five can give you a solid footing so you can effortlessly find metabolic balance without relying on exogenous medications. That's the power of the Foundational Five!

1. BLOOD SUGAR MATTERS, CALORIES DON'T

If there is one concept that will change the course of your health more than any other, it's understanding the impact food has on your blood sugar. When I refer to "sugar," I don't mean the refined highly processed sugar we find in food. I mean the glucose levels that are measurable in your blood. Every time you eat, your food gets broken down into glucose molecules. Some foods break down into many glucose molecules, while others break

THE HORMONAL HIERARCHY

Hormones don't work in a silo. They act as a community. If one hormone spikes high or suddenly drops low, all the other hormones adapt. Understanding how each hormone responds to one another is important. This is why I repeat in many of my books a critical concept called the Hormonal Hierarchy. Here's how the hierarchy works: Your sex hormones—estrogen, progesterone, and testosterone—are greatly influenced by insulin production. If there's too much insulin, your sex hormones can quickly go out of whack. Your insulin system is also dramatically impacted by the presence of cortisol. If your stress levels are chronically high, cortisol will constantly be in your bloodstream, and your cells will stay in an insulin-resistant state. At the top of the hierarchy is oxytocin. When your body makes oxytocin, it stops cortisol spikes, which moves you out of an insulin-resistant state and puts your sex hormones back into a more natural, balanced state.

Luckily, oxytocin is a fun hormone to produce. You make oxytocin when you laugh, connect with others, hug your favorite human, pet your dog, have an orgasm, or when you go into a relaxed state during a massage. Building in oxytocin moments throughout your day calms all your hormones and puts you back into hormonal balance.

down into only a few. When glucose levels go up after a meal, it triggers your pancreas to make a hormone called insulin. Insulin is your glucose storage hormone, and it helps move glucose into your cells for use. Once inside your cells, glucose fuels your mitochondria so they can make energy.

Your cells thrive with *small* bursts of glucose. Large amounts overwhelm them. Repetitively eating foods that spike large amounts of glucose will force your pancreas to make large amounts of insulin. When a huge influx of insulin and glucose comes rushing in, a cellular traffic jam occurs. This jam makes it so all the glucose and insulin swimming in your bloodstream can't get into your cells. The excess will then get stored as fat. Think about that for a moment: Your body stores what it can't get into the cell as fat. Fat isn't something your body accumulates to punish you. It's the opposite: Fat is a survival mechanism.

Excess glucose destroys the tissues of your vital organs. Your body knows this, so it puts the excess glucose in fat first. One reason so many women are experiencing a dysregulation in their metabolic systems is because they've been trained to count calories to lose weight. A low-calorie diet can still create mayhem in your metabolic system. Focusing on blood sugar puts not only your metabolic system back into harmony but it can also calm a raging nervous system and regulate even the craziest of hormonal challenges.

2. EAT NATURE'S FOOD, NOT HUMANMADE FOOD

Chemical-laden, hormone-disrupting foods are all around you. Often referred to as *obesogens*, these humanmade chemicals destroy both your metabolic and hormonal systems. Some obesogens are intentionally added to foods, while others enter our food system through environmental pollution and other means. When we are exposed to these chemicals, they increase our appetite and encourage fat production in all the wrong places. Many experts will tell you that these chemicals are the root cause of skyrocketing obesity rates.[3] We can no longer turn a blind eye to the harsh reality that, as of 2022, one in eight people in the world is living with obesity. Adult obesity has more than doubled worldwide since 1990, and adolescent obesity has quadrupled, while 35 million children under the age of five are diagnosed as overweight. As chemicals are poured into our food system, the human body has responded by storing them as fat.[4]

Why do these chemicals wreak so much havoc on our bodies? First, they signal specific stem cells in your body to make fat cells.[5] Stem cells are a universal cell that can make and repair any tissue in your body. When you are exposed to these obesogens, you trigger these stem cells to start making fat cells. Think about the ramifications of this for a moment. You eat one of your favorite foods, and maybe it's even a "diet" food because you don't want to gain weight. But many of these diet foods are packed with obesogens. The irony! So you think that you are helping yourself lose weight, but the opposite is actually happening—you've stimulated your stem cells to make more fat. Crazy frustrating, right? Can you see why so many people are struggling to lose weight?

Unfortunately, that's not the end of the obesogens story. They also act as estrogen mimickers. An estrogen mimicker is a fake version of estrogen that is not naturally produced by your body. Once this toxic estrogen enters your body, it binds to your estrogen receptor sites. These are hormonal receptor sites on the outside of your cells that insulin also uses to move glucose into your cells. If these sites get a massive influx of both estrogen and insulin, all those excess hormones get moved to the pantry closet of your body: fat. Often the body's preferred fat storage place is breast and abdominal tissue. Now you are not only setting yourself up for more belly fat, but also increasing your chances of hormonal cancers like breast and ovarian cancers. All from a diet food you thought was going to help you lose weight! Are you mad yet? I know I am!

But this bodily destruction doesn't stop there. These chemicals can also throw off your hormonal system, leading to changes in your menstrual cycle, affecting your fertility, creating painful periods and erratic premenstrual moods, and adding to the turbulence of the perimenopausal years. For all my fellow post-menopausal women, these obesogens can be why you can't lose the menopausal weight and end the hot flashes that started in your perimenopausal years. It's massively important we get these chemicals out of our bodies and our food system. You can find a list of common obesogens found in food on page 294.

How to Locate Hormone-Disrupting Chemicals on Nutrition Labels

Too many of us look first at the calorie content of a food, but that number tells you nothing about the impact that food will have on your hormones. The ingredient list, however, will. This is why the recipes in this book do not include calorie information.

Ingredient lists are organized in order from greatest to least amount, meaning that the first ingredient makes up most of that food product. One food rule that my mom had

1. Serving Size

Based on the amount the FDA believes people usually eat, based on people aged four years old and older. This is not always accurate to how you're eating today or how much you should eat per serving.

2. Total Fat

Includes all fat in a serving, refined, trans, etc., in addition to natural fats in ingredients.

3. Trans Fat

Can list 0% if it has less than 0.5g per serving! Always check ingredients lists to avoid trans fats as this can be misleading.

4. Total Carbohydrate

Measure of all carbohydrates. Doesn't separate out refined carbs or added sugars.

5. Dietary Fiber

Fiber count is key for metabolizing hormones. The more fiber the better. When calculating net carbohydrate amount you will take the total carbohydrates and subtract the fiber. This gives you the true carbohydrate load.

Nutrition Facts

1 servings per container

① Serving size   **1.6oz (45g)**

Amount per serving

Calories   **230**

%Daily Value*

② Total Fat 19g	**24%**
Saturated Fat 14.7g	**74%**
③ *Trans* Fat 0mg	
Cholesterol 0mg	**0%**
Sodium 35mg	**2%**
④ Total Carbohydrate 17g	**6%**
⑤ Dietary Fiber 1g	**4%**
Sugars 10g	
⑥ Includes 9g Added Sugars	**19%**
Protein 4g	
Vitamin D 0mcg	**0%**
Calcium 65mg	**4%**
Iron 1.44mg	**8%**
Potassium 235mg	**4%**

* The % Daily Value (DV) tells you how much a nutrient in a serving of food contributes to a daily diet. 2,000 calories a day is used for general nutrition advice.

⑦ INGREDIENTS: Shredded Coconut, Blended Almonds, Coconut Palm Nectar, Dark Chocolate Chips (Cocoa Beans, Evaporated Coconut Palm Nectar, Cocoa Butter, Sunflower Lecithin), Espresso, Coconut Oil, Ground Vanilla Beans.

⑧ CONTAINS: Coconut, Almonds

6. Added Sugars

This will clue you in that there are sugars added to this product, besides those naturally occurring in ingredients. Check the ingredients list to determine whether they are refined or not.

7. Ingredients

The most important part of a nutrition label. Foods are listed in descending order. This means the first few ingredients make up the majority of the food. Golden rule: Ingredient lists should be short and all ingredients should be ones you recognize and can pronounce.

8. Contains

Includes ingredients or protein from one of the eight common food allergens: milk, eggs, fish, crustacean shellfish, tree nuts, peanuts, wheat, and soybeans, but NOT gluten. May also just be listed in bold type in ingredients list rather than listed separately.

was that sugar couldn't be listed in the first four ingredients—she was a woman ahead of her time and knew that keeping our sugar intake low would benefit us. So first look at the order of ingredients. Does it mostly list whole foods or chemicals? Then ask yourself, *Can I pronounce all these ingredients?* If you can't pronounce them or have never seen that ingredient in whole form in a grocery store or on a recipe page, it is most likely a chemical that can disrupt your hormones. Then decode the sneaky ways food companies tuck these chemicals into our foods. Look for words like *artificial flavors*, *artificial sweetener*, *natural flavor*, *preservatives*, and even *added sugars*—these all indicate where these chemicals can be hidden.

3. EAT FOR YOUR MICROBES, NOT YOUR TASTE BUDS

How do you decide what foods you are going to eat? I'm guessing most would say, "It depends on what I am in the mood for," and by this, we usually mean what tastes good to us. Pacifying our taste buds is all too often the deciding factor when it comes to our food choices. Enter your microbiome. Did you know that your gut bugs can change your taste buds? These smart little microbes all have different food preferences. Knowing how to feed the good microbes and starve out the bad ones will not only change your cravings but also your overall health. Let's talk about how to best feed them.

There are a few steps to consider when making sure you have a diverse set of microbes. The first is to feed your microbes a variety of fiber-rich plant foods. A high-fiber dietary regimen has been consistently shown to increase the diversity of your microbiome.[6] In Chapter 3, I will go deeper into the food choices your microbes love. For now, think fiber, fiber, fiber. Fiber up your diet and you will see your taste buds start craving healthier foods.

The second step is to stop eating foods that destroy these powerful microbes, like gluten. Gluten is a protein found in wheat, barley, and rye. These grains are now all genetically altered to contain a toxin called Bt (short for *Bacillus thuringiensis*). These new grain versions were created to help protect crops from insects. When a bug tries to eat these crops, this toxin causes it to die. This is great for the farmer, but not so great for the bugs in our gut. Unless you live in a country like France that outlaws glyphosate, most of the gluten available to you comes from plants that have been sprayed with this pesticide that not only is an endocrine disruptor, but also kills many of the helpful microbes in your gut as well.[7]

Other chemicals that destroy your gut microbes are antibiotics and pesticides. Antibiotics are designed to kill bacteria in your body, including the good ones in your gut. This means that any food product that has been treated with antibiotics or sprayed with pesticides is also damaging to your gut microbes. You will find antibiotics mostly in animal products like meat, dairy, and eggs. Whenever you consume animal-based foods,

you are now eating whatever that animal ate. Cows, pigs, and chickens are often given antibiotics to prevent infections, so when you eat these animals, you are ingesting those antibiotics. This is why I am a huge fan of grass-fed, antibiotic-free dairy and meat.

Pesticides are sprayed mostly on our fruits and vegetables. Exposure to pesticides has been shown to disrupt gut microbiota composition—specifically the microbes that make neurotransmitters that help support a healthy brain. Studies have shown that repeated exposure to pesticides can have a negative impact on our cognitive processes.[8] An easy work-around to this is to buy organic whenever possible.

One last thought about eating for your microbes: Your gut microbes thrive when you eat a diverse range of plants. You can starve out helpful microbes when you don't get a lot of variety in your diet. Eating the same foods over and over again creates what we call a monoculture, where certain microbes grow stronger while others starve. The more diverse your plant foods are, the larger variety of microbes you feed. If you see some unique foods you haven't eaten before in the following recipes, be curious about eating these. Your microbes will thank you! I specifically encouraged the chefs to diversify the ingredients they used so we can keep all your good microbes healthy and strong.

4. PROTEIN IS THE HERO MACRO INGREDIENT

For way too long now, protein has been the province of men, but we women really miss out when we don't prioritize this hero macronutrient. Too many of us have been so focused on counting calories to stay thin that we forgot

FOODS THAT DESTROY YOUR MICROBIOME

Artificial sweeteners: Studies suggest that artificial sweeteners like aspartame, sucralose, and saccharin may disrupt the gut bacteria balance, potentially leading to glucose intolerance and increased risk of metabolic diseases.

High-sugar diets: Consuming large amounts of sugar can promote the growth of certain harmful bacteria and yeasts in the gut, such as *Candida*, while reducing the diversity of beneficial bacteria.

Processed and high-fat foods: Diets high in processed foods and unhealthy inflammatory fats can decrease microbial diversity and promote the growth of bacteria associated with inflammation and chronic disease.

Antibiotics: While sometimes medically necessary, antibiotics can have a broad impact on the gut microbiome, killing off beneficial bacteria along with harmful ones. Frequent or unnecessary use should be avoided.

Alcohol: Excessive alcohol consumption can disrupt the gut barrier function, leading to a condition known as leaky gut syndrome, where bacteria and toxins can enter the bloodstream and negatively affect the balance of gut bacteria.

Pesticide-contaminated foods: Residues from pesticides such as glyphosate, found on nonorganic fruits and vegetables, may be harmful to gut bacteria and contribute to dysbiosis.

Fried foods: High in unhealthy fats, fried foods can contribute to inflammation and negatively impact gut health.

Emulsifiers and preservatives: Common in processed foods, these substances can alter gut bacteria and increase intestinal permeability, contributing to inflammation and associated health issues.

Refined carbohydrates: Foods made with refined grains, such as white bread and pastries, can rapidly spike blood-sugar levels and favor the growth of harmful bacteria over beneficial ones.

(or never even knew) about the importance of protein. A daily low protein intake contributes to metabolic dysregulation.

Protein is the one macronutrient that builds muscle. Women need muscle for a variety of health reasons, one of the most important being that the more muscle you have, the more insulin receptor sites you will have. Since muscle needs glucose to perform at its best, it houses a vast number of insulin receptor sites to serve as entry points for that glucose. When you build muscle, your body will be more insulin-sensitive, allowing you to use glucose better instead of storing it as fat.

Protein is partly made up of a compound called amino acids, which are key nutrients not only for building muscle but also for making hormones and neurotransmitters. Without enough protein, all three of these can diminish.

You can get protein from both plant and animal foods. While animal food sources do give you a more complete amino acid profile, eating a variety of plant foods can provide you with all 20 amino acids that humans need as well. One amino acid that is getting a lot of attention right now is called leucine. It triggers a sensor that signals our muscles to grow stronger. The World Health Organization (WHO) even acknowledges that we need 39 grams of leucine per kilogram of body weight each day.[9]

I've seen many people spreading the misinformation that animal-based foods like eggs, chicken, and beef are the best place to get leucine. But did you know many plant-based foods also have leucine in them? Legumes like lentils and navy beans contain large amounts of leucine. This is why it was so important to me to create a cookbook that honors both plant-based and omnivore eaters. Women need protein—no matter what their dietary preferences are.

It's my goal to help you understand the principles of food that will help you and your hormones thrive, so that you will know how to successfully navigate your preferred food style. Later in the book I will take you deep into the nuances of protein so you can understand how to eat the right proteins to balance hormones, improve neurotransmitter production, and build muscle.

5. FAT DOESN'T MAKE YOU FAT

There is so much cultural shame around the fat that lives on our bodies, but fat seriously needs a rebrand. It's simply the storage closet for excess glucose, toxins, and hormones. Yet when we look in the mirror, we villainize fat. We don't see it as a lifesaving mechanism. Once you start eating foods that don't cause high spikes of glucose, your body will stop storing fat.

What stops glucose spikes? Healthy dietary fats. Healthy fats put the brakes on your blood sugar. Add or pair fat with any meal, especially our carbohydrates, and you will experience fewer fluctuations in blood sugar.

If you are scared to eat too much fat, let me walk you through how this works. Knowing the *why* behind your food choices helps greatly. You have three macronutrients: carbohydrates, protein, and fat. Each one of these macronutrients affects your blood sugar differently. Generally, carbohydrates spike your blood sugar the highest, protein second highest, and fat last. If you pair a fat with your carbohydrate, you slow the spike. As mentioned above, the fat on your body is just a place where it stored the excess. So, if you don't want to store more fat, you need to stop the excess from coming. The best way to do that is to always dress carbs up with fat.

Counting calories, leading with our taste buds, neglecting fiber-filled foods, skimping on protein, and avoiding fat—can you see how we have become so metabolically dysregulated? With the Foundational Five, we now have a map to guide us back to a coherent metabolic state. We have been muscling our way to better health all while moving into a more dysregulated state. It's time to turn the tide and take our power back.

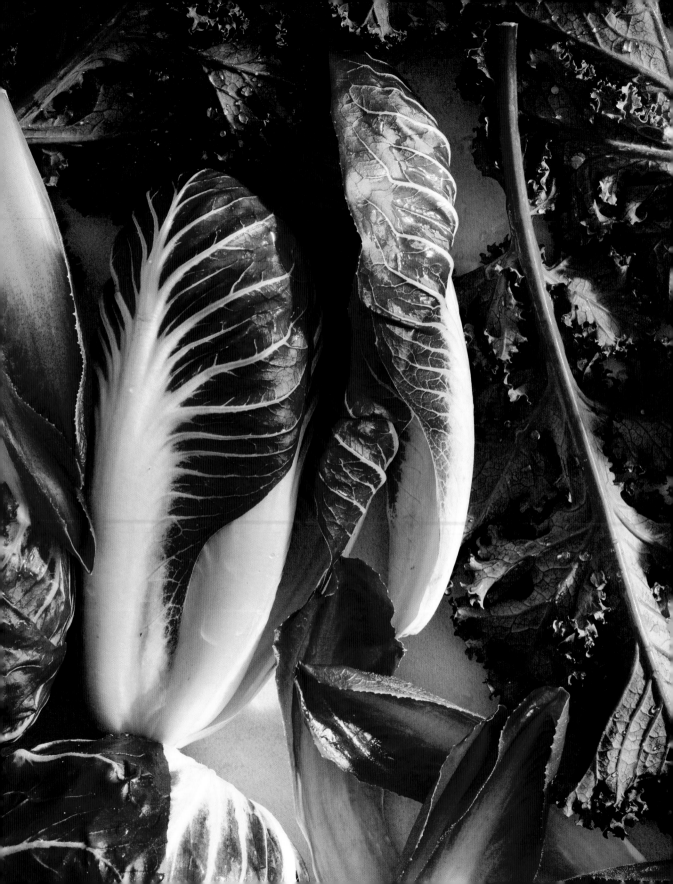

2

The Wisdom of Your Hormones

I STILL REMEMBER the day our high school health class was divided into boys and girls and our male physical education teacher, who was really the track coach, taught us about our female bodies. He knew absolutely nothing about what it was like to live in a hormonally driven female body. It wasn't exactly the most comprehensive, insightful, or even comfortable lesson, and it certainly didn't teach me much about my changing body.

I'm sure the experience looks different for each of us, but I am willing to bet that for the overwhelming majority of us, it's not much better. The education we get about our bodies and our hormones is incredibly anemic. For too many women, the only message we get when our cycles start is "You can get pregnant now, be careful." This lack of hormonal education leaves many of us lost and confused at a time when we are starting to experience our bodies in a whole new way. And because we are not taught how to adapt our lifestyle to meet the ebbs and flows of our hormones, our moods become erratic, cravings for sugary foods begin, our skin spontaneously breaks out, fat starts forming in unwanted places,

and the hatred for our bodies begins. At a time when we are stepping into our hormonal brilliance, we feel like we've been cursed. A beautifully profound hormonal moment is hijacked by ignorance.

Despite what my high school track coach said (or didn't say) that day, something magical happens when our hormones show up. It is the time in our lives when we are being crowned with our shiny new hormonal superpowers—powers that spark our creative brains, give us the power to multitask, make us articulate, pull us to connect with others, fire up our motivation, turn on our cognitive skills, and allow us to access a wide spectrum of emotions. Without proper education, we miss understanding the power and the potential of this moment. We are left bewildered as to why in one moment, we feel so joyful, and in the next, we are a ball of tears.

Your hormones do so much more than orchestrate your menstrual cycle. There are hormone receptor sites in every single organ system in your body. That means that once a hormone is released, it does its primary reproductive job and then moves onto its secondary role in your body. This secondary job is the part of the hormonal story that is not being talked about enough. Outside of reproduction, your sex hormones have seven other major job responsibilities: bone health, muscle function, brain function, cardiovascular health, metabolism, skin and hair health, and immune system regulation. These neurochemicals are powerful! Which is why I lovingly think of them as wisdom molecules—molecules that connect us back to the generations of women who came before us.

The Foundational Five, along with fasting, are the most powerful way I know of to heal the metabolic dysregulation most of us are suffering from in this modern world. We also want to individually and collectively stop the hormonal dysregulation that causes us to feel out of sync with the natural rhythms of our female bodies. To build a lifestyle that honors the natural rhythms of your female body, you need to understand your hormones and the roles they play. Your hormones run you in all the right ways. Understanding their personalities is as important as learning how to care for a child. Without your assistance, patience, and care, they will struggle. So, let's roll up our sleeves and dive in as I walk you through a short master class on your hormones.

Estrogen

Estrogen is your wild, outgoing, at times rambunctious, extroverted hormone. This is largely because she stimulates some powerful neurotransmitters like dopamine, serotonin, acetylcholine, and glutamate that activate your brain. Her presence also stimulates oxytocin, the wisest hormone of them all, which gives us access to deep levels of compassion and desire for connection with others. And if that isn't juicy enough, she has the power to upregulate brain-derived neurotropic factor (BDNF), a protein that stimulates neuronal growth in your brain so you can integrate new skills into your life. You have some serious neurochemical power surging through your body when estrogen shows up!

The wisdom that estrogen carries with her as she works her neurochemical magic is the wisdom of happiness, motivation, connection, focus, creativity, learning, and memory. Yet her influence on your brain is not her only job— she also protects your cardiovascular system, influences your respiration rate, strengthens your immune system, and ramps up collagen production to give you glowing skin and great musculoskeletal flexibility and strength. Makes you want to take great care of her, doesn't it?

Estrogen comes surging into your life between Days 1 and 15 of your menstrual cycle. In these 15 days, she slowly builds until she peaks at ovulation. Estrogen comes in three different flavors: estrone (E1), estradiol (E2), and estriol (E3).

Estrone is the dominant form of estrogen during menopause but is considered the least potent estrogen. Her role is less powerful than (but similar to) estradiol. As a post-menopausal woman, I like to think of estrone as the crone of hormones. In *Women Who Run with the Wolves* and *The Power of the Crone*, Dr. Clarissa Pinkola Estés writes that the word *crone* means "crown." I love thinking that our young and mighty—and sometimes even erratic—estradiol shifts into the calmer, wiser, more stable version of estrogen we call estrone as we move from our diva years to our crone years. It's in this crowning of ourselves through this estrogen conversion that we often find more peace, stability, inner wisdom, and lasting joy. Although historically, the transition from estradiol to estrone has caused so many menopausal women to struggle with brain function, bone density, immune function, and cardiovascular health, if you learn how to eat like a girl, that handoff will be much smoother. It can be a beautiful journey that extends well into your post-menopausal years.

Estradiol is your diva hormone. She is the rock star of all hormones! She is most potent and prevalent during the reproductive years, playing a critical role in releasing an egg at ovulation. She is responsible for the development of breasts and the distribution of body fat, and she also has a significant effect on the seven responsibilities listed earlier. Estradiol is the type of estrogen that goes away in your menopausal years.

Estriol, the weakest of the three estrogens, shows up primarily during pregnancy. She is produced by the placenta and used as an indicator of the fetus's well-being and the placenta's functioning. She plays a part in preparing the uterus for delivery and promoting the growth of the milk ducts in the breasts for lactation.

Progesterone

Progesterone is your sweet, nurturing, quiet, loving, and introverted hormone. Whereas estrogen will tell you to get up and go, progesterone will lovingly nudge you to stay cuddled up on the couch a little longer. You get a small amount of progesterone at ovulation, and in the week before your period, progesterone comes roaring in to activate the shedding of your uterine lining. As you will learn in later chapters, progesterone perishes in the presence of the stress hormone cortisol. So, if you

raise your cortisol levels by pushing life too hard at either of these phases, you may find that your progesterone levels tank. This can lead to strong premenstrual symptoms like irritability, cramping, spotting, and anxiety.

Progesterone has one unique secondary job that your other sex hormones don't: She activates gamma-aminobutyric acid, or GABA. GABA is the neurotransmitter that calms you. Without progesterone's stimulation, you may find yourself in an anxious state. Why would progesterone stimulate calm? Hormones stimulate other neurochemicals for specific reasons. Progesterone peaks somewhere around Day 21 of your cycle, and she has to hit a certain level to initiate the shedding of your uterine lining. This is a really important note for those of you who are in your fertility years and have lost your cycle. Catering to progesterone's needs can bring your period back.

Culturally, our periods have been thought of as a hassle. And yes, let's just call out the elephant in the room—managing blood flowing out of you every month is not a lot of fun! Yet, this a magical moment that your body uses to get rid of what no longer serves you. Old cells, mucus, and even toxins are found in menstrual blood. It's a shedding of the old that is moving into the rebirthing of a new cycle. All too often, we look at reproductive health from a mechanistic point of view, like it's a bunch of parts and stages. But there is something powerful about thinking of it as a flow—a monthly movement in and out of neurochemicals all working together for our greatest good. When progesterone peaks, your body is preparing to shed the old and making room for the new. A good dose of GABA in this moment serves you!

The other interesting quality of progesterone is that she needs glucose to make her appearance. This is why you crave carbohydrates, especially sugar, the week before your period. Progesterone needs glucose to hit her monthly high. How many times have you been on a diet, only to struggle the week before your period? This can happen because progesterone wants stress to be low and glucose to be high. She sends subtle clues. When we honor them, our cycles balance out.

For my fellow menopausal friends, the loss of progesterone can throw a wrench into our lives. As you move through your perimenopause years, you may notice your ability to handle stress, calm your body and mind, and stay asleep all night long become luxuries of the past. In Chapter 8, I will show you how to use different foods to ease the slow exit of progesterone and bring calm back to your menopausal life.

Testosterone

Testosterone peaks mid-ovulation, around Day 12, and yes, it increases libido during that time. Why would your body come equipped with a surge of testosterone at ovulation? Well, in the hope that you will have sex to reproduce. Whether you decide to have children or not, your body is built for reproduction. Adding in a surge of testosterone during the time an egg is released ensures that reproduction. Testosterone's secondary role outside of reproduction is to ramp up your motivation and drive. This makes ovulation a great time to start a new project, increase the intensity of your workouts, or launch a new business plan. Your motivation and drive will be at its highest when testosterone is around. Testosterone also helps you build muscle. This makes your five-day ovulation window a

phenomenal time to power up on protein and lift heavy weights.

An interesting aspect of testosterone is that it is made from a steroid hormone called dehydroepiandrosterone, or DHEA. DHEA is also needed to make cortisol and progesterone. This is important because if you are chronically stressed, you may find both your progesterone and testosterone are depleted. This happens largely because DHEA has prioritized making cortisol over sex hormones. Of the thousands of urinary hormone tests we've run on women in my clinic and online community, almost every test has come back low in DHEA, progesterone, and testosterone. Sadly, this reflects the stress too many women are under, which dysregulates our hormones, especially testosterone and progesterone, and gets us out of sync with our bodies.

A great way to remember the personalities of your sex hormones is to think about how they would operate at a party. Estrogen would be the life of the party, dancing on tables and getting everyone to join in. Testosterone would want to make sure that the party kept going all night long, while progesterone would be asking when it is time to go home and go to sleep. I love thinking of our hormones from this lens, because it helps us understand why at different times of our cycle, we feel more outgoing, motivated, or introverted than others. It also explains many of the mood and behavior changes we see during our menopausal years.

Now that you've got the in-depth explanation of your hormones that you deserved to get in high school health class (or even earlier!), let's build on the Foundational Five by applying this information to how to eat for your hormonal thriving in what I call the "eat like a girl philosophy."

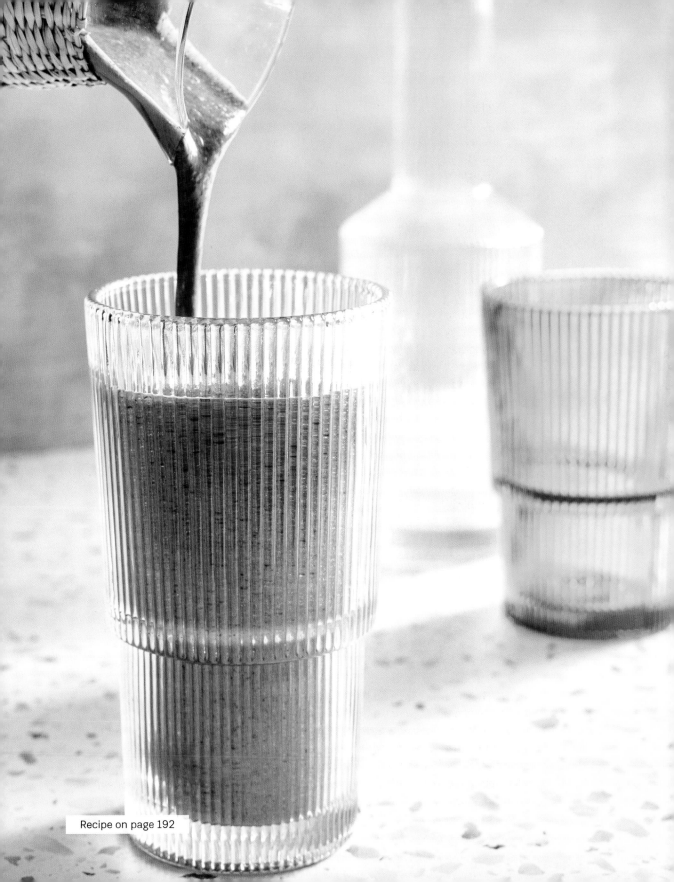

Recipe on page 192

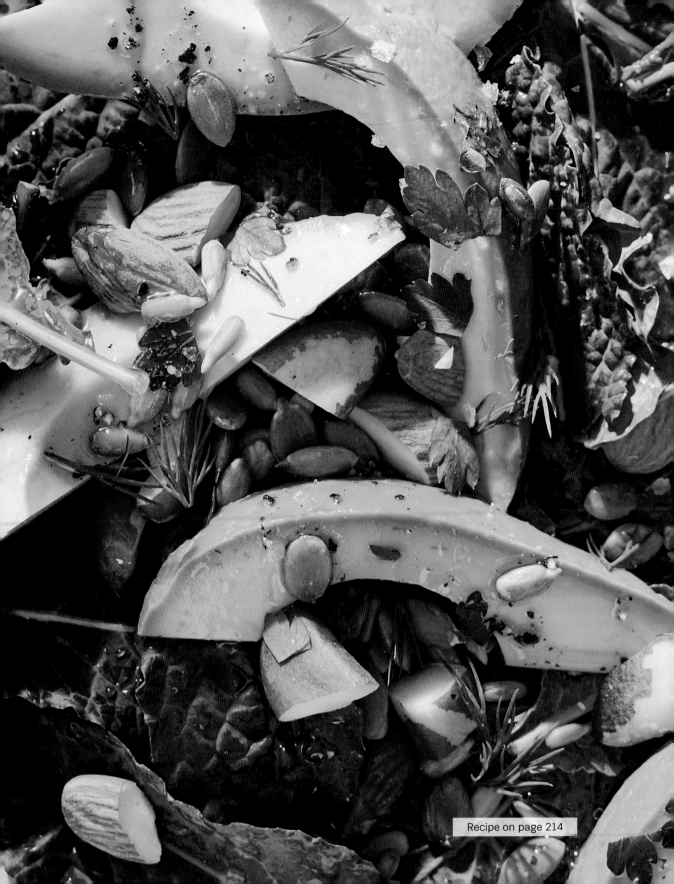

Recipe on page 214

3

The Eat Like a Girl Philosophy

THERE ARE THREE pivotal phases to a woman's hormonal journey. I call them the warm-up, the main act, and the cooldown. You may know these as your puberty years, childbearing years, and menopausal years. No matter where you are on this hormonal journey, learning *what* and *when* to eat will smooth the bumps hormones can often provide.

Our hormonal system works very much like a symphony, with several instruments coming together to play beautiful music in our bodies. When we are teenagers, it takes about 10 years from our first period for this symphony to find its perfect, cohesive rhythm. This means that we have some months where we feel in control of our bodies, and other months where everything in our bodies and minds feels out of control. Once we hit our childbearing years, the hormonal music that gets played in our bodies should smooth out. The biggest challenge we face during these years is stress. When physical, emotional, and chemical stressors increase, our hormonal symphony plays out of tune. This can lead to missed periods, painful premenstrual symptoms, and wild mood swings. When these stressors calm, the symphony clicks back into harmony.

When we enter our perimenopausal years, our hormonal symphony begins to wind down, taking another 10 years to move from a regular menstrual cycle into its post-menopausal rhythm. Much like our teenage years, this is another moment when most of us don't understand the changes happening within us. The closing down of our hormonal music can leave us feeling disconnected from our bodies, as every organ system has to learn to live without the hormonal notes that have been playing within us for decades. Once we are well into our post-menopausal years, however, our hormonal symphony should be quietly playing in the background of our lives. Softer hormonal surges should mean fewer mood swings and body changes. Our hormones are sensitive, though, and no matter where you are on your hormonal journey, your hormones will always be responding to the stressors you are faced with.

At every phase of your journey, chemical stressors from the wrong foods can contribute to the dysregulation of the music of your hormonal symphony—something will be out of time or tune, or there may be an aggressive rock song instead of a gentle ballad, or no music at all. The right foods will perfectly tune your hormones and allow them to make beautiful music.

So how do we attune our food choices with the changing rhythms of our hormones? This is where my Three Food Rules for eating like a girl come in handy. If you keep these three rules in mind, you will find less turbulence within you. These are the food rules your health-class teacher should have taught you in your teens, what the doctor should have given you when you said you were depressed and having difficult periods, and what your ob-gyn should have informed you about during your menopausal years when hot flashes, anxiety, and insomnia appeared. One of the greatest hormone-regulating tools already exists in our daily lives: the food we eat. Food is a major fuel source for our hormones. If you learn to eat like a girl—in a way that helps you produce, metabolize, and detox your hormones—you will find yourself living in a body you love.

Three Food Rules for Eating Like a Girl

Not only will these three rules ensure that your hormones are always working for you, they can also be a guiding light in helping you organize a meal.

RULE #1: EAT TO MAKE HORMONES

The first step of a hormone's journey is production. It doesn't matter if you are 20 or 60—the control tower of all our hormone production lives in a part of our brain called our hypothalamus. If you are a cycling woman, your hypothalamus receives hormonal communication from three endocrine organs: ovaries, adrenals, and fat cells. An endocrine gland is an organ in your body that can produce a hormone. And yes, our fat cells make estrogen. Once your hypothalamus receives chemical information from these organs, it tells your pituitary gland to send instructions to all the necessary endocrine organs for sex hormone production. It's a feedback loop, where your body is informing the brain of its needs and the brain is responding by sending signals back to the body.

In our menopausal years, this feedback loop starts to shift communication from the ovaries to the adrenal glands. This is the moment chronic stress can overload your hormonal system. Taking on the added load of producing both sex hormones and cortisol can challenge your adrenals. For a perimenopausal woman, this can be when she starts experiencing signs of low progesterone and estrogen, leading to anxiety, depression, inability to focus, and new cognitive challenges. In your post-menopausal years, your adrenals have figured out how to navigate the extra load. Although stress can still greatly impact a post-menopausal woman's body, the sex hormone demands on the adrenals are much lighter. This can be why many women feel that their menopause symptoms level out in their post-menopausal years.

Just like a recipe, the making of hormones requires certain ingredients. All three of your sex hormones need some basic nutrients—I call them the Key 24. They come in four major categories: vitamins, minerals, fatty acids, and amino acids. Think of these as categories of ingredients you would need to make bread. Regardless of what type of bread you are making, all recipes require a handful of necessary ingredients: flour, yeast, water, etc. Without one of these key ingredients, your bread won't turn out the way you want it. The 24 nutrients operate in the same way. Regardless of what stage of life you are in, you need adequate amounts of these nutrients to make your sex hormones. If one of these nutrients is low, it can have a massive impact on your sex hormone production.

Now you may look at the list on the next page and think *Wow! How can I ever get all those ingredients into my body daily?* A key component of eating for hormone production is diversification of foods. We need to eat a good variety of nutrient-rich foods to ensure our bodies get all 24 nutrients. When we consume a highly processed, refined-food diet, not only is it void of these 24, but these toxic foods also pull nutrients out of our bodies. Eating a diverse range of healthy foods ensures that you are getting all 24 of these nutrients. You will see that variety built into the recipes my chefs have provided in this book. In Part III, I have taken these recipes and mapped them to my 30-Day Fasting Reset. This makes it easier for you to get all 24 nutrients into your diet in 30 days.

It's not just toxic food that depletes you of vitamins and minerals—certain medications can too. Ironically, the birth control pill is one of those medications. If you are actively on an oral birth control pill or have spent years on this medication, I highly recommend that you supplement your diet with the following vitamins and minerals, as research shows that these key nutrients are depleted with the use of oral contraceptives.[1]

- Folic acid
- Vitamins B2, B6, B12
- Vitamin C
- Vitamin E
- Magnesium
- Selenium
- Zinc

RULE #2: EAT TO METABOLIZE HORMONES

Once a hormone is produced, it must be broken down into a simple, usable format for your cells. It's similar to what we must do to a large electronic file we want to send through e-mail; we often have to compress that file into a different format so that it can easily be delivered. Your hormones operate in the same way. Once you have produced a hormone, you must change its format to make it available to your cells. We call this process metabolizing a hormone.

Two organs help you metabolize your hormones—your liver and gut. If your liver is overloaded with toxins or your gut microbiome is depleted, you may not have the resources to reformat that hormone. Without a change in format, it doesn't matter how well your brain and body are coordinating the production of that hormone; it is rendered useless to your cells.

This is a very common scenario for both cycling and menopausal women when it comes to taking exogenous hormones. Whether it's hormone replacement therapy or the birth control pill, these outside sources of hormones still have to metabolize, or change formats, to be rendered usable by your body. If your liver and gut are not functioning at their best, these exogenous hormones may not make it all the way to your cells and the excess will be stored as fat. How many women have gone on hormone replacement therapy only to complain that they gained weight? That can be a sign the body is struggling to

THE KEY 24

Vitamins

1. **Vitamin B6 (pyridoxine):** This vitamin aids in the regulation of estrogen, progesterone, and testosterone levels in the body. It's also important for liver function, which is crucial for hormone metabolism. It's also involved in the synthesis of neurotransmitters and can help alleviate symptoms of premenstrual syndrome, or PMS. It is found mostly in meat, legumes, nuts, seeds, dairy, and fruits.

2. **Vitamin B9 (folic acid):** Folic acid works closely with B12 in the production of DNA and is important for overall hormone balance. It is found in leafy green vegetables, cruciferous vegetables, beets, asparagus, nuts, and seeds.

3. **Vitamin B12 (cobalamin):** B12 is essential for cell division and the synthesis of DNA, which are important for maintaining healthy hormone levels. B12 is also vital for energy metabolism, and its deficiency can lead to low energy levels and reduced testosterone production. It's found mostly in animal foods like meat, eggs, and dairy, as well as in fermented foods.

4. **Vitamin C:** This vitamin helps in the synthesis of estrogen and progesterone. It's also a powerful antioxidant that supports the overall health of hormonal systems.

5. **Vitamin D:** Often referred to as a steroid hormone, vitamin D is essential for maintaining healthy testosterone levels. Sun exposure is a primary source, but it can also be obtained through diet and supplements.

6. **Vitamin E:** Known for its antioxidant properties, vitamin E is thought to help regulate estrogen levels and alleviate some symptoms of menopause. This vitamin is known for its role in improving luteal blood flow, which is essential for progesterone production in the second half of the menstrual cycle. It also has powerful antioxidant properties.

Minerals

7. **Zinc:** Zinc plays a role in hormone production, including estrogen and progesterone, and is essential for enzyme function that aids in hormone metabolism.

8. **Magnesium:** Magnesium is involved in numerous biochemical reactions in the body, including those that regulate the balance of estrogen and progesterone. Magnesium contributes to progesterone production by supporting the pituitary gland. It also helps reduce muscle cramps and mood symptoms associated with the menstrual cycle.

9. **Iodine:** While more commonly associated with thyroid function, iodine also influences estrogen metabolism.

10. **Selenium:** This mineral is important for the proper functioning of the thyroid gland, which indirectly influences progesterone levels due to the interrelation of endocrine hormones.

11. **Boron:** This trace mineral, although required in only small amounts, has been shown to impact testosterone levels positively.

12. **Calcium:** While primarily known for its function in bone health, calcium also plays a role in hormonal secretion and function.

13. **Copper:** Copper, in balance with zinc, is important for hormone production and overall health. It plays a role in various enzymatic reactions in the body.

14. **Manganese:** This trace mineral is involved in various body processes, including the metabolism of cholesterol, carbohydrates, and proteins, all of which are important for hormone production.

15. **Iron:** Iron is essential for producing hemoglobin in red blood cells, which transport oxygen around the body. Adequate oxygenation is important for all bodily functions, including hormone production.

Fatty Acids

16. **Omega-3 fatty acids:** While not a vitamin or mineral, omega-3s are essential fats that can influence hormone production and may help in balancing estrogen levels.

Amino Acids

17. **L-arginine:** An amino acid that is important for improving blood flow and may indirectly support hormone balance and progesterone levels.

18. **Tyrosine:** It's a precursor for the synthesis of dopamine, norepinephrine, and epinephrine, which are all neurotransmitters that can influence the release of sex hormones. Additionally, tyrosine is involved in the synthesis of thyroid hormones, which indirectly affect sex hormone levels.

19. **Phenylalanine:** This amino acid can be converted into tyrosine in the body, and thus it indirectly contributes to the synthesis of sex hormones.

20. **Tryptophan:** This essential amino acid is a precursor to serotonin, a neurotransmitter that can influence mood and sexual behavior. Serotonin levels can indirectly affect sex hormone production.

21. **Glutamine:** While not directly involved in the synthesis of sex hormones, glutamine supports overall immune and gut health, which can indirectly influence hormonal balance.

22. **Lysine:** Important for overall protein synthesis and hormone production, lysine can play an indirect role in hormonal health.

23. **Leucine, isoleucine, and valine (branched-chain amino acids or BCAAs):** These are important for muscle protein synthesis and overall physical health, which can indirectly support healthy hormonal levels.

24. **Glycine:** It supports detoxification processes in the liver, which are important for hormone balance, including sex hormones.

break that hormone down, because it stores it in fat (remember, fat is where your body stores excess everything). This is why Rule #2 for eating like a girl is to eat so that you metabolize your hormones.

This is such a key part of the hormone conversation. Everyone wants to focus on getting more of a hormone, but that is only one part of the hormonal equation; you need a healthy liver and gut to metabolize that hormone so that your cells can use it.

With that in mind, let's get to know these organs and how you can keep them healthy so that they provide great hormonal health.

Meet Your Estrobolome

Ready for this? Your gut health is so pivotal to metabolizing hormones that you have a specific set of good gut bacteria whose job is to break down estrogen. That's how important your microbes are for your hormonal health. Together, these good bugs are called your estrobolome. Without these key microbes, estrogen can't get reformatted for cellular use. To support these hormone-metabolizing bacteria, you need to avoid the following things that destroy them:

- A highly processed diet
- Alcohol
- Antibiotics
- Birth control pills
- Environmental pollutants

It's easy to see every woman's lifestyle in this list. Our goal is to eat foods that bring back the health of the microbes that metabolize our hormones. These foods fall into three categories that I call the three Ps: probiotics, prebiotics, and polyphenols.

Probiotic-Rich Foods

Probiotic-rich foods add new healthy bacteria into your gut. Be sure that all the foods listed here are organic and raw. When these foods undergo pasteurization, the good bacteria are destroyed. Here's a list of the 12 most powerful probiotic-rich foods:

1. **Yogurt:** One of the most well-known sources of probiotics. Look for yogurt labeled with "live and active cultures" for the best probiotic benefits.
2. **Kefir:** A fermented probiotic milk drink, similar to a thin yogurt, which is made by adding kefir grains to milk.
3. **Sauerkraut:** Fermented cabbage rich in probiotics and vitamins. Ensure that it's unpasteurized, as pasteurization kills the beneficial bacteria.
4. **Kimchi:** A Korean dish made from fermented vegetables, primarily cabbage, along with a variety of seasonings. It's rich in probiotics and often spicy in flavor.
5. **Miso:** A Japanese seasoning made by fermenting soybeans with salt and a fungus called koji. It's used in miso soup and other dishes.
6. **Tempeh:** A fermented soy product from Indonesia that's a great source of probiotics and a good protein source for vegetarians and vegans.
7. **Pickles (in brine):** Cucumbers fermented in saltwater brine (not vinegar) are good probiotic sources. Ensure that they are naturally fermented by checking the ingredient label to make sure they are saltwater-brined, not vinegar-brined.
8. **Traditional buttermilk:** The liquid left over after making butter, particularly the traditional type (cultured buttermilk

usually doesn't have probiotics). Be sure to read the label to recognize the difference.

9. **Natto:** A traditional Japanese food made from fermented soybeans, known for its strong flavor and slimy texture; it is a great source of probiotics.
10. **Kombucha:** A fermented tea drink that has become increasingly popular for its probiotic benefits.
11. **Cheese:** Certain types of cheese like Gouda, cheddar, Swiss, and Parmesan are fermented and can contain probiotics. Raw cheese has the richest probiotic content.
12. **Lassi:** A traditional Indian drink made from fermented yogurt, often enjoyed before meals for its digestive benefits.

Prebiotic Foods

Prebiotic foods feed your healthy microbes so they get stronger and multiply. To reap the maximum power from these foods, make sure they are organic and come from a regenerative farm. Here's a list of 19 powerful prebiotic foods:

1. **Garlic:** Contains high levels of the prebiotic inulin and fructooligosaccharides (FOS), which support the growth of beneficial bacteria.
2. **Onions:** Rich in inulin and FOS, onions are great for gut health and also have antioxidant properties.
3. **Leeks:** Similar to garlic and onions, they are high in inulin and FOS.
4. **Asparagus:** Contains inulin, which helps promote healthy gut bacteria.
5. **Bananas:** Unripe (green) bananas are high in resistant starch, a type of prebiotic fiber.
6. **Barley:** A whole grain rich in beta-glucan, a type of soluble fiber with prebiotic benefits.
7. **Gluten-free oats:** Contain large amounts of beta-glucan and are also a good source of resistant starch.
8. **Apples:** Rich in pectin, a prebiotic fiber that promotes healthy gut bacteria and reduces harmful bacteria.
9. **Cocoa:** Contains flavanols that have prebiotic benefits. Dark chocolate is a good source of cocoa.
10. **Flaxseed:** Loaded with soluble fiber that acts as a prebiotic.
11. **Seaweed:** A great source of prebiotic fibers, including fucans and galactans.
12. **Chicory root:** One of the best sources of inulin.
13. **Jerusalem artichokes (sunchokes):** Extremely high in inulin.
14. **Dandelion greens:** Contain inulin fibers and are also a rich source of antioxidants.
15. **Jicama:** High in inulin and very low in calories.
16. **Peas:** Contain soluble fiber that feeds beneficial bacteria.
17. **Soybeans:** Rich in oligosaccharides, which act as prebiotics.
18. **Lentils:** Provide a variety of fibers, including prebiotic types.
19. **Konjac root (glucomannan):** Known for its high glucomannan content, a form of prebiotic fiber.

The Soil Your Food Is Grown in Matters

In this modern world we are living in, a new awareness around the soils our food is grown in is emerging. Traditional agriculture practices have left our soils bereft of nutrients. Soil that is depleted of vitamins, minerals, and good, healthy microbes will yield nutrient-depleted foods. Remember the Key 24? You need to eat foods that are nutrient-dense to ensure you have all the ingredients necessary to make hormones. This is why knowing if your food came from a conventional farm or a regenerative one is important.

Conventional farms tend to be larger farms that slant more to monocropping. This means they focus on growing one type of food in that soil. When that crop is done, they till the soil and plant that same crop again. Often in this process, many chemicals are sprayed to prevent the crop from being destroyed by insects. This process not only depletes the soil of nutrients, but also exposes your produce to harmful endocrine-disrupting chemicals.

A regenerative farm views soil from the lens of creating an ecosystem. Its focus is to bring as many different plants and animals together around a crop to diversify its nutrient profile. These farms do not spray with harsh chemicals. In this type of soil environment, fruits and vegetables contain more nutrients. Knowing the type of farm where your food is grown will help ensure you are getting the vitamins, minerals, and healthy microbes that keep your microbes healthy and happy.

Polyphenol Foods

Polyphenol-rich foods are plant-based foods that are known for their antioxidant properties. These compounds are often responsible for the color, flavor, and bitterness in fruits, vegetables, and other plant-based foods. A diet rich in these foods regrows the microbes that metabolize hormones for you, helping you feel more hormonally balanced and avoid storing unmetabolized hormones as fat. To get the maximum polyphenol power from these foods, make sure they are organic and come from a regenerative farm.

Here's a list of 18 polyphenol-rich foods:

1. **Cloves:** One of the richest sources of polyphenols.
2. **Star anise:** High in polyphenols and used as a spice in various cuisines.
3. **Cocoa powder:** Raw, unprocessed cocoa powder is very rich in polyphenols.
4. **Dark chocolate:** Contains significant amounts of polyphenols, especially in higher cocoa content varieties.
5. **Berries:** Blueberries, blackberries, strawberries, and raspberries are all rich in polyphenols.
6. **Black olives:** Particularly high in polyphenols, especially when unprocessed.
7. **Green olives:** Similar to black olives, they are a good source of polyphenols.
8. **Nuts:** Nuts, in general, are good sources of polyphenols. Hazelnuts and pecans are among the richest sources.
9. **Artichokes:** Particularly rich in certain types of polyphenols like chlorogenic acid.
10. **Red onions:** High in quercetin, a type of flavonoid polyphenol.
11. **Spinach:** Contains several different polyphenols.
12. **Black elderberries:** Known for their high polyphenol content.
13. **Green tea:** A major source of catechins, a type of polyphenol.
14. **Black tea:** Similar to green tea but with different polyphenol profiles due to the fermentation process.
15. **Black chokeberries** (*Aronia*)**:** Extremely high in polyphenols.
16. **Flaxseed meal:** Rich in lignans, a type of polyphenol.
17. **Cherries:** Both sweet and sour cherries are good sources of polyphenols.
18. **Plums and prunes:** Especially high in chlorogenic acids.

Your Liver: Estrogen's Bestie

Not many women know this, but your liver is your hormones' greatest friend! Any behavior, food, or drink that taxes your liver will have a consequence on the metabolism of a wide array of hormones because the list of hormones the liver metabolizes is long. Everything, from the hormones that control your menstrual cycle to those that help you manage stress and oversee the process of burning fat, is processed through your liver. If your liver is overloaded, not only will its ability to metabolize hormones be impaired, but the unmetabolized hormones will be stored in fat.

The good news is that your liver is a powerful organ. It detoxes all day long and can handle a huge amount of chemical stress if you treat it right. Depending on how much of a toxic load has been thrown at it, your liver cells can regenerate themselves within days to weeks. You first want to start avoiding anything that taxes your liver, including (sorry) alcohol. Alcohol is a toxin that the liver has to break down to get it out of your system. If it didn't do that, this poison would accumulate in your body and brain and eventually kill you. For many alcoholics, this is exactly what it does. But for social drinkers, what is important to note is that when you drink, you temporarily halt your liver's ability to metabolize hormones. Once your liver has cleared the alcohol, it will go back to the business of breaking down hormones. Where I see this challenging women the most is during their perimenopausal years. This is a tough one because, as progesterone declines, anxiety goes up. For many women, this is the moment they reach for a glass of wine. The nightly glass of wine now turns off hormone metabolism for hours, leading to belly fat, increased menopausal symptoms, and erratic moods. The

suggested dose of alcohol for menopausal women is no more than two glasses per week. More than that and you may find yourself in a bit of a hormonal jam. Here are the top lifestyle habits that tank your liver's ability to efficiently metabolize your hormones:

- Excessive alcohol consumption
- Recreational drug abuse (primarily opioid abuse and cocaine)
- Exposure to environmental toxins like heavy metals
- Eating a diet packed with sugar, refined flours, and inflammatory fats
- Drinking soda and fructose-rich beverages
- Taking medications: acetaminophen (Tylenol), nonsteroidal anti-inflammatory drugs (NSAIDS), methotrexate, amiodarone, and some antiviral drugs

---

WHAT CAUSES BLOATING?

It's common for women to experience bloating after ovulation, and perimenopausal women often experience bloating as their hormonal landscape changes. This bloating is often due to the body's need to detox estrogen. If you want to make the bloat go away, you need to break down the estrogen that is surging through your system. The easiest way to do that is to increase your intake of the foods listed in this chapter. Power up your estrobolome with enough probiotic, prebiotic, and polyphenol foods, and they will be able to break down estrogen more efficiently, and the bloat will go away. Your liver is also key for detoxing estrogen. If bloating becomes a persistent problem post-ovulation, it may behoove you to support your liver with the principles I lay out here.

The liver's ability to efficiently metabolize these hormones is essential for overall hormonal balance and health. Disorders of the liver can lead to imbalances in hormone levels and contribute to various health issues.

What Is Belly Fat?

Belly fat is a huge burden for many women, especially menopausal women. As our hormones shift, fat definitely settles right in the belly region. Ugh! It's frustrating, I know! Perhaps the worst part about belly fat is that you can't diet or exercise your way out of it. That's because this is one of the areas where your body stores all the excess hormones it can't metabolize and detox out of you, especially cortisol and estrogen. If you want to get rid of belly fat, approach it from a hormonal lens. Be sure you are following the rules of eating like a girl, paying extra special attention to Rules #2 and #3.

Foods That Support Great Liver Health

Since the liver is constantly detoxing, it is best to make sure these foods haven't been heavily sprayed with pesticides. To optimally support the liver, get these foods in organic form from a regenerative farm. Here are my top 20 best liver-supporting foods:

1. **Garlic:** Contains sulfur compounds that aid in liver detoxification.
2. **Leafy green vegetables:** Spinach, kale, and Swiss chard are high in chlorophyll, which can help detoxify the liver.
3. **Beets and carrots:** Both are high in flavonoids and beta-carotene, which can improve liver function.
4. **Green tea:** Contains catechins, antioxidants known to improve liver function.
5. **Olive oil:** A healthy fat that provides a lipid base to absorb harmful toxins, thereby relieving the liver of some burden.
6. **Walnuts:** High in omega-3 fatty acids and glutathione, supporting liver detoxification.
7. **Turmeric:** Its active ingredient, curcumin, is known for its liver-protective and anti-inflammatory properties.
8. **Citrus fruits:** Lemons, limes, and oranges are high in vitamin C and antioxidants, aiding the detoxifying process.
9. **Apples:** High in pectin, a type of fiber that can cleanse the liver and the digestive tract.
10. **Grapefruit:** Contains antioxidants that naturally protect the liver.
11. **Cruciferous vegetables:** Broccoli, brussels sprouts, and cauliflower increase the liver's detoxifying enzymes.
12. **Berries:** Blueberries, raspberries, and strawberries are rich in antioxidants, which can protect the liver from damage.
13. **Avocado:** Helps the body produce glutathione, a compound necessary for the liver to cleanse harmful toxins.
14. **Fish:** Rich in omega-3 fatty acids, which are beneficial for liver health.
15. **Radicchio:** My personal fav! Contains inulin, a type of prebiotic fiber that aids in detoxification processes in the liver.
16. **Raw nuts:** Especially almonds and hazelnuts, which are good sources of vitamin E, a nutrient beneficial for liver health. Keep in mind that raw nuts are not heated up like dry-roasted and therefore pack the greatest nutrient punch.
17. **Artichokes:** Known to improve liver health and aid digestion.
18. **Dandelion leaves:** Used as a liver tonic in traditional medicine.

HORMONES THE LIVER METABOLIZES

Estrogen: The liver breaks down estrogen into less active forms. Efficient estrogen metabolism in the liver is crucial for maintaining hormonal balance, especially in women.

Testosterone: The liver helps in the metabolism of testosterone, converting it into more water-soluble forms for excretion.

Insulin: The liver aids in regulating insulin levels in the blood. It can also degrade insulin, helping to maintain appropriate blood-sugar levels.

Cortisol: This stress hormone is metabolized in the liver. Cortisol is broken down into inactive forms that are then excreted.

Thyroid hormones: The liver converts thyroid hormones into their active (or inactive) forms. For instance, the liver converts thyroxine (T4) into its more active form, triiodothyronine (T3).

Growth hormone: The liver metabolizes growth hormone and is also a key site for the production of insulin-like growth factor 1 (IGF-1), which is stimulated by growth hormone.

Adrenaline (epinephrine): The liver plays a role in breaking down this stress-related hormone.

Aldosterone: This hormone, which regulates sodium and potassium balance, is also metabolized in the liver.

Progesterone: The liver helps in breaking down this hormone, which plays a role in the menstrual cycle and pregnancy.

---

19. **Asparagus:** A natural diuretic that helps cleanse the liver.
20. **Watermelon:** Its high water content helps flush toxins from the body, supporting liver health.

RULE #3: EAT TO DETOX HORMONES

Once a hormone has been produced and metabolized and has served its purpose in your body, it needs to exit your system. If it doesn't, it will be stored in fat. The last eat-like-a-girl rule to properly fuel your feminine body is to eat foods that support your detox pathways. Your body has six key pathways to detox these hormones—liver, kidneys, gastrointestinal tract, skin, lungs, and lymphatic system—and the first three are easily supported by the food you eat.

Several lifestyle behaviors deplete these powerful detox organs, and certain foods you can eat support these hard-working organs. Supporting these organs with proper health and nutrition will allow your body to effortlessly clear out these hormones. We've already talked about your liver and your gut health, so let's look at your kidneys.

Your Kidneys

Once a hormone is broken down by your liver, it gets sent to your kidneys for excretion.

Hormones must undergo the liver's metabolic processes to become more water-soluble so they can freely move through the kidneys' filter system. We call this water-soluble version of a hormone a metabolite. If you ever have done a urinary hormone test, you are familiar with the estrogen metabolites. Estrogen breaks down into three specific metabolites—2-OH, 4-OH, and 16-OH. Knowing the ratios of these metabolites is critical for your health. In my Reset Academy, we run urinary hormone tests all the time. This test is truly a lifesaving tool, as it can tell you how much toxic estrogen your body is exposed to. Toxic estrogens come from chemicals in our food, beauty products, and environment. It doesn't matter how clean your lifestyle is; you will still have some toxic estrogen in you. Your liver and kidneys remove this toxic estrogen, and this is why nourishing these organs with good nutrition is so imperative. Toxic estrogen that doesn't detox out of your body can lead to hormonal cancers like breast and ovarian.

Toxins That Harm Your Detox Organs

- Artificial sweeteners
- Alcohol
- Heavy metals (lead, mercury, cadmium, arsenic)
- Over-the-counter painkillers and non-steroidal anti-inflammatory drugs (NSAIDs), like ibuprofen and naproxen
- Illicit drugs (heroin, methamphetamine, and cocaine)
- Environmental pollutants (persistent organic pollutants, or POPs, which can be found in some industrial and agricultural settings, may have harmful effects on kidney function)
- Tobacco (smoking can impair blood flow to the kidneys and exacerbate kidney disease)
- Air pollution
- Pesticides and herbicides
- Polychlorinated biphenyls (PCBs)
- Perfluoroalkyl and polyfluoroalkyl substances (PFAS)
- Bisphenol A (BPA)
- Being in a state of body dehydration

You may be thinking it's too hard to avoid many of the above toxins. I hear you! Most of them are in our environment and we are exposed to them daily. So once again, we must use the power of food to give our kidneys the extra nutrients to handle the ongoing load of toxins they are exposed to.

Foods That Support Your Detox Organs

- **Leafy greens (e.g., spinach, kale):** High in antioxidants and chlorophyll, which can help the liver detoxify the blood.
- **Garlic:** Contains sulfuric compounds that support the liver in producing detoxification enzymes.
- **Lemons:** High in vitamin C, which aids the body in turning toxins into digestible material.
- **Beets:** High in antioxidants and nutrients, including betalains, which support liver detoxification.
- **Green tea:** Contains antioxidants known as catechins, which assist liver function.
- **Turmeric:** Contains curcumin, which is believed to have liver-protecting and regenerative properties.
- **Apples:** High in pectin, a soluble fiber that helps remove toxins and cholesterol from the blood.
- **Ginger:** Helps with digestion and nausea and supports the detoxification process by speeding the movement of food through the intestines.
- **Broccoli sprouts:** High in antioxidants and glucosinolates, which support the liver's detoxification enzymes.
- **Avocados:** Promotes liver health by protecting it against toxic overload and boosting its cleansing power.

- **Flaxseed and chia seeds:** Rich in omega-3 fatty acids and fiber, which help flush toxins from the intestinal tract.
- **Grapefruit:** High in antioxidants and vitamin C, it helps the liver flush out carcinogens and toxins.
- **Dandelion greens:** Known to support digestion and liver detoxification. They can stimulate the liver to eliminate toxins.
- **Artichokes:** High in cynarin and silymarin, which improve liver health and promote bile production, helping to digest fats.
- **Asparagus:** A natural diuretic, which helps flush toxins out of the body, supporting kidney function.
- **Cilantro:** Helps remove heavy metals from the body, which can hinder the body's natural detoxification processes.
- **Seaweed:** Binds to heavy metals and radioactive particles to help remove them from the body.
- **Walnuts:** High in omega-3 fatty acids and glutathione, walnuts support liver cleansing.
- **Cabbage:** Contains sulforaphane, a compound that helps the liver break down toxins.
- **Carrots:** High in beta-carotene and fiber that support liver and digestive health.
- **Watercress:** Acts as a diuretic and digestive aid and provides liver protection.
- **Berries (e.g., blueberries, raspberries):** Rich in antioxidants, they support the liver and protect it from damage.
- **Lentils:** High in fiber, which is essential for healthy digestion and aiding in the detoxification process.
- **Almonds:** Rich in fiber, magnesium, and vitamin E, almonds support liver detoxification and digestive health.
- **Tomatoes:** High in lycopene, which protects the liver from damage by toxins.

Eating like a girl is all about eating for your hormonal health, and as you can see, there are many delicious ingredients that go into that.

Now that you understand the ground rules for eating like a girl, let's put these all together into one easy-to-use lifestyle—a lifestyle where you use food to support both your fasting and eating windows. I am also excited to introduce you to two eating styles, **ketobiotic** and **hormone feasting**, that support *all* your hormones. In the following chapters, I will show you how to effortlessly build this lifestyle for yourself.

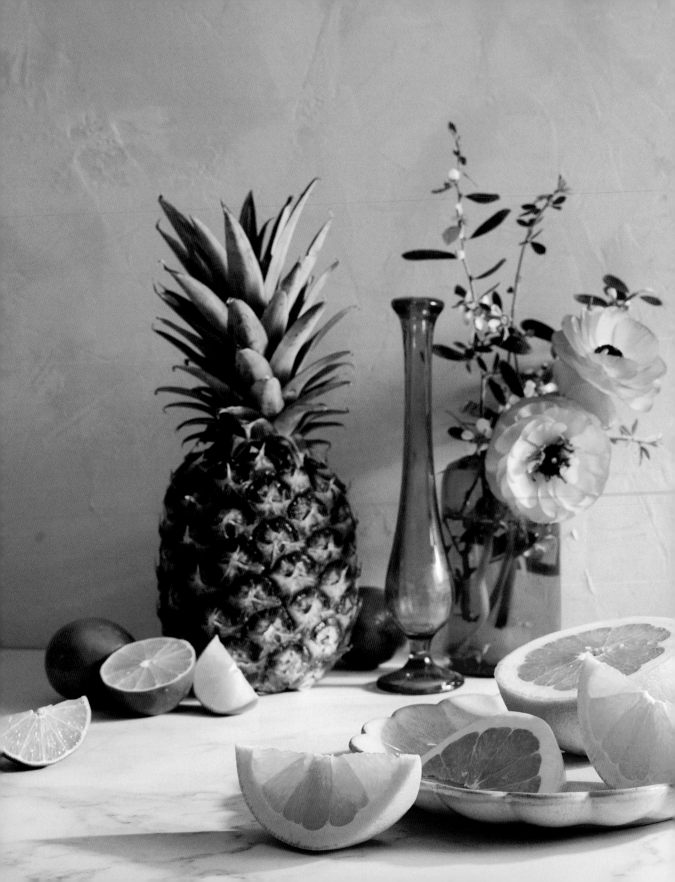

PART II

Using Food to Support Your Fasting Lifestyle

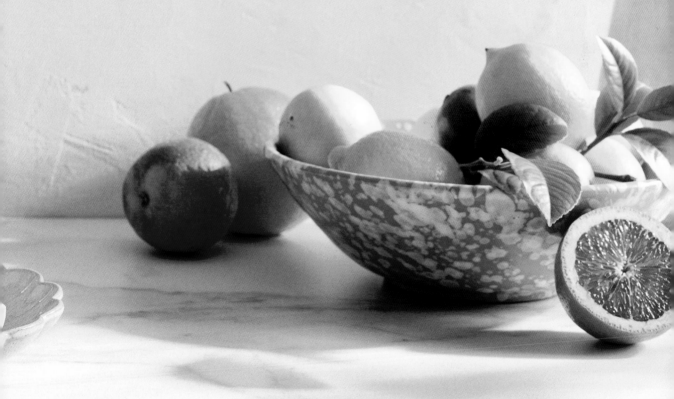

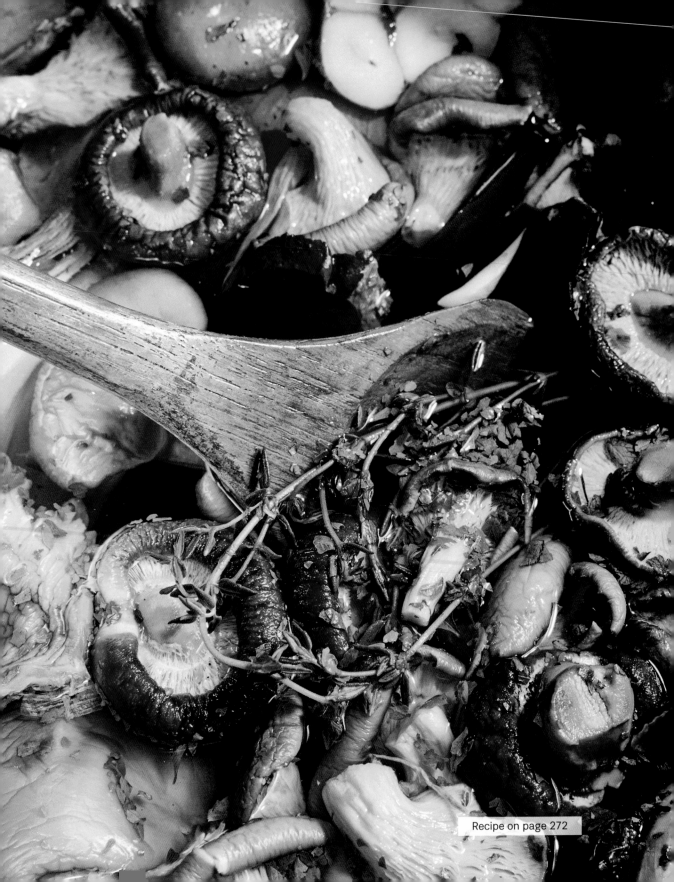

Recipe on page 272

4

Creating Fasting and Eating Windows

THE OLD-SCHOOL approach to speeding up your metabolism was to eat more often. Remember how we were told that eating six small meals a day speeds up our metabolism? How'd that approach work for you? Yeah, it didn't work for me either. In fact, most people saw no evidence of weight loss when they ate all day long. Believe me, I have scoured the research looking for evidence that eating small meals throughout the day speeds up your metabolism. I can't find any scientific evidence that eating more often helps you burn fat. But I *can* find a tremendous amount of research showing that metabolic switching helps us release weight. What we now know is that you can dysregulate your metabolic system by eating the wrong foods all day. If there is anything the research on fasting has taught us, it's that the body repairs during longer periods of rest without food. Just like animals turn away from food when they are sick so they can heal, our bodies operate in a similar fashion. In the absence of food, your body gets a unique opportunity to turn on several healing processes it can't access when you eat.

Does that mean you should fast often if you want to create an amplified healing state? Not necessarily. The top goal for your health should be to regulate your metabolic system. I call this your metabolic switch. Learning how to activate your metabolic switch is the door into a healthy metabolic system. You can accomplish this by creating a window of time when you eat and a window of time when you fast each day. This will bring you back into the natural 24-hour rhythm for which your body was built. When you create these windows, you begin to watch your body effortlessly drop weight, stabilize your hunger, tap into limitless energy, and sharpen your cognitive powers. That's how a regulated metabolic system is meant to feel!

While *Fast Like a Girl* taught you everything you need to know about embracing a fasting lifestyle by adding a regular fasting window to your life, and this book is primarily about finding healing within your eating window, there's still an elephant in the fasting room that I want to address. It's the question I received from thousands after the release of *Fast Like a Girl*: "What can I eat or drink in my fasting window?"

Fundamentals of Your Fasting Window

At its core, the goal of your fasting window is to make sure you don't elevate your blood-sugar levels. In fact, your blood sugar often drops while fasting. Whatever you want to eat or drink within your fasting window (and there are a handful of items you can have), you must not elevate your blood sugar. Depending on how metabolically fit you are, your fasting window will usually start around eight hours without food. At this eight-hour fasting mark, your body starts to switch over into fat burner mode. This switch can take up to four hours, which is why you will see that ketones—a chemical your liver produces when it breaks down fat instead of glucose for energy—start to kick in somewhere around twelve hours in the fasted state. Ketones are an organic acid that are a required fuel source for both the mitochondria of your cells and your brain. The longer you stay in a fasted state, the more your body will fuel itself with ketones, energizing you and amplifying the healing that needs to take place in your body, all while killing hunger. Ketones are largely why fasting gets easier with time.

WHAT IF YOUR BLOOD SUGAR RISES IN THE FASTED STATE?

There are two ways your blood sugar could rise during your fasting window: from endogenous or exogenous sources. An endogenous increase of blood sugar happens when your body releases stored sugar from your tissues. This can happen with exercise, stress, or at night when your body needs to release more glucose.

An exogenous increase in blood sugar happens when you put something in your mouth like food or a drink. Exogenous blood sugar increases are the only ones that pull you out of a fasted state. If you are fasting and decide to go for a run and your body releases stored sugar, you are not breaking a fast. If you drink a cup of coffee before that run and it spikes your blood sugar, it does break your fast.

Although there are some popular foods and drinks that I know will pull you out of a fasted state, ultimately your blood-sugar response is personal. Your gut microbiome controls how high your blood sugar will spike after a meal. We all have a different collection of bacteria in our guts, so one drink may not spike my blood sugar, thus keeping me in a fasted state, while for another person, that same drink pulls them right out of their fasting window. Because of this, even with the fasted-snack guidelines I have provided here, you will want to use the tips in this chapter to tell if you've been pulled out of a fasted state.

HOW CAN YOU TELL IF SOMETHING PULLS YOU OUT OF A FASTED STATE?

The best way to tell if a food or drink has pulled you out of a fasted state is to measure your blood sugar before and after you ingest that food or drink. This is best accomplished with a glucose monitor. If you have a blood-sugar reader (continuous glucose monitor or finger-prick blood-sugar reader), did your blood sugar rise more than 10 mg/dl from the premeal amount? If so, that is a good indicator that what you ingested has pulled you out.

If you can't get a monitor, you can familiarize yourself with some proven symptoms that will help you navigate a fasted snack. If you say yes to any of these questions, most likely it's pulled you out:

- Are you hungrier after that food or drink?
- Are you tired after that food or drink?
- Do you have brain fog after that food or drink?

READING YOUR TONGUE WHEN YOU FAST

A really interesting barometer of healing when you fast is your tongue. Your tongue will often show you how your gut is detoxing while in the fasted state. White, yellow, and black colorations in your tongue while fasting are signs that you are killing off a fungus called *Candida*. I am very familiar with it, as I spent most of my 20s battling it. This fungus lives in your gut; gives you brain fog, fibromyalgia, rashes, and yeast infections; and makes you crave sugary carbohydrates and alcohol to keep it alive. When you fast, you begin to kill off this damaging fungus. That will reflect in your tongue. The longer you fast, you will start to see this discoloration only in the center of your tongue and that fresh pink flesh appears along the edges. That's your body healing! Many people will stay in their extended fast until their tongues are fully pink. That's a sign that most of the nasty microbes in your gut have died off and you are ready for food again.

WHAT IS A FASTED SNACK?

For a good solid seven years, I scoured the research on fasting, grabbing every study I could find on the topic. One day I came across a study that mentioned a fasted snack. It was in a journal produced by the same company that publishes the very well-respected science publication *Nature*, which especially caught

RULES FOR A FASTED SNACK

- < 200 calories
- < 18 grams of fat
- < 5 grams of protein
- < 4 grams of carbohydrates

my eye. This study looked at a 14:10 window, meaning 14 hours of fasting with a 10-hour eating window.[1] What the researchers wanted to see is if people who ate a fat bomb at Hour 12—allowing them to go two hours longer with their fast—got the same benefits as the people who powered through to Hour 14. What they found is that those who ate a fasted snack at Hour 12 did have the ability to go 2 more hours and got a better weight-loss result than the people who stopped fasting at 12 hours.

Why did a pure fat bomb work? Well, fat is a macronutrient that doesn't typically spike your blood sugar. And it kills hunger, which is a faster's dream. I started to experiment with this tool during the monthly Fast Training Weeks that I lead on my socials. Guess what?! The fasted snack worked like a charm! When people hit that point, whether it was Hour 12 or 20, if they ate a fasted snack, they were able to continue longer in a fasted state. And that fasted snack didn't elevate their blood sugar!

The trick then became to decipher the parameters of a fasted snack. The fasted snacks in the *Nutrition & Diabetes* study had some clear metrics; the researchers specifically used mixed nuts that contained 200 calories, 18 grams of fat, 5 grams of protein, and 4 grams of carbohydrate. This is great news because there are many foods you can eat to match those nutritional requirements! To make the fasted snack as easy and delicious as possible, I asked one of my chefs to make a series of possible fasted snacks for you all that will make extending your fasting window that much easier. You will find them in the recipe section of this book.

TRAINING YOURSELF TO STAY IN THE FASTING WINDOW LONGER

When I first started teaching the principles of fasting on my socials, my team and I experimented with all the different types of fasts that were emerging in the research. We started our Fast Training Week, and we had millions of people fasting, trying out all types of fasts. What I learned from that experience is fasting is like running a marathon. If you are training for a marathon, you don't just throw on some running shoes and hope you can make it 26.2 miles. You start with a few miles, then build yourself up. The same goes for fasting. If you want to fast longer, you start with shorter-length fasts and then work yourself up to longer ones. The best approach is to find a fasting length that works for you, do that five days out of the week, then one day a week slowly stretch your fast. Once you can go 24 hours of fasting, you are ready for the fat burner, dopamine reset, and immune reset fasts.

TIPS FOR FEELING BETTER IN THE FASTING WINDOW

As amazing as many people feel in their fasting windows, some will experience negative side effects, especially when they are first learning. Going an extended period without food can cause your body to go into an accelerated healing state. Healing doesn't always feel great. For instance, a fever is your body's way of healing an infection. In the presence of an infection, your body will raise its temperature to burn it out. You feel horrible, yet your body is working

SIX DIFFERENT-LENGTH FASTS

Not all fasts are created equal. With that in mind, let's break down the six different fast lengths:

- Intermittent fasting: 12–16 hours
- Autophagy fasting: starts at 17 hours
- Gut reset fast: 24 hours
- Fat burner fast: 36 hours
- Dopamine reset fast: 48 hours
- Immune reset fast: more than 72 hours

magic in you so that it can destroy that infection. The same thing can happen in your fasting window. As your body repairs itself, you can experience some of the following symptoms:

- Nausea
- Headache
- Bloating
- Light-headedness
- Dizziness
- Feeling weak
- Brain fog
- Insomnia
- Bad breath
- Rashes

As challenging as some of these symptoms may be, they are normal healing responses from your body. Just like when your body is healing from a cold, they are temporary.

Here is a trick you can do to ease these symptoms: Add minerals. We live in a time when our soils are massively depleted of minerals, which means we are eating foods that are the same way. Mineral depletion can give you many of the symptoms listed above. Adding minerals to your water when you're fasting can not only help the cravings for something other than water but also help mitigate these symptoms.

FOOD AND DRINKS THAT CAN PULL YOU OUT OF A FASTED STATE

Perhaps the question I answer the most about fasting is "Will this pull me out of a fasted state?" Although we all have subtle differences in the blood-sugar responses to the foods we eat, there are clearly some I would tell you to avoid in your fasting window. The following are the most common foods and drinks that people think will keep them in a fasted state but often don't. As always, make sure you do the blood-sugar test or pay attention to your symptoms to confirm if it pulls you out.

- Diet drinks
- Gum
- Fruit juices
- Green juices
- Green powdered drinks
- Coffee with pesticides and other chemicals
- Cream in your coffee
- Mushroom coffee
- Kombucha
- Sweet-flavored herbal teas
- Protein drinks

FOOD AND DRINKS THAT TYPICALLY WON'T PULL YOU OUT OF A FASTED STATE

There are some tried-and-true drinks that will not pull most people out of a fasted state. In fact, some of these drinks are used to make fasting easier. This is definitely true with coffee. Many fasters depend on that coffee with a splash of MCT oil to help kill hunger in the fasting window. I can confidently say

that the following drinks and snacks will most likely keep you in a fasted state:

- Water
- Sparkling water
- Organic, mold-free coffee
- Cinnamon and nutmeg in coffee
- Organic unsweetened tea
- Unsweetened mineral packets
- Salt water
- Lemon and ginger juice
- MCT oil in coffee or tea
- Apple cider vinegar
- Some supplements (minerals, algae, spirulina)
- Fasted snacks (see Chapter 11)

Fasting is a great way to heal metabolic, hormonal, and nervous-system dysregulation because it targets your cellular health, cleaning up old, malfunctioning parts and building new, clean, optimally functioning parts. You can use food to help you fast—and extend your fasts—as long as you're not raising your blood-sugar levels, which you can monitor with subjective measures like how you feel and watching for symptoms on your tongue. Keep in mind the most accurate way to monitor your blood sugar is with a blood-sugar reader or continuous glucose monitor.

Now that the fundamentals of using food to support your fasting are firmly under your belt, let's move deeper into a conversation about the importance of food when you go from your fasting window into your eating window. Although this entire book is about navigating your eating window, the first meal you eat after fasting is incredibly important. Fasting is healing and food is healing. Understanding how to strategically move into your eating window will dramatically help you with all your health goals.

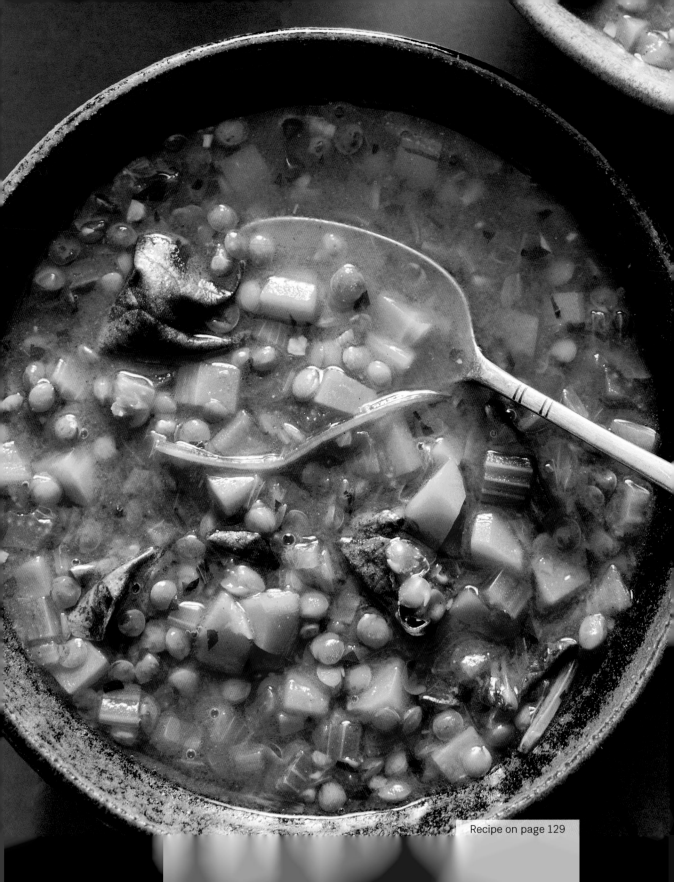

Recipe on page 129

5

Your First Meal Matters
The Art of Breaking Your Fast

A FEW YEARS AGO, I customized a fasting life-style for Jesse Itzler, who is the co-founder of Marquis Jet, a partner in ZICO Coconut Water, co-owner of NBA's Atlanta Hawks, and husband to Sara Blakely, founder of Spanx. He asked me a surprising question: "If I fast, then eat really bad food, have I undone the benefits of the fast?" As I sat with his question, I realized that the answer is actually no. You don't undo the healing benefits of the fast if you eat junk food as your first meal. However, you do stop the healing process that began in your fasting window.

I know Jesse isn't the only person with that question. In fact, I very often see critics of fasting make a similar mistake. Fasting is only one side of the healing equation. We can't just look at absolutes and say fast or don't fast. We need to look at the whole picture. Fasting isn't just about not eating; it's also about the art of breaking your fast.

There's a way to take care of your body in this transition from fat burning to glucose burning, a way to support your microbiome through this journey, and a way to gently and therapeutically move yourself into your eating window. There's an art to it, a rhythm that supports your body's own rhythms and cycles. Just like it's difficult to go from complete and total stress to sitting on the couch relaxing, it can be hard on your body to go from fasting to eating. Your nervous system would still be on high alert and in fight-or-flight mode if you went directly from a high-stress situation to sitting on the couch. It takes a moment to rest and digest before you can really down regulate and relax. We also need to have the right tools to lovingly support the body to go from a fat burner to sugar burner state.

Why Your First Meal Matters

The art of breaking your fast matters for many reasons, but three of the most important have to do with key healing processes your body undergoes when you fast—microbiotic, metabolic, and cellular shifts that occur in the fasted state. For your gut microbiome, fasting changes the whole ecosystem for the better. During your fast, bad bacteria die, good microbes spread out, and depending on the length of your fast, stem cells that repair your intestinal lining wake up and are rejuvenated. Why would the body do this when fasting? Well, it makes perfect evolutionary sense. Your body is preparing for the reintroduction of food. It needs a better terrain inside the lining of your gut so that when food does come in, it's ready to move into the action of using it to keep you functioning at your best. This makes that first meal massively important because your microbes are now ready to serve you. If you feed those microbes foods that support the growth of good bacteria, you will grow them even stronger. Fasting is out with the old, and eating is in with the new.

Your cells also do important work while you fast. Remember the process of becoming insulin-resistant? Your cellular receptor sites get flooded with insulin and glucose. Well, when you are fasting, you stop the flood. This allows both the cellular membranes and insulin receptors to rest and repair. This is the beginning of becoming insulin-sensitive again, where your cells are able to respond appropriately to the gentle surges of glucose and insulin that come at them from your meals. Once your cells reach this new healthy state, if you eat a high-sugar diet, you overwhelm them and put them right back into a state of resistance. Making sure that first meal has a moderate glucose surge is important.

When you fast longer than 17 hours, you also stimulate a cellular healing process called autophagy. This is where the cell registers that no energy from food is coming in, and it starts to clean up the cellular parts that no longer function well. It will also remove bacteria or viruses that may be inside it. In some

cases, if it registers complete dysfunction, the cell will even kill itself in a process called apoptosis. This is important work because dysfunctional cells can turn into cancer cells or zombie aging cells. Autophagy is a wickedly powerful process!

On the other end of autophagy is a cellular process called mTOR, which is a growth process. Whereas autophagy breaks down worn-down cellular parts, mTOR builds them back up new again. You can't be in both autophagy and mTOR at the same time, so if you know that fasting is how your body stimulates autophagy, you can use food—specifically protein—to stimulate mTOR.

Many people have asked, "Doesn't fasting make you lose muscle?" My response to that is only if you don't stimulate mTOR with protein—especially in that first meal. Think of autophagy as getting rid of the cellular parts that no longer serve you, much like the microbiome does. If you follow a fast with protein, you will activate mTOR and build your muscles even stronger than before.

Now that we know that we want to support the health of our gut microbes, keep our cells healthy and in their insulin-sensitive state, and build muscle, let's talk about the principles for your first meal after a fast.

Since your approach should be a little different depending on the length of your fast, I have broken your first-meal guidelines into those two categories—short fasts and long fasts. With longer fasts, your digestion is in pause mode for a longer period, so a more methodical approach to that first meal is important. With shorter fasts, you most likely will do those more often, so putting the right combination of foods together to continue the healing state is important.

Shorter Fasts (12–24 Hours)

I like to think of shorter-length fasts as pulses of healing. When you approach your day through the lens of having a fasting window and an eating window, the first meal of your eating window should serve a healing purpose. Two of the more common fasting lengths that I have watched my community gravitate to on a regular basis are the 17- and 24-hour fasts. Since these fasting lengths tend to be done more frequently, the reentry back into food needs to be simple and easy to follow.

There are three ways to approach breaking these shorter fasts. You can put these three together in one meal or separate them out, depending on what works best for you. Whatever strategy you go with, the most important concept here is to be intentional about your first meal. Here are three strategies for breaking shorter fasts:

- Feed your microbes.
- Slow the blood-sugar spike.
- Power up your muscles.

FEED YOUR MICROBES

This is where the three Ps (polyphenol, probiotic, and prebiotic foods) that I mapped out in Chapter 3 come into play. If you want to rebuild your microbiome after you fast, you are going to want to make sure that you incorporate the three P foods. I often break my fast with a fermented yogurt with blueberries. Fermented yogurt adds new bacteria to my gut and the blueberries fuel all the good microbes. Another favorite is an avocado with sauerkraut and hemp seeds. Sauerkraut is also packed with helpful new probiotics, while the hemp seeds feed those microbes.

It's incredibly powerful to add new bacteria into your gut after a fast. The new gut terrain you created with your fast is primed for new microbe friends! We want those good microbes to have a party in your gut so they can work their magic on your health. Good microbes make important neurotransmitters like serotonin, help you break down estrogen, and power up your immune system. Let's give them what they want so they can thrive! This strategy can repair even the most depleted gut microbiome in a matter of days.

For years in my clinic, I recommended supplements to my patients to repair their guts. Once I found the hack of a 24-hour fast followed by a meal packed with the three Ps, I found supplements were no longer needed. Fasting and food alone repaired their guts! Breaking your fasts with these foods is also powerful for the following conditions:

- Leaky gut
- *Candida*
- Constipation
- Chronic diarrhea
- Post-antibiotic treatment

I also love to break a fast with the healing power of bone broth. The inner lining of your gut loves bone broth! Bone broth contains a key amino acid called glycine. Glycine can help repair a leaky gut, where the integrity of the inner gut lining has been compromised. When this happens, undigested food and toxins can get into your bloodstream and create inflammation. In my clinic, when I had someone with chronically low energy combined with a severe gut dysbiosis, I would have them consistently break their fast with bone broth first. After a cup of bone broth, I had them then get a good dose of the three Ps. That worked like magic!

Sometimes the added fiber that comes with the three Ps can cause you to bloat. If this is you, I recommend you break every fast with bone broth and do more 24-hour fasts to allow the gut more time to heal. Slowly add in sauerkraut after that. When that combo doesn't bloat you, your gut is now ready to go back to more of the foods on the three Ps list.

SLOW THE BLOOD-SUGAR SPIKE

Many people build fasting lifestyles to overturn their metabolic challenges. It is one of the fastest ways I know to turn around insulin resistance. Learning how to metabolically switch can be magic for the person who is weight-loss resistant, has prediabetes, or is diabetic. Whether you are using a fasting lifestyle to overturn a metabolic condition or just want to improve your metabolic markers like fasting glucose or hemoglobin A1c, I highly encourage you to include fiber and fat in your first meal.

Fiber acts like a net for glucose. It catches all the glucose as food enters your stomach, slowing down its absorption into your bloodstream. Adding something very simple like chopped veggies or a bowl of salad to your first meal will help minimize the glucose spike from that meal.

Fat is another powerful food tool that can keep your glucose spikes low. I think of fat as a brake for glucose. You may have heard the recommendation, such as from the Zone Diet, to always put butter on your bread. This works for our metabolic health because butter is a high-fat food that slows down the glucose response that a high-glycemic food like bread can often trigger.[1] In an interview on my *The Resetter Podcast* with Jessie Inchauspé, author of *The Glucose Goddess Method*, she

brilliantly called this "putting clothing on your carbs." Never leave your carbs naked—always dress them up with a fat and you will get a better glucose response to that meal.

You'll notice that the makeup of a fasted snack is largely fat. There is a reason for that. Fat rarely pulls you out of your fasted state. I have used this trick when training people to fast longer. Instead of having them suffer through a longer fast, we start by giving them some fat bombs like those one of our chefs has provided later in the book. It's a great way to kill hunger and not get a glucose spike. It works much like our fasted-snack research showed: Eating a meal rich in fat may help you get the benefits of lower blood sugar hours after you have technically broken your fast. When you are coming out of your fasting window and opening your eating window, fiber and fat can be magical for filling you up, stopping your hunger, and stabilizing your blood sugar.

POWER UP YOUR MUSCLES

The last thing to consider when breaking a shorter fast is mTOR. I have noticed that so many fasters are "in it" for autophagy, a natural cellular process where unnecessary or dysfunctional cellular parts get removed. The minute the world heard that stimulating autophagy meant slowing down aging, preventing cancer, and rejuvenating tired, worn-down cells, it became obsessed. Dr. Yoshinori Ohsumi, the Japanese scientist who discovered the autophagy capabilities of our cells, became a hero, winning the Nobel Prize in Medicine or Physiology for this cellular repair concept. But just like many aspects of the human body, we need *both* repair (autophagy) and growth (mTOR).

LEUCINE-RICH FOODS

Leucine is an essential amino acid, meaning it must be obtained through the diet as the body cannot produce it. It's particularly important for muscle synthesis and repair. Foods high in protein generally contain significant amounts of leucine.

Here are some foods that are particularly rich in leucine:

Whey protein: Whey, a by-product of cheese-making, is one of the richest sources of leucine and is commonly found in protein powders.

Lean meats: Chicken, beef, and pork are excellent sources of leucine. Leaner cuts tend to be preferred for their lower fat content.

Fish: Types like salmon and tuna are not only high in leucine but also rich in omega-3 fatty acids.

Dairy products: Milk, cheese, and yogurt are good sources of leucine. Greek yogurt, in particular, is higher in protein.

Eggs: Eggs are a complete protein source, meaning they contain all nine essential amino acids, including leucine.

Soy products: Tofu, tempeh, and edamame are rich in leucine and are great options for vegetarians and vegans.

Legumes: White beans, navy beans, and lentils contain leucine, although in smaller amounts compared to animal products. They are also a good source of fiber and other nutrients.

Nuts and seeds: Brazil nuts, almonds, peanuts, pumpkin seeds, and chia seeds contain leucine, along with healthy fats and other beneficial nutrients.

Gluten-free grains: Quinoa and oats contain more leucine than most other grains and are also rich in fiber.

Protein-rich vegetables: Peas and mushrooms, for example, contain a fair amount of leucine compared with other vegetables.

The greatest way to stimulate the growth response of the mTOR cellular pathway is with protein. This is key for the faster who wants to build muscle. Once you have stimulated autophagy with fasting, stimulate mTOR with protein. According to the current research, you need to have at least 30 grams of protein in every meal to stimulate the growth of your muscles.[2] You also want to make sure that protein contains the amino acid leucine. Leucine triggers your muscles to open their amino-acid sensors and pull all the other amino acids into them to build them stronger.[3] There are both plant-based and animal-based ways to get leucine into your diet, so pick your sources according to your food philosophy.

Longer Fasts (24+ Hours)

I remember jumping right back into food with scrambled eggs after my first three-day water fast. That seemed like an easy thing for my body to digest, but it wasn't. Two things happened: I felt like a bowl of tar was sitting in my tummy, and I was really tired. What I learned

THE BOOMERANG EFFECT

The four-step process I recommend for your first meal after a longer fast is key if you suffer from the boomerang effect, which I'm pretty sure happens to every beginning faster. When you open up your eating window, you go crazy with food. As I told Jesse Itzler, it doesn't undo the healing that happened while you were fasting, but it does abruptly halt the healing state you created in your fasting window. The more experienced you get with your fasting lifestyle, the less the boomerang effect will happen to you.

If you feel like this is a huge hurdle for you, be sure your first meal follows either the three principles I laid out for you with the shorter fasts, or do the four-step process for longer ones. A helpful trick to tell your mind is that the first meal is a healthy one, then you can go crazy eating what your taste buds are calling for. What I have noticed with our community is that after they have an intentional healthy meal first, the cravings for the junky food tend to go away. So task yourself with one good meal first, then see what your taste buds want. You may be surprised to find that your craving for processed foods goes away. This is the beginning of how you start to change your taste buds.

in that failed experiment was that while protein is incredibly powerful for ending shorter fasts, it is the wrong thing to add back in first after three days of not eating. I needed a different approach.

When you fast longer than 24 hours, you have all these cellular and microbial healing processes going on, and your digestive system has been on pause mode. This means you want to be a little slower in how you reintroduce food. To best help your digestion, I created a four-step process you can use to slowly warm up your digestive system as your eating window opens.

This process was originally developed for a three-day water fast. But one thing I noticed with the launch of *Fast Like a Girl* was how many women gravitated to the 36-hour fast. Perhaps it's because of the science showing this fast length's ability to burn belly fat or because of its simplicity, but either way, I began to see that, for these women, the reentry back into food was a little challenging after they hadn't eaten for 36 hours. That's when I started recommending the four-step process to anyone who does more than 24 hours. Wait 30 to 60 minutes between each step.

- **Step #1:** Drink a cup of bone or vegetable broth.
- **Step #2:** Eat a probiotic-rich meal with a good fat.
- **Step #3:** Consume nature's carbs (steamed veggies, fruits, and potatoes).
- **Step #4:** Eat protein-rich foods (animal meats and high-protein veggies).

Here's why it works: Broth coats the gut, probiotic foods give your gut more good bacteria, the fiber of nature's carbs feeds those bacteria, and protein gives you the amino acids needed to build muscle. It works like a charm for letting your body ease back into food, all while honoring your good gut bacteria and stimulating mTOR for growing muscle, hormones, and neurotransmitters.

WHAT TYPE OF BROTH DOES IT NEED TO BE?

Many in our plant-based community have asked if they can use vegetable broth instead of bone broth, and the answer is resoundingly yes. In fact, one of my chefs has provided a functional mushroom broth for those of you who prefer plant-based.

Please note, though, that while functional medicinal mushrooms hold lots of healing power and are a great way for those of you who are plant-based to get back into food, they are missing glycine. Glycine makes up around 33 percent of the collagen in the human body. Not only is it key for gut repair, but it can also help regulate your nervous system, lift your moods, improve your memory, bind to toxins, and help assist you in a good night's sleep.[4] It is such a powerful nutrient that I have added a list of foods that contain glycine. Be sure that somewhere along your entry back into eating, you incorporate these foods into your meals.

For those who are omnivores, my other chef has created two amazing bone broths. Both are great for breaking your fast. How you choose which one to break your fast is up to you, but keep in mind that the poultry broth will have more tryptophan, which is terrific for moods, whereas beef broth has more glycine, which, as I pointed out above, can have a huge upside for your body.

FOODS HIGH IN GLYCINE

Gelatin: Derived from animal collagen, gelatin is one of the richest sources of glycine.

Bone broth: Made by simmering bones for a long time to extract nutrients.

Skin and connective tissues of poultry: Chicken skin, turkey skin, and other poultry connective tissues are high in glycine.

Fish and seafood: Ones with their skin on, such as salmon, are especially good sources of glycine.

Meat cuts with connective tissue: Meats that contain more connective tissue, such as oxtail, chuck roast, and other tougher cuts, are higher in glycine.

Spirulina: This blue-green algae is a superfood due to its high nutrient content and a good plant-based source of glycine.

Eggs: The white parts are a particularly good source of glycine and other amino acids.

Dairy products: Animal-based milk, cheese, and yogurt contain glycine, with whey protein being particularly rich in this amino acid.

Legumes: Beans, lentils, and other legumes contain glycine, although in lower amounts compared to animal-based sources.

Nuts and seeds: Certain nuts and seeds, such as pumpkin seeds, are good plant-based sources of glycine.

WHY DO I NEED TO STEAM THE VEGGIES IN STEP #3?

As much as I love the fiber that raw vegetables provide, when you are coming out of a longer fast, it can be too much fiber. That's why I like to just lightly steam them. You still want them crunchy, so don't steam them too long. Sometimes raw vegetables after a fast can bloat you, so steaming them will help minimize the bloat.

HOW LONG DO I HAVE TO WAIT IN BETWEEN EACH STEP OF BREAKING A LONGER FAST?

With longer fasts, there is definitely an excitement that comes over you when you realize you get to eat again. My general rule for how much time you wait between each step is 30 to 60 minutes. This allows you to see how your body did with that step. If you are tired, bloated, or feel brain-foggy after a step, wait a little longer before you move to the next step. These symptoms can mean that your body just needs a slower reentry into food. If you do a step and feel great, keep going—your body is assimilating it well.

WHAT IF I DON'T FEEL WELL WITH CERTAIN FOODS AFTER I DO A LONGER FAST?

Fasting can act like an elimination diet. Before we had food allergy tests, doctors would do elimination diets to see which foods people reacted to. Elimination diets entailed pulling the suspected offending foods out of a person's diet and slowly reintroducing each food one at a time. If you reacted badly to a food, then there was a large possibility that you were allergic to it. Longer fasts can provide you this same experiment. Only in this case, you took all food out of the equation. So, for the days following a longer fast, take special note as to which ones make you tired, give you brain fog, cause your muscles to ache, or make you gain weight. This is a unique opportunity to see how your body reacts. If a food causes you any discomfort, take it out of your diet for some time. Remember, over time, fasting will help you repair your gut.

One of my favorite foods that I loved for years was cereal. Yep, you heard that right! Cereal was my go-to meal. But when I first started experimenting with building myself a fasting lifestyle, I tried breaking my fast with cereal. Wow! Was I a hot mess! Brain fog, sleepiness, and heavy limbs flooded me within an hour of eating a bowl of my favorite cereal—and that was with a shorter fast. It was such a profound experience that I never ate cereal again. Often, when we experience the consequence of a certain food, we find the motivation to avoid it. That's what happened to me with cereal.

Now that you understand the Foundational Five, the Three Food Rules for eating like a girl, and the fundamentals to moving between your fasting and eating windows, the moment has arrived to chat about how we align all this to the rhythm of your hormones.

Recipe on page 266

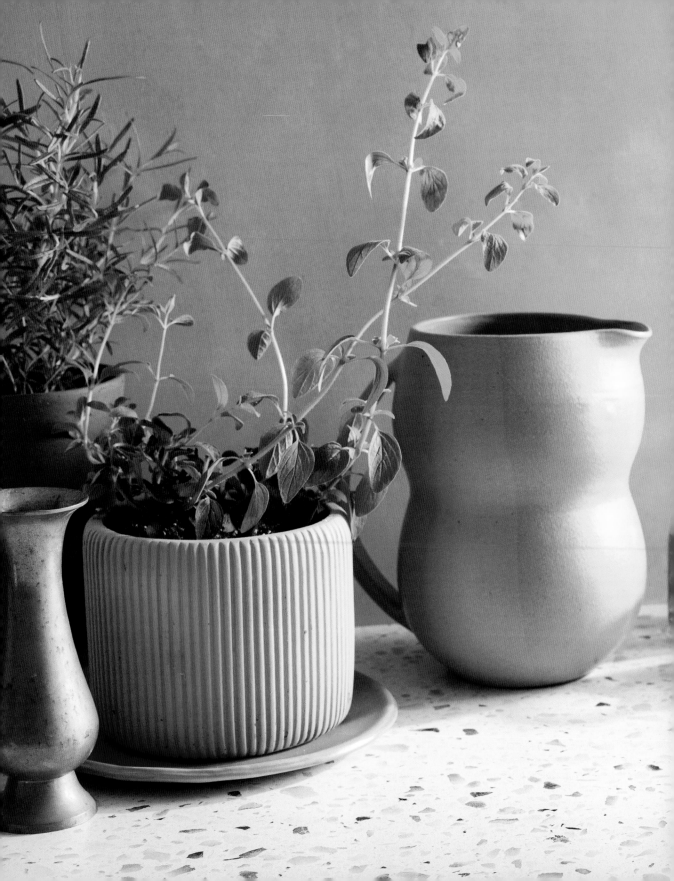

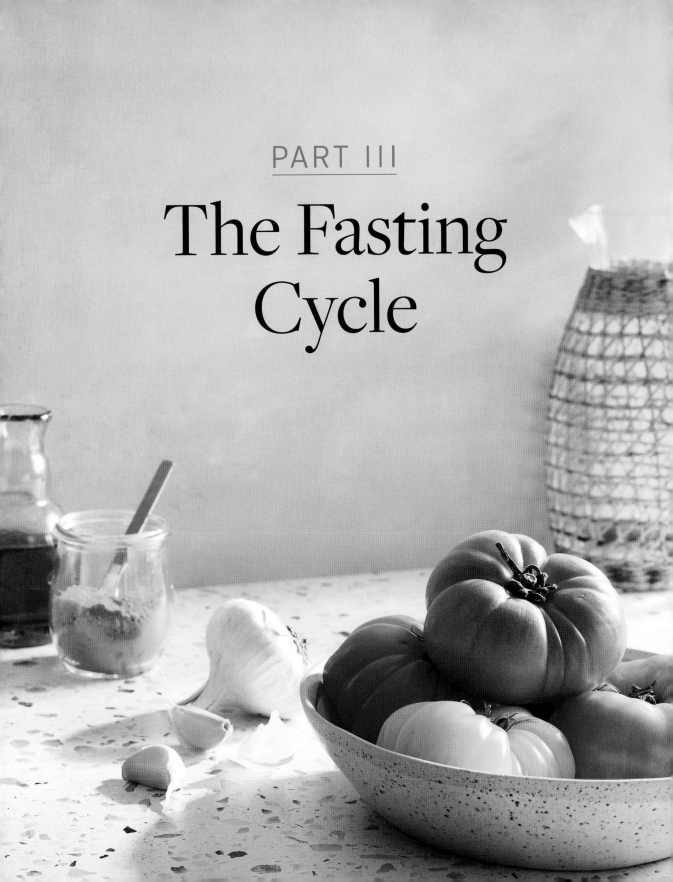

PART III

The Fasting Cycle

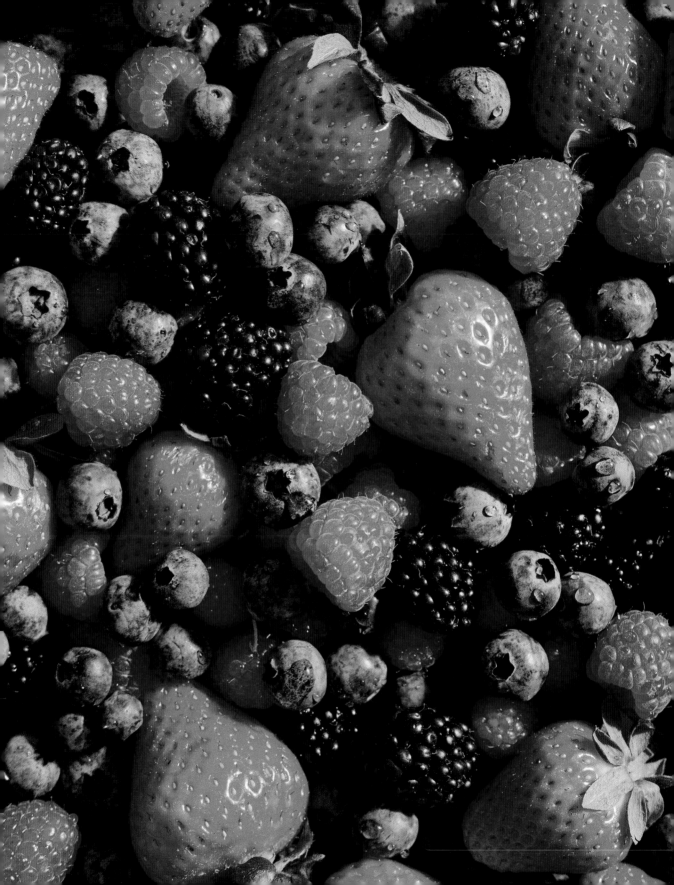

6

Your Power Phases

FOLLICULAR PHASE, LUTEAL PHASE, luteinizing hormone, follicular-stimulating hormone, estrogen metabolites, estradiol, estrone, estriol, pregnenolone, DHEA—hormones are complicated enough, but when you add sophisticated language to the discussion, it can be even harder to grasp these molecules that are so central to who we are and how our bodies operate. My friend and fellow hormone expert Dr. Carrie Jones once told me that we really need to give our hormonal system nail polish names. I love this idea! It made me realize that if we could make the language of hormones fun and approachable, more women might be able to understand these incredible wisdom molecules that affect so

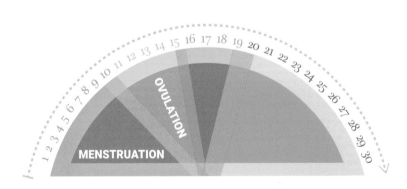

THE POWER OF FASTING AND YOUR CYCLE

DAYS 1–10	DAYS 11–15	DAYS 16–19	DAYS 20–BLEED
POWER PHASE 1	MANIFESTATION	POWER PHASE 2	NURTURE PHASE
(MENSTRUATION)	(OVULATION)		
FASTING:	FASTING:	FASTING:	NO FASTING
13–72 HOURS	13–15 HOURS	13–72 HOURS	
FOOD:	FOOD:	FOOD:	FOOD:
KETOBIOTIC	HORMONE FEASTING	KETOBIOTIC	HORMONE FEASTING

FEMALE HORMONE CYCLE

■ Estrogen   ■ Oxytocin   ■ Testosterone   ■ Progesterone

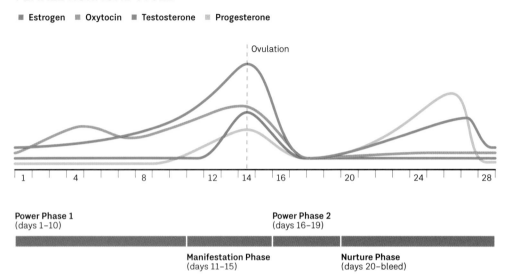

Ovulation

1   4   8   12   14   16   20   24   28

Power Phase 1
(days 1–10)

Power Phase 2
(days 16–19)

Manifestation Phase
(days 11–15)

Nurture Phase
(days 20–bleed)

many of us. This led me to develop easy-to-understand names for the ebbs and flows of our hormones throughout our monthly menstrual cycle so that we can more easily align our lifestyle choices with our bodies' rhythms.

I call this the Fasting Cycle, which breaks down the menstrual cycle into four parts. The first 10 days of your menstrual cycle are considered Power Phase 1—the time when you go from low hormones to estrogen surging in. The second phase of your cycle is your Manifestation Phase—the moment of ovulation when estrogen, testosterone, and progesterone all come together to give you some wicked hormonal superpowers. The third phase of your cycle is Power Phase 2—another low-hormone moment when detoxing hormones becomes your focus. And the fourth and last phase is the Nurture Phase, when progesterone peaks before you bleed again. The following chapters explore each phase in depth from a food perspective and what to do if you have lost your cycle or are a menopausal woman.

You'll notice that the Fasting Cycle incorporates two food styles: ketobiotic and hormone feasting. The major difference between these styles of food is the carbohydrate amounts. With hormone feasting, you eat more carbohydrates to ensure that you are accomplishing all Three Food Rules for eating like a girl. With ketobiotic, you bring your carbohydrate load down to ensure that you stay insulin-sensitive, which helps with weight loss and estrogen production. In the recipe section of this book, my chefs have created delicious recipes that fit the guidelines of each style.

About the Power Phases

Let me introduce you to the parts of your menstrual cycle I call your power phases. If you are a menstruating woman, you have two times in your cycle when your hormones are at their lowest. The first is the day your period starts, or Day 1 of your cycle. It's the time when you need feminine care products to manage the blood flow. The other low-hormonal time is right after ovulation—around Day 16 of your cycle. When a released egg is not fertilized, all your hormones come crashing down again.

When your hormones are low, your health habits can go high. That's why I named these your power phases. Whether it's a new, more restrictive diet, an intense workout, or an elite biohack, your power phases are a time to tackle your biggest lifestyle tools. This works because when your hormones are low, your body is more resilient to the cortisol surges that tough workouts and longer fasts bring. Many of the intense health strategies popular today can temporarily increase cortisol in your body, especially when it's new for you and your body is forced to adapt in a big way. You don't have to avoid major health challenges, just use them strategically—and using your power phases as opportunities to lean into big, bold, and intense lifestyle choices can be helpful.

Power Phase 1 (Days 1–10)

For many of us, once our period starts, there seems to be a moment of relief and release. That's because it's a time when our hormones go low.

Power Phase 1 is also a time when a hormonal tag team comes together to start to build up estrogen, specifically estradiol, for releasing an egg during the following phase, which is ovulation. Knowing that your hormones are low and slowly building in these first 10 days enables you to focus on longer fasts, lower-carbohydrate diets, and more challenging workouts. In addition to focusing on leveling up your health strategies during

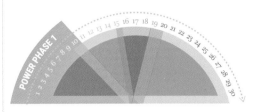

THE POWER OF FASTING AND YOUR CYCLE

DAYS 1–10
POWER PHASE 1 (MENSTRUATION)
FASTING: 13–72 HOURS
FOOD: KETOBIOTIC
POWER PHASE 1

this time, you can also prioritize eating foods to support estrogen's needs.

HOW DOES YOUR BRAIN RESPOND TO AN INCREASE IN ESTRADIOL?

Your brain functions differently during different parts of your cycle. As estradiol increases in your first power phase, so will your moods and cognitive powers. Estradiol stimulates five key brain neurochemicals: dopamine, serotonin, glutamate, acetylcholine, and brain-derived neurotrophic factor (BDNF). This surge of neurochemicals can elevate your moods, increase your energy levels, and give you an overall sense of well-being. You may also notice that the closer you get to the peak of estradiol at ovulation, you have enhanced verbal fluency, memory, and focus.

NUTRITION FOR YOUR FIRST POWER PHASE

Think of your first power phase as a time to create an environment inside your body that will effortlessly allow for estrogen production.

There are five key strategies to follow in Power Phase 1:

1. Keep glucose levels low and stable.
2. Avoid processed carbs.
3. Eat more of nature's fiber-rich carbs.
4. Choose healthy oils, not inflammatory oils.
5. Avoid obesogens.

Estrogen thrives in an insulin-sensitive body! This makes this first power phase a beautiful 10-day period where a lower-carbohydrate diet will favor both your metabolic health and your hormonal health. Avoiding humanmade, processed carbohydrates during this time is pivotal. That doesn't mean you have to completely give up carbs—you just want to switch your carbohydrate load to nature's fibrous carbohydrates. This is best done by eating a modified version of the ketogenic diet called ketobiotic. The reason the ketogenic diet failed so many women is because in order to go extremely low carb, you had to give up fruits and vegetables. Long term, this is horrible for a woman's hormonal system. With ketobiotic, you have a higher carbohydrate amount than a typical keto diet, plus all your carbohydrates are coming from plant-based sources.

Total Carbohydrates Versus Net Carbohydrates

All carbohydrates are not made equal. The best way to choose the right carbohydrate for you is to know the difference between a total carbohydrate and a net carbohydrate. Net carbs (as the keto world lovingly refers to them) means the total carbohydrate minus the fiber. You will see that when you eat lots of vegetables, they contain so much fiber that you can eat a large amount and still stay

CARBOHYDRATES
Blood Glucose Levels over Time

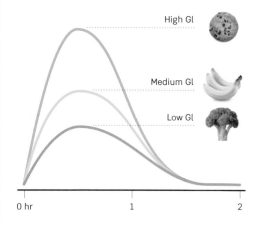

within the recommended carbohydrate load of 50 net carbs. For example, the typical total carb load of a piece of whole-wheat bread is 17 grams with 2 grams of fiber. That gives you a 15-gram-net-carb expense for one piece of bread. That's expensive! Whereas a half cup of broccoli is 5.6 grams of total carbohydrates, with 2 of the grams coming from fiber, giving it a net carb load of 3.6 grams. The high fiber in vegetables and some fruits makes the net-carb load low. This means you can eat a lot of them in your power phases!

How Much Protein Should You Have When Eating Ketobiotic?

Protein is trendy right now in the nutritional world, and rightly so! There are so many reasons for women to eat more protein, perhaps the biggest being its amino acid profile. Amino acids are key nutrients needed to make hormones.

Many experts recommend consuming 1 gram of protein for every pound of ideal body weight. That means if your ideal body weight is 130 pounds, you would eat 130 grams of protein in a day. I like this approach, but I

THE KETOBIOTIC FOOD STYLE

- < 50 grams net carbohydrates; nature's carbs only
- No humanmade carbohydrates (breads, pastas, desserts, crackers, etc.)
- 75 grams of protein
- Fat with every meal

have found that if you are extremely insulin-resistant with a depleted gut microbiome, your body will convert high amounts of protein into excess glucose that can then be stored as fat.

Remember that the purpose of your power phases is to ensure your body stays insulin-sensitive. These are two unique times in your cycle when you can make great strides in improving your metabolic health without hurting your sex hormones. For many women, this means potentially keeping protein intake to a recommended 75 grams of protein rather than protein loading. Mixing a lower-than-usual protein and carbohydrate load with some longer fasts during your power phases will train your body to become insulin-sensitive again. Once you become insulin-sensitive, you can begin to bring your protein loads up to match your ideal body weight.

EXAMPLES OF KETOBIOTIC CARBOHYDRATES

Vegetables (serving size equals 1 cup unless otherwise noted)

Spinach (raw): Net carbs: 1 gram

Lettuce (romaine): Net carbs: 1 gram

Zucchini: Net carbs: 2 grams

Asparagus: Net carbs: 2 grams (for 6 spears)

Avocado: Net carbs: 2 grams (for ½ avocado)

Broccoli: Net carbs: 4 grams

Cauliflower: Net carbs: 3 grams

Cabbage: Net carbs: 2 grams

Mushrooms: Net carbs: 2 grams

Green beans: Net carbs: 4 grams

Fruits (serving size equals ½ cup unless otherwise noted)

Raspberries: Net carbs: 3 grams

Blackberries: Net carbs: 4 grams

Strawberries: Net carbs: 4 grams

Blueberries: Net carbs: 9 grams

Cantaloupe: Net carbs: 6 grams

Peaches: Net carbs: 7 grams (for ½ peach)

Watermelon: Net carbs: 5 grams

Avocado (also listed as a vegetable due to its culinary uses): Net carbs: 2 grams (for ½ avocado)

Lemon: Net carbs: 4 grams (for 1 whole lemon, but usually consumed in smaller quantities)

Kiwi: Net carbs: 8 grams (for 1 medium kiwi)

THE *N*-OF-1 THEORY

N of 1 is an incredibly important concept for women. It comes from the research world: Whenever a study is performed, the researchers tell you the number of people in the study. They do that by phrasing it as *n*. So if there are 3,000 people in the study (which would be an impressive number!), it would say *n* = 3,000. The *n*-of-1 theory means that there is only one person to study: YOU! This matters for our feminine bodies because our hormones demand we personalize our lifestyle choices.

The *n*-of-1 theory emphasizes the importance of individualized treatment plans based on direct evidence of how a single patient responds to a specific intervention. This *n*-of-1 concept is being used more often for women,

and it represents a shift away from a one-size-fits-all approach toward more personalized healthcare. When you take health information and test it on yourself to decide if it's right for you, you take your power back—a power that gets pulled from you every time you try a new trendy diet, take medication researched only on men, or try to follow the herd when it comes to health. You are unique! Be curious about how different health concepts work for you. Finding what is effective for your feminine body is a critical component of lasting health. Don't fear tapping into your own intuitive sense to find the best macronutrient needs for your body and the different phases of your cycle.

How Much Fat Should You Eat?

When it comes to the amount of good healthy fat you need in a day, there is no real proven gram amount to follow. If you are tracking your macronutrients on an app like Carb Manager, it will give you a percentage of the total fat that you ate in a day. During your power phases, this is important because fat kills hunger. Remember, we are using these low-hormone moments to train your body to become metabolically healthy. I often say shoot for 60 percent of your food coming from good fat. That can be hard to measure, so I use it loosely as a target. Some days you will hit it, some days not. A good rule is to just have fat with every meal. When the keto diet first became popular, many thought it was a high-fat diet. Nothing could be further from

the truth. The major concept of the keto diet is to eat to stabilize your blood sugar. There are many ways you can do this, and increasing your healthy fat load is one of them.

If hunger is an issue as you make changes to your food choices, always remember that good fat is an incredible tool to control hunger. Adding a little bit of healthy fat to a meal will stop the blood-sugar spikes and kill your cravings for more food. Keep in mind that choosing the right amount of fat in a day is what we call an *n*-of-1 experience. Decide how much fat in a day works best for your body.

Are There Specific Foods You Can Eat to Improve Estrogen Production?

In addition to eating the ketobiotic way in Power Phase 1, you may also want to emphasize specific foods that will help you build

FOODS THAT SUPPORT ESTROGEN

Organic soy products: Items such as tofu, tempeh, soy milk, and edamame contain phytoestrogens that can mimic the effects of natural estrogen.

Flaxseed: High in lignans, which are another type of phytoestrogen.

Sesame seeds: Also contain phytoestrogens, with the added bonus of essential minerals.

Garlic: Can help in maintaining balanced levels of estrogen in the body.

Chickpeas: A good source of plant-based protein and phytoestrogens.

Alfalfa sprouts: Known for their rich content of phytoestrogens.

Beans: Various beans, like kidney beans and black beans, contain phytoestrogens and are also high in fiber.

Peas: Another legume with phytoestrogen content.

Nuts: Especially almonds, walnuts, and pistachios, which have phytoestrogens.

Apples: High in fiber, which helps in regulating estrogen levels. Green ones are best.

Carrots: Their fiber content can aid in estrogen metabolism.

Pomegranates: Contain compounds that may have estrogen-like effects.

Plums: They have some level of phytoestrogens and are also high in antioxidants.

Berries: Strawberries, raspberries, and cranberries all have phytoestrogenic properties.

Brussels sprouts: Can promote estrogen metabolism and are high in vitamins.

Bok choy: Contains phytonutrients that may influence estrogen metabolism.

Kale: As a cruciferous vegetable, it supports hormonal balance.

Cauliflower: Another cruciferous vegetable that aids in estrogen metabolism.

Broccoli: Contains compounds that help in the detoxification of estrogen.

your protective estrogen levels. Years ago, the term *estrogen dominance* got thrown around a lot, but as in many aspects of health, the nuance was left out. When you hear someone talk about being estrogen-dominant, they are often referring to the fact that they have too much toxic estrogen. One way of protecting yourself from toxic estrogen is to build up your protective estrogen stores. You can increase this helpful form of estrogen by eating the foods listed in the chart above.

WHAT'S THE BEST TIME IN YOUR CYCLE FOR LONGER FASTS?

Fasting is a wonderful healing tool for women. We just need to time it right, especially the longer fasts. Another incredible insight I gained from the success of *Fast Like a Girl* was how many women wanted to try longer fasts. If you are one of those who are called to the longer fasts, keep in mind that the power phases are the moments in your cycle where

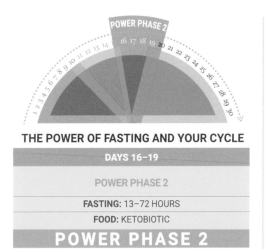

THE POWER OF FASTING AND YOUR CYCLE

DAYS 16–19
POWER PHASE 2
FASTING: 13–72 HOURS
FOOD: KETOBIOTIC
POWER PHASE 2

you can successfully do that. When I am working with a patient, I use their power phases to dip into longer fasts so that we can start to get their bodies insulin-sensitive again. Then, when they go into the other phases of their cycle, we tighten up their fasting windows and lean into the healing power of food. One hack to keep in mind if you are going into longer fasts is to be sure to power up on electrolytes like sodium, magnesium, potassium, and calcium while you are fasting. These electrolytes are the ones you lose while you are bleeding at the start of your menstrual cycle.

Power Phase 2 (Days 16–19)

The second low-hormonal moment in your menstrual cycle is right after ovulation, around Day 16. Although your actual ovulation day may vary from month to month, around Day 16 you can pretty much guarantee you are entering a four-day period where your hormones will be at another monthly low. Just like with Power Phase 1, this little four-day window can be a great time to go

back to the ketobiotic diet and hop on some longer fasts to help you stay metabolically healthy. In my clinic, I would often use this moment of a woman's cycle to help her overturn weight-loss resistance. Additionally, there are a few unique things about the second power phase—most importantly that you want to lean into foods that will help you detox the estrogen that peaked during ovulation.

YOUR MENSTRUAL CYCLE WEIGHT-LOSS MOMENTS

You are *not* meant to eat the same foods all month long. When you go on a weight-loss "diet," usually you eat one specific style throughout the month to lose weight. There is no variation according to your hormonal ebbs and flows. But two major hurdles occur with this approach. First, many weight-loss strategies spike cortisol. High cortisol all month long can cause your hormones to tank. This can cause too many women to lose their menstrual cycles. Being your ideal weight but not having a regular menstrual cycle is not healthy. You need that uterine lining to shed every month to release excess toxins; this also creates a new healthy environment in your uterine lining. You also need to not be in a fight-or-flight state all the time. You need to rest, digest, and flow with your natural hormonal rhythms.

The second problem with most weight-loss diets occurs when a diet stops working. Ever wonder why that happens? It's because your hormones demand food variation. If you go into a restrictive diet that keeps a diversity of food choices and perhaps even calories at an all-time low, your body starts to think that it's in a crisis. It worries that no more food is

FATS AND OILS

Healthy Noninflammatory Fats

- Extra-virgin olive oil
- Flaxseed oil
- Avocado oil
- Walnut oil
- Chia seed oil
- Hemp seed oil
- Algae oil
- Pumpkin seed oil
- Krill oil
- Sesame seed oil
- Coconut oil
- MCT oil
- Grass-fed dairy (butter, cheese, yogurt)
- Raw nuts and seeds
- Raw nut butters
- Avocado

Harmful Inflammatory Oils

- Soybean oil
- Corn oil
- Cottonseed oil
- Canola oil
- Sunflower oil
- Peanut oil
- Safflower oil
- Grapeseed oil
- Margarine and vegetable shortening

coming in, so it slows down the burning of fat. And without the variety of good nutritious nature's food, the microbes that balance your blood sugar can perish.

On the contrary, the key to lasting weight loss is learning how to metabolically flex in and out of your sugar burner and fat burner metabolic systems. If you are embarking on a low-calorie or low-carb diet, the best part of your cycle to do this is your power phases. Pair it with a fasting window and you will accelerate weight loss. Between the two power phases, you have 14 days to concentrate on losing weight. During other times of the month, focus on higher-carbohydrate food as your medicine for hormonal health.

This is what it means to eat like a girl! You get your cake and eat it too. Parts of the month are reserved for weight loss, while other parts of the month you should focus on keeping your sex hormones at their best.

YOUR MENSTRUAL CYCLE DETOX MOMENTS

Think of your second power phase as a moment you want to focus on detoxing. Remember how estradiol peaks to release an egg during ovulation? Well, after that egg is released and estradiol has worked her magic in many parts of your brain and body, she needs to be detoxed out. Just like excess glucose gets stored as fat, if you don't detox estrogen, she will be stored as fat. And guess where your body likes to store that excess estrogen? Your belly and boobs! Knowing this makes the ketobiotic way of eating a great tool for this short four-day period. Pay especially close attention to powering up on foods that support your gut and liver. These foods will help you detox estrogen the best:

- **Fermented foods:** sauerkraut, raw kefir, and yogurt
- **Bitter foods:** radicchio, dandelion greens, ginger, and lemon
- **Cruciferous foods:** broccoli, cauliflower, and brussels sprouts
- **Leafy greens:** spinach, Swiss chard, and kale
- **Sulfur-rich foods:** garlic, onions, and leeks
- **Citrus fruits:** lemon, grapefruit, and oranges
- **Nuts and seeds:** chia seeds, hemp seeds, and walnuts
- **Green tea**

AREN'T SOY PRODUCTS HARMFUL TO WOMEN?

Soy has definitely gotten a bad rap. So much so that women seem to completely forget that nature has provided an incredible plant version of estrogen called a phytoestrogen. Soy has a high content of isoflavones, a class of phytoestrogens that can mimic or modulate the body's natural estrogen.[1] These natural estrogens are not carcinogenic; in fact, they actually protect the female body. Soy is also high in antioxidants and is a complete protein source (rare for plants). My only note of caution with any soy product is to make sure it's organic so that you don't get a dose of estrogen-mimicking pesticides.

Here are some of the key health benefits of soy products for women:

- Menopause symptom relief[2]
- Bone health[3]
- Heart health
- Reduced risk of breast cancer
- Fertility
- Reduced risk of endometrial cancer
- Weight management[4]
- Improved skin health

WHAT IF YOU ARE TRYING TO GET PREGNANT?

A note of caution: If you are actively trying to conceive a baby, when you come out of ovulation, don't move into the ketobiotic food style. Keeping carbs low can add stress to your body, even with the more generous carb amounts that the ketobiotic food plan offers. Instead, you will want to move immediately into hormone feasting, which is a style of eating I explain in detail in the next chapter. This style supports progesterone in a better way.

WHAT'S IN YOUR MENSTRUAL BLOOD?

Too many of us spend our menstruating lives hassled by our periods. But if you understand what is happening in the first few days of your cycle, you might reevaluate how you look at this time. The week before your period, progesterone surges and then estrogen makes a momentary appearance. This combo triggers your uterine lining to shed. The bleeding that happens to you every month is not useless. It's a detox moment. Your body is excreting what no longer serves it. It is getting rid of the uterine lining and giving you a fresh new one for an egg to implant. Your menstrual blood consists of more than a thousand different proteins, including proteolytic enzymes, cytokines, a host of proteins from diverse types of immune cells, and discarded, worn-out cellular parts.[5] But that is not all that is in menstrual blood. Many women are shocked to hear that it is one way the female body detoxes harmful chemicals we are exposed to on a daily basis. Research is revealing that it contains toxins, parabens, pesticides, BPA plastics, and phthalates.[6] This makes it massively important to have a period every month so you can get these toxins out so that they don't build up in your system and cause disease.

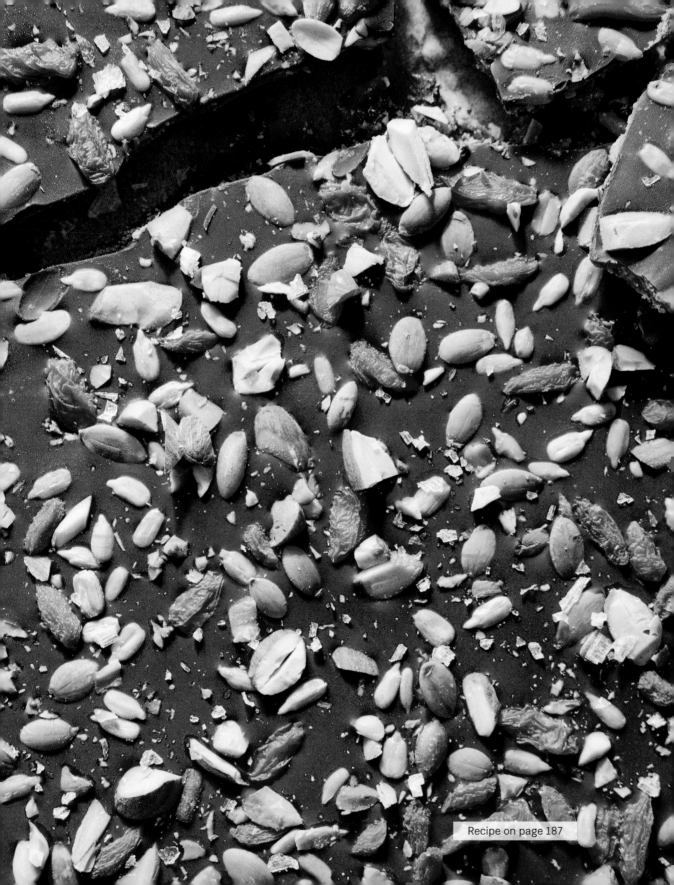

Recipe on page 187

7

The Manifestation Phase

WHY DO WE LOOK AT a woman's hormonal swings as being a negative? If a woman is super emotional, she is often referred to dismissively as "hormonal." The week before our periods, if we are feeling irritable and agitated (which is totally normal!), comments like "She's PMS-ing" or, for the older crowd, "Is she on the rag?" get thrown our way. These pervasive comments may seem harmless at first glance, but they are doing women a disservice. Here's why: Your hormones are not a negative part of your humanness; they are your superpowers. The fact that you can be happy one moment, then crying the next is part of your authentic feminine nature. Your hormonal landscape is intricate and sophisticated. These wisdom molecules give you access to a wide range of emotions. It's what makes you a woman. Let's celebrate this, not condemn it.

If there is one moment where your hormonal superpowers come together in all their glory, it's at ovulation. At this unique moment in your cycle, the most neurochemicals will flood your brain and body. These magical molecules brighten your mood and memory and give you an immense capacity to love. Estradiol is not the only hormone you're blessed with during your ovulation window; you also get a huge surge of testosterone at this time,

the largest you will receive all month. While it is often thought of only as your libido hormone, testosterone does so much more than ramp up your sex drive; she also helps you build muscle and increases your motivation and general drive. But wait—your hormonal magic doesn't stop there! You also get a tiny pulse of progesterone during ovulation to keep you calm. Happiness, motivation, focus, drive, cognition, connection, and calm—that's what your hormonal superpowers offer you during ovulation. That's why I call this moment the Manifestation Phase. You are locked and loaded with an arsenal of neurochemical superpowers. You can manifest anything you want!

Your Manifestation Phase (Days 10–15)

Before I dive into the food focus for this powerful moment, there is some nuance to know about ovulation. First, every woman ovulates at a different time. Some women ovulate on Day 10, while others ovulate on Day 14. Some women even ovulate outside this typical six-day window. Second, you may not ovulate on the same day every month. In some months, your body will release an egg on Day 10 and

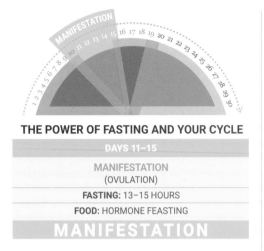

THE POWER OF FASTING AND YOUR CYCLE

DAYS 11–15
MANIFESTATION (OVULATION)
FASTING: 13–15 HOURS
FOOD: HORMONE FEASTING

MANIFESTATION

other months it may be on Day 13. Confusing, isn't it? This is why successfully fertilizing an egg can be such a moving target.

In the first 10 days of your cycle, estradiol is building. Each day she gets stronger and stronger until she peaks somewhere in the middle of your ovulation window. When she peaks, she brings with her a serious neurochemical team, special molecules that keep you happy, mentally clear, motivated, and cognitively sharp.

There are five primary neurochemicals that estradiol stimulates, igniting some serious brainpower. Here they are:

1. **Dopamine:** Dopamine plays a crucial role in regulating pleasure, motivation, and reward in the brain, influencing how women experience joy, satisfaction, and emotional well-being.
2. **Serotonin:** Serotonin regulates mood, appetite, sleep, memory, and sexual desire, playing a key role in supporting a woman's emotional well-being and overall mental health.
3. **Glutamate:** Glutamate supports cognitive functions such as learning

and memory in women by facilitating synaptic transmission and neuronal communication.

4. **Acetylcholine:** Acetylcholine plays a vital role in muscle contraction, arousal, attention, memory, and motivation, impacting both the central and peripheral nervous systems in women.
5. **Brain-derived neurotrophic factor (BDNF):** BDNF supports the survival and growth of neurons, playing a crucial role in learning, memory, and mood regulation in women.

Pause and process all this for a moment. Reread the above list. That's one heck of a powerful team of neurochemicals that estradiol brings with her. See why she's the diva? Making sure you get the right foods to support her needs allows *five* other powerhouse neurochemicals to appear. Think of estradiol as the main star during ovulation, with her five supporting stars going wherever she goes.

During your manifestation phase, you are also getting the most testosterone you will get all month long. Testosterone helps you build muscle strength and bone density and positively influences your mood and energy levels. She fires up your motivation and can give you that drive to accomplish a big goal. You also get a small dose of progesterone that stimulates the neurotransmitter GABA, giving you an overall peaceful feeling of calm.

When you put all three of these hormones together with the other neurochemicals they stimulate, you start to see why we never want to curse these wisdom molecules. You have every neurochemical resource during this time to manifest a new job, a raise, birth a new business idea, or use that testosterone to build extra muscle. Let's make sure we dial in your food to support this powerhouse moment!

FIBER-RICH BITTER GREENS PERFECT FOR THE MANIFESTATION PHASE

- Dandelion greens
- Arugula (rocket)
- Endive
- Radicchio
- Kale
- Mustard greens
- Swiss chard
- Collard greens
- Chicory
- Escarole

WHAT'S THE FOOD FOCUS FOR YOUR MANIFESTATION PHASE?

Let's go back to the Three Food Rules of eating like a girl: You need to make a hormone, metabolize a hormone, and detox a hormone. Your manifestation phase is when you want to put a *huge* focus on metabolizing hormones.

Metabolizing is a fancy term for breaking down into usable parts. Two major organs help you do that—your liver and gut. Both of them love when you eat lots of fiber-rich bitter greens. See the boxed list for my favorites. A guiding principle to apply to your manifestation phase is to make sure you have a salad at every meal. This one simple step ensures that both your liver and gut are nutritionally supported and ready to break down your hormones so they can supercharge you.

Another unique food focus during your manifestation phase is to increase your protein amount. Choosing the amount of protein that is right for you depends on how much muscle you are trying to build. With all the testosterone surging through you at this time, it's a fabulous menstrual cycle moment to build muscle. To best accomplish that, you will want to increase your protein amounts to the suggested 1 gram to 1 pound of body weight. You will also want to obtain protein from a variety of sources to ensure you are getting a complete dose of amino acids. On the next two pages are 20 great plant-based and omnivore protein sources for this phase of your cycle.

NUTRITION DURING YOUR MANIFESTATION PHASE: HORMONE FEASTING FOODS

The food style that best works in your manifestation phase is called hormone feasting. You will notice that this style of eating increases both your protein and carbohydrate amounts. When hormones go high, you need more glucose, amino acids, fiber, and nutrients. Thus, your macronutrient target will change. Along with adding in more diverse protein choices and increasing your fiber, you should increase your amount of nature's carbohydrates.

Nature's Versus Humanmade Carbohydrates

In recent years, a very clear conversation has been happening in the health world about the difference between good fat and bad fat. By now, most of us know that not all fats are the same—we can't put all fats in one category and avoid them. We needed to separate the good from the bad. The same now goes for carbohydrates. Carbs are not all bad—in fact, many carbs are key for your hormonal health. The trick is choosing the right ones. This is why I started using the term *nature's carbs*, as opposed to humanmade carbs. Nature's

BEST OMNIVORE AND ANIMAL-BASED PROTEIN SOURCES

Chicken Breast (cooked, 100 grams)

Protein: Approximately 31 grams
Amino acids: Rich in all the essential amino acids and particularly high in leucine, isoleucine, and valine, which are critical for muscle building and repair.

Turkey Breast (cooked, 100 grams)

Protein: Approximately 29 grams
Amino acids: Similar to chicken, turkey is rich in BCAAs (branched-chain amino acids) and provides a complete amino acid profile.

Egg (large, about 50 grams)

Protein: Approximately 6 grams
Amino acids: Eggs are a complete protein, meaning they contain all nine essential amino acids in the right proportions for human dietary needs.

Salmon (cooked, 100 grams)

Protein: Approximately 25 grams
Amino acids: In addition to providing a complete amino acid profile, salmon is rich in omega-3 fatty acids, which are beneficial for heart and brain health.

Beef (lean, cooked, 100 grams)

Protein: Approximately 27 grams
Amino acids: Beef is another excellent source of all essential amino acids, particularly creatine and carnosine, which support muscle function and performance.

Pork Loin (cooked, 100 grams)

Protein: Approximately 27 grams
Amino acids: Provides a complete amino acid profile, with high levels of threonine and lysine.

Greek Yogurt (full-fat, 100 grams)

Protein: Approximately 10 grams
Amino acids: Contains all the essential amino acids, with a particularly high amount of isoleucine.

Cottage Cheese (full-fat, 100 grams)

Protein: Approximately 12 grams
Amino acids: Like other dairy products, cottage cheese is rich in leucine, which is crucial for protein synthesis.

Whey Protein Powder (30 grams)

Protein: Varies by brand, approximately 20 to 25 grams
Amino acids: High in BCAAs, especially leucine, making it popular for muscle repair and growth after exercise.

Tuna (cooked, 100 grams)

Protein: Approximately 28 grams
Amino acids: Tuna offers a complete amino acid profile, with a significant amount of methionine, which is essential for various metabolic processes.

BEST PLANT-BASED PROTEIN SOURCES

Soybeans (and soy products like tofu and tempeh): Soybeans are a complete protein source, meaning they provide all the essential amino acids. Tofu contains 10 to 20 grams of protein per ½-cup serving, depending on its firmness.

Lentils: Lentils pack about 18 grams of protein per cooked cup and are a great source of fiber, iron, and potassium.

Chickpeas (and other beans like black, kidney, and pinto beans): Chickpeas offer about 14.5 grams of protein per cooked cup, along with fiber and essential nutrients.

Green peas: A cup of cooked green peas provides about 8 grams of protein, plus vitamins A, C, and K, and fiber.

Quinoa: Quinoa is a complete protein with about 8 grams of protein per cooked cup, including all nine essential amino acids.

Nutritional yeast: Often used as a cheese substitute, nutritional yeast can provide up to 14 grams of protein per ounce, along with a range of B vitamins.

Seeds (hemp seeds, chia seeds, and flaxseed): Hemp seeds offer about 9 grams of protein per 3 tablespoons, making them a rich source of protein as well as omega-3 and omega-6 fatty acids.

Nuts (almonds, peanuts, and cashews): Almonds provide about 6 grams of protein per ounce, along with healthy fats, fiber, and vitamin E.

Spirulina: This blue-green algae packs about 8 grams of protein per 2 tablespoons, along with a full spectrum of essential amino acids, vitamins, and minerals.

Edamame: Young soybeans are served steamed or boiled and contain about 17 grams of protein per cup, along with fiber and vitamins.

---

carbs can heal your hormonal health, while humanmade carbs destroy it. Both are considered carbs, but they have drastically different effects on your body.

Nature's carbs have two qualities. First, they come from the earth. This means they had to be harvested from the soil or a tree. Second, foods provided by nature also tend to contain more fiber, which is gold for metabolizing hormones. All fruits and vegetables fall into the nature's carbs category.

Humanmade carbs are those that have been highly processed and refined by humans. Wheat is an excellent example of this. Although wheat comes from the ground, many of the modern strains have been genetically modified, sprayed heavily with pesticides, and highly altered into a refined state. These alterations rob it of nutrients, causing it to spike your blood sugar incredibly high. Does that mean you should avoid all breads? Absolutely not! Whole grains, when left unaltered by humans, can be a great fuel source for your hormones. These unaltered whole grains are usually referred to as *ancient grains* or sometimes called *sprouted grains*. This means that the grain has been left as close to its original state as possible before being milled into

FOOD FOCUS FOR THE MANIFESTATION PHASE

- Eat lots of fiber-rich bitter greens to detox hormones.
- Eat more protein to build muscle.
- Avoid alcohol.

HORMONE FEASTING FOODS

- Consume no more than 150 grams of net carbs per day.
- Focus on fiber-rich nature's carbs.
- Consume 1 gram of protein for every pound of ideal body weight per day.
- Consume healthy fats as desired.

flour. It's a nuttier-tasting grain that has a lot more nutrients and enzymes that support both the production and metabolization of your hormones.

What about Gluten?

Although removing gluten is a process done by a human, for some women it is necessary. Gluten is a family of proteins found in grains like wheat, barley, and rye. It gives dough its elasticity and provides a chewy texture to baked goods. For many, consuming gluten causes health issues. This is largely because gluten grains are heavily sprayed with pesticides like glyphosate, and many are genetically engineered to have a toxin called Bt built into them, which destroys the microbiome of your gut. Gluten can lead to all kinds of challenges, including the following:

- Diarrhea
- Bloating
- Constipation
- Fatigue
- Brain fog
- Weight-loss resistance
- Contributes to autoimmune conditions

All the recipes in this book are completely gluten-free. Many of us feel better when we avoid gluten, so I asked my chefs to keep gluten out of the recipes.

Choosing the Right Amount of Protein for Your Manifestation Phase

Since the writing of *Fast Like a Girl*, our collective conversation around protein for women has continued to emerge and shift. What that means is that we have some differing opinions and a bit of experimentation going on with this topic. So, once again, you are going to need to put on your *n*-of-1 glasses and see what feels right for you during this phase of the month when you increase your protein. Here's the current research and expert wisdom:

- We need at least 1 gram of protein for every pound of ideal body weight.
- When you consume protein, make sure you are getting at least 30 grams per meal.
- Post-workout protein is critical for muscle growth.
- For some, too much protein will convert to excess glucose and thus be stored as fat.

With all that in mind, the way I currently look at protein is that it is incredibly helpful to the female body. Trying to get 1 gram of protein per pound of ideal body weight is a good idea throughout your cycle. Having said that, if you up your protein and start gaining weight, then I would use your power phases to bring your protein down to a lower amount. The

75 grams I recommend in Chapter 6 would be a good next step.

Add in Gut Soothers

In addition to adding fiber-rich foods during this phase, eating foods that heal your gut can be very helpful for metabolizing hormones. One of the best ways to heal a damaged inner gut lining is with broth.

Remember that bone broth, made by simmering bones, marrow, skin, feet, tendons, and ligaments of animals for an extended period, is rich in several nutrients that heal your gut: minerals, amino acids (particularly glycine), and collagen. Glycine repairs the integrity of your thin gut lining. When consumed before bed, it leads to more restful sleep.[1]

Mushroom broth is helpful for your gut largely because it acts like an incredible prebiotic. Mushrooms contain natural fibers and polysaccharides, such as beta-glucans, which feed the beneficial bacteria in the gut microbiome, promoting their growth and activity. Compounds in mushrooms such as ergothioneine, triterpenoids, polyphenols, selenium, and vitamin D can help reduce inflammation in the gastrointestinal tract.

Bieler's broth is a nutrient-rich vegetable broth created by Dr. Henry Bieler to support detoxification and restore the body's balance. It consists primarily of green vegetables, which are simmered in water until soft. The broth's list of health benefits is impressive, making it an excellent choice for your manifestation phase. Not only is it packed with nutrients, but its fiber-rich vegetables keep the microbes in your gut flourishing. It is also very hydrating and helps with detoxification. It's such a therapeutic broth that I asked one of my chefs to create a tastier version of it for you to sip during your ovulation time.

CREATING AN OXYTOCIN-RICH MEAL

One of the more fascinating attributes of estradiol is that when she peaks during ovulation, she brings oxytocin with her. Two days before your body has enough estradiol to trigger the release of an egg, this lovely bonding hormone comes screaming in. I have often wondered why our bodies would orchestrate such a hormonal symphony at ovulation. High estradiol to release an egg, peaking levels of testosterone to increase libido, and oxytocin makes her splash to connect you to a mate. No doubt this hormonal confluence is to ensure that we have all the neurochemicals needed to reproduce. That's how magic we are!

The whole premise of fasting and eating like a girl is knowing how to sync your lifestyle choices with your hormones. If we get a natural influx of oxytocin during ovulation, then we want to learn how to accommodate her presence. Let's give oxytocin a seat at the dinner table by making sure that during your manifestation phase, you create a warm, nourishing food environment.

Remember the Hormonal Hierarchy? Oxytocin calms cortisol. If you find yourself incredibly stressed during your ovulation time, how about using your meals to increase oxytocin? This could manifest as slowing down, putting on your favorite music, and truly enjoying your food. Invite someone to join you. Oxytocin loves company! Most important is honoring your body's need for oxytocin during this time.

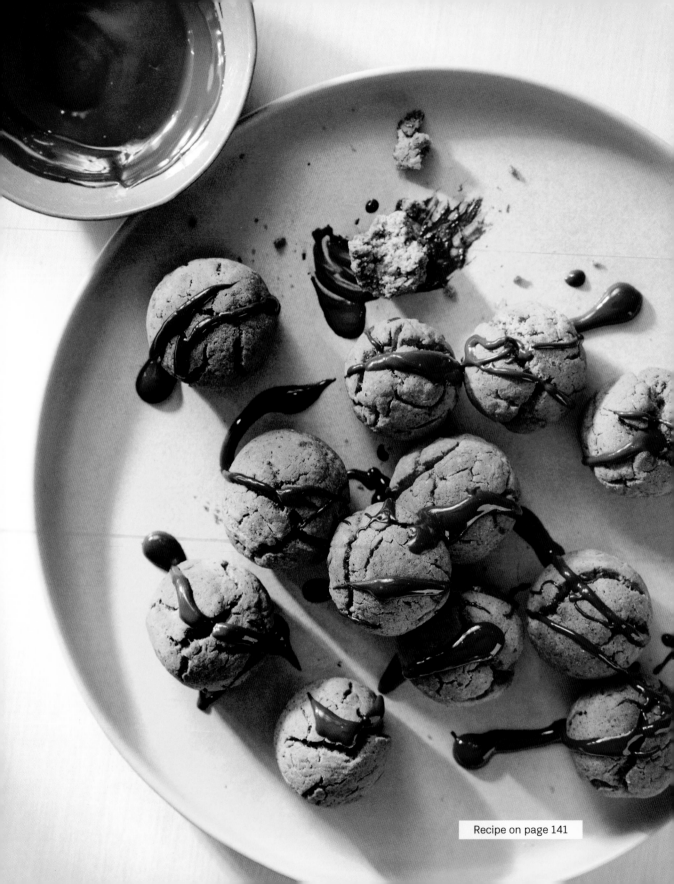

Recipe on page 141

8

The Nurture Phase

THIS IS THE PART OF YOUR CYCLE that every woman gets wrong.

It's not your fault, I promise. Since many of us were taught about our periods by a male gym teacher, I am not surprised that we didn't get the memo that our lifestyle choices should change during this week. Yet, even though this lack of information may not be our fault, I strongly believe that once we're informed, it is our responsibility to do this week differently.

Not understanding the physiological needs of our bodies at this menstrual moment causes all kinds of challenges. Conditions like premenstrual dysmorphic disorder, mood disorders, insomnia, chronic fatigue, and even several autoimmune challenges can be linked to this misunderstanding. Common menstrual symptoms like heavy periods, intense cramping, tender breasts, bloated bellies, fatigue, and brain fog can also be signs that your lifestyle choices are out of sync with your hormonal needs during the week before your period.

Collectively, as women, our health is perishing because we haven't been properly taught how to take care of ourselves during this stage in our cycle. Let's change that now!

Your Nurture Phase (Day 20–First Day of Your Period)

Let's recap your hormonal journey up to this point. During the first 10 days, your body is focused on making hormones, specifically estrogen. Then you hit ovulation, when your body ramps up testosterone and turns its resources toward breaking these hormones down into usable parts. In the days immediately following ovulation, your body works hard to detox those hormones out of your body. By the time you hit Day 20 of your cycle, your body needs a rest. It's worked hard to coordinate this complex hormonal system. It wants to recover before it does it all again, and it accomplishes this by ramping up progesterone. Progesterone has many superpowers, but one of her greatest attributes is to calm you. She does this by activating your calming neurotransmitter GABA.

This is the part of your cycle I call the Nurture Phase. It's the moment in your cycle when you get to slow down and nurture yourself. Notice I said you nurture *yourself*. This is pivotally important. As women, we often

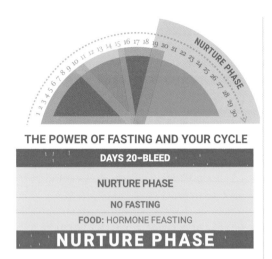

THE POWER OF FASTING AND YOUR CYCLE

DAYS 20–BLEED
NURTURE PHASE
NO FASTING
FOOD: HORMONE FEASTING

NURTURE PHASE

look at self-care as a luxury we don't have. That might serve you at other moments in your cycle, but not during the week before your period. This is the moment your body is begging you to slow down and nurture yourself.

This is a hard concept to fully grasp for so many of us in this modern world. We live such busy lives. We live in a world of achievements. To keep up with the production pace of the patriarchal world, we've had to suck it up and ignore our body's internal instinct to rest. In doing that, we have destroyed our health. We have dysregulated our hormonal system. We often criticize ourselves for not being able to do it all. When our bodies scream at us to rest, we try to push through instead. Then we don't understand why we struggle to stick to the discipline of a diet. We start believing that we are somehow at fault when rigid food programs fail us. This leads us right into the hands of guilt, shame, and frustration.

It's time to let all that go. You have a natural hormonal rhythm that at times works well with a more intense lifestyle, but at other times, it desperately needs a softer, gentler approach. When you don't honor that softer side, you feel as if you are failing with your health. It's time we bring back this softer side of you.

To fully understand the needs of your body during your nurture phase, let's go back to the concepts of the Hormonal Hierarchy. Two hormones that dramatically affect our sex hormones are insulin and cortisol. Estrogen doesn't mind if cortisol is high, but she wants you to keep the insulin low. Progesterone is the opposite. She wants you to keep cortisol low and will actually make you more insulin-resistant this week so that she has enough glucose to make her appearance. Your nurture phase is progesterone's moment. You need progesterone to peak for your uterine lining to shed. If you are working out too hard, fasting too long, or dieting too much at this time, progesterone will perish. This can manifest as you stop losing weight, you lose your menstrual cycle, or you are incredibly irritable and cranky this week. These are all signs you are not giving progesterone what she needs.

WHAT IS YOUR FOOD FOCUS FOR YOUR NURTURE PHASE?

How many of us crave carbohydrates this week? Each time I give a speech, I ask this question to the audience, and every woman in the room raises her hand. That is because your body needs more glucose the week before your cycle. To best accomplish this, your brilliant body gives you carbohydrate cravings. How smart is that? Yet when those cravings come, we villainize them. This is the moment that low-carb diets, calorie-restriction plans, and designer weight-loss

EXCITOTOXIN ADDITIVES TO AVOID

Aspartame: An artificial sweetener found in many diet sodas, sugar-free gum, low-calorie desserts, and certain medications.

Monosodium glutamate (MSG): A flavor enhancer commonly added to Asian food, canned vegetables, soups, low-sodium foods, and processed meats.

Hydrolyzed vegetable protein (HVP): Often used in processed foods to enhance flavor, similar to MSG.

Autolyzed yeast extract: Found in many savory processed foods, like soups, snack foods, and sauces, it enhances flavor similarly to MSG.

Sodium caseinate: A food additive derived from casein in milk, it is used in many non-dairy and dairy products for its texture and protein content.

Soy protein isolate and concentrate: Used in a wide range of products, including meat alternatives, protein bars, and dietary supplements, these can contain excitotoxins due to their processing.

Whey protein concentrate: Not all whey protein is harmful, but some processing methods can result in excitotoxin formation; it is used in protein supplements and various processed foods.

Glutamic acid: An amino acid used as a food additive for its flavor-enhancing properties, similar to MSG.

Calcium caseinate: Found in many "diet" foods, sports drinks, and protein supplements, it is used for its texture and nutrient content.

Yeast nutrient, yeast food, or yeast extract: Often found in baked goods and beer, these ingredients can be sources of free glutamic acid.

Isn't it ironic that many of these are found in "diet" foods? It's another moment to acknowledge how our food system has led us astray. Excitotoxins raise cortisol levels, causing your progesterone levels to tank. The diet culture has set you up to fail long term. What's beautiful is that when you understand your rhythm of eating like a girl, you start to take your power back. You see the moments in your menstrual cycle that call for a more disciplined food approach and the moments when you can lean into ease.

programs fail us. Progesterone needs your blood-glucose levels to be higher than they are the rest of the month. But before you rush out and grab a box of donuts, remember you need to keep your cortisol low. The highly processed foods that many women eat today are not only packed with obesogens that turn stem cells into fat cells, but they also contain excitotoxins that raise cortisol levels. Making sure you avoid these chemicals is massively important all month long, but *especially* the week before your period.

FOODS THAT SUPPORT PROGESTERONE

Sweet potatoes: High in vitamin B6 and magnesium.

Avocados: Rich in healthy fats, magnesium, and vitamin B6, which can support overall hormonal balance.

Bananas: Provide vitamin B6, which is important for progesterone synthesis.

Spinach: High in magnesium, which plays a role in hormone balance.

Broccoli: Contains diindolylmethane (DIM), which helps metabolize estrogen and may support progesterone levels by improving estrogen-progesterone balance.

Salmon: Rich in omega-3 fatty acids, which can reduce inflammation and support hormonal health.

Walnuts: Another excellent source of omega-3 fatty acids.

Chicken: Lean protein source that supports the adrenal glands and hormone production.

Eggs: Provides vitamin B6 and vitamin D, both important for hormone synthesis.

Pumpkin seeds: A good source of magnesium and zinc, supporting the endocrine system.

Quinoa: Contains protein, magnesium, and phosphorus, supporting overall hormone balance.

Beans: Provide fiber and B vitamins, supporting gut health and liver function, crucial for hormone metabolism.

Lentils: Rich in fiber and folate, supporting methylation, a biochemical process important for hormonal health.

Papaya: Contains vitamins and minerals that support the endocrine system.

Sunflower seeds: High in vitamin E, which can play a role in hormone synthesis and balance.

Kale: Provides a wealth of nutrients, including magnesium, to support hormone health.

Almonds: Rich in vitamin E and magnesium.

Turkey: A good source of lean protein and vitamin B6.

Sesame seeds: Contain lignans and essential fatty acids that can help in hormone balance.

Shellfish: Provides zinc, which is crucial for hormone production and overall reproductive health.

Chickpeas: High in fiber and protein, supporting detoxification and hormonal balance.

Yogurt (full-fat): Contains probiotics, supporting gut health and hormone metabolism.

Flaxseeds: Rich in fiber and lignans, which can help balance estrogen and progesterone levels.

Brussels sprouts: Like broccoli, they help in the metabolism of estrogen, potentially supporting progesterone balance.

Red peppers: High in vitamin C, which is essential for corpus luteum function and progesterone production.

CREATE A PERSONAL FOOD VALUE SYSTEM

You know how there are bumper rails to help beginner bowlers keep their ball from going into the gutters? I discovered a mindset hack that acts like bumper rails to ensure that as I raised carbohydrates the week before my period, they were health-supporting carbohydrates. It's called the personal food value system. This is an exercise often used in goal setting: Identify what you value in life and then create a life around those values. Let's take that same idea and now apply it to food.

My food value system has three key values: quality, taste, and functionality. I want to make sure that every meal I eat is made up of clean, chemical-free food that tastes amazing and leaves me feeling at my best. Carbohydrates are an interesting beast, largely because once you open your mind to eating carbs, you can quickly step into eating bad carbs. A traditional donut is a perfect example of this (my apologies to the donut lovers out there). What makes it so harmful is that it contains the deadly combo of refined sugar, refined flour, and bad oils. But what if I'm craving a donut? This is when I put my food value system into action. I want clean, quality ingredients. I want to not only enjoy this donut, but I also want to feel good afterward. And I want it to taste good. This can be tricky, but I've included a fabulous recipe on page 141 in this book that ticks all these boxes. So if you have a craving for a good donut, I highly recommend you try it!

As you learn to raise your carbohydrate levels the week before your period, I encourage you to create your own food value system. That way, you can pick the right carbohydrate for you. You can never go wrong with nature's

FOOD FOCUS FOR YOUR NURTURE PHASE

- Bring your carbohydrate load up.
- Focus on progesterone-supporting foods.
- Avoid synthetic ingredients with excitotoxins.
- Create a personal food value system.

carbohydrates. The box on the left contains a list of foods that progesterone loves, including several of nature's carbohydrates. You will see that a sweet potato is at the top of that list. I love sweet potatoes! Believe it or not, they have a lighter net carbohydrate load than white potatoes, but taste sweeter. Perhaps sweet potatoes are a kiss to us from nature.

Hormone Feasting Foods for Your Nurture Phase

Because your body needs more glucose during this week, it's the perfect time to dip back into hormone feasting foods. Consuming hormone feasting foods at this moment not only gives progesterone the extra glucose it needs, but if you eat nutrient-dense foods, you also provide all your hormones the necessary fuel they require to flourish. Chocolate is a terrific example of this. It will help progesterone levels by raising your glucose while at the same time providing your body with a good dose of magnesium, a mineral all your hormones require. Just make sure it's high-quality, organic, nutritionally dense chocolate, ideally at least 70 percent cacao and grown on a regenerative farm. Both of my chefs prepared delicious chocolate recipes for you to enjoy during this week.

THE EMOTIONAL SIDE OF FOOD

Food is so much more than nourishment. It can be a state-changer. It can momentarily lift us when we are sad and can amplify our joy when we celebrate. We come together and connect around food. Family recipes are passed down, linking us to the generations that came before. Certain foods take us immediately back to a sweet memory from the past. Others remind us of a troubling time in our lives. We gather around food, whether it's in the cooking or eating process of a meal. Our memories, our stories, and our connections with others often have food at their heart. Because of this, I can't write a book about food for women without addressing this emotional relationship we have with it. There are two major ways I have seen food used as mood changers and connectors.

The negative relationship many women have with food often gets all the press. I deeply understand the physical and emotional challenges that disordered eating creates for so many women. Experience has taught me that as many women start to build fasting lifestyles, surprisingly their relationship with food changes. If you have been clinically diagnosed with a disordered eating condition, the following ideas may not apply to you, and please know that it is always wise to consult your doctor before embarking on a fasting lifestyle. If you haven't been diagnosed with a disordered eating condition and perhaps are just looking to positively change your relationship with food, consider the following thoughts.

Food as a Mood Changer

One message I got about food as a child was that if you are having a bad day, eating something yummy will make it all better. It became a strategy for momentarily taking me out of pain.

If I didn't like the emotions I was experiencing, I ate. It wasn't until I dedicated my career to understanding the neurochemical system of the body that I realized I used food to give me a dopamine hit. But dopamine is the molecule of more, not the molecule of enough. The more I leaned into that dopamine hit from food, the more food I wanted. It became a vicious cycle.

When I first started learning how to build myself a fasting lifestyle, going for longer periods without food, I had to develop new state-changers. A huge benefit of fasting for me was to help me redefine my relationship with food. I remember the first 24-hour fast I did. About 15 hours in, I was cranky. I didn't have food to pull me out of the mood I was in, and I had another 9 hours to go! That's the moment I started to discover all the state-changers I had access to. This was the beginning of freeing myself from the emotional hold food had on me.

After that 24-hour fast, I started looking differently at my hunger. I started to ask myself, *Am I hungry or am I bored?* Add whatever emotion you want into the "bored" part, but ultimately, I wanted to acknowledge to myself *why* I wanted to eat. If it was to change a current mood I was in, I started to try other state-changers. Sometimes, I would answer this question with a *Yes! I am bored! And I am going to eat anyway.* This is where my personal food value system came in handy because I knew the food I was going to use to change my state was healthy food.

Asking myself *Why am I hungry?* helped me reestablish the relationship I wanted with food. Once I realized that I ate to change my emotions, I could decide if that was how I wanted to relate to food on that day. As with any healthy relationship, knowing how you show up in the relationship is important.

Food as a Connector

Like most of us, I have many fond memories around food: Holidays spent cooking with my mom, sister, and grandmother; favorite restaurants we ate at for our birthday celebrations; endless hours in the kitchen cooking with my kids when they were young; and exposing my taste buds to new flavors and new food experiences on excursions to foreign countries. So many great times. Food can be a beautiful way to connect with others. Wherever there is connection, there is oxytocin. And oxytocin balances all your other hormones.

I have also seen the connection we have with others take us down a bad food path. When coaching patients back to health, I have witnessed time and time again when well-intentioned loved ones keep us stuck in bad food choices. We can bond over toxic food. I remember one patient who had a Starbucks habit with her girlfriends. After they dropped their kids off at school, they would gather at the local coffee shop and get a whole host of sugary treats. It was their mommy moment where they could talk about the struggles in their lives while eating dopamine-rich foods. When I started to work with my patient to change her food choices, this morning moment became an issue. When she made different food choices around her friends, they felt threatened. This happens all too often. If we have connected with others around poor food choices and then decide to make healthier ones, it acts like a mirror for them. They start to feel bad about the choices they are making. It is all very subconscious, and most the time, they don't realize that you are triggering in them something they know they need to work on. If you find yourself in a position like that as you start cleaning up your diet

HEALTHY STATE-CHANGERS

- Physical exercise
- Deep breathing or meditation
- Listening to music
- Spending time outdoors
- Engaging in a hobby
- Laughing
- Connecting with friends or loved ones
- Practicing gratitude
- Aromatherapy
- Sunlight exposure
- Doing a good deed
- Taking a short nap
- Dancing
- Taking a warm bath or shower

and eating like a girl, realize that any negative feedback you get is most likely a reflection of the person giving you that feedback. It's their issue, not yours.

In a fast-paced culture where nutrient-deficient, quick-fix meals are at your fingertips, keep in mind that the environment you eat in can be as important as the food itself. When you commit to eating healthy meals, you commit to connecting to your body in a deeper, more meaningful way. It's an honoring of the beautiful home you get to live in all day long. When you eat that meal with people you love, you amplify its healing effect. As you dive into these recipes, keep that in mind. Surround yourself with people you love. Maybe one of the recipes in this book will become a family favorite that gets passed down through the generations. However you choose to connect with these recipes, do it with love and kindness. That's an energy that both your body and the world will benefit from.

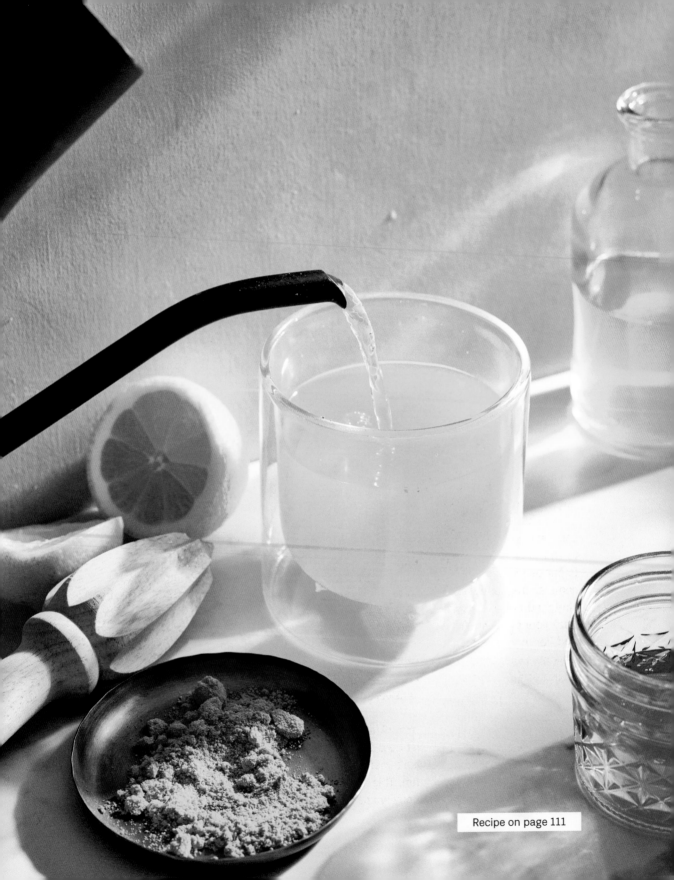

Recipe on page 111

9

What to Do If You Have No Cycle

NO DOUBT WHAT SHOCKED me the most with the release of *Fast Like a Girl* was the number of messages I received from 20- and 30-year-old women who didn't have a regular period. As nice as it is to not have to deal with your period each month, it's not good for your health if you are of childbearing age. Remember that your menstrual blood is one way your body detoxes.

Another common message was from the peri- and post-menopausal women wanting to know how to cycle their foods and fasting. In our perimenopausal years, our periods can come as frequently as every two weeks or as stretched out as every 60 days. How do you track your cycle when it's that unpredictable? And for my post-menopausal women who have no cycle, do you need to still cycle your foods and fasts? If so, what do you track it to? These are all questions I will answer in this chapter.

Keep in mind that your feminine body has a cyclic rhythm to it, so just because you don't bleed each month doesn't mean you don't still have a natural rhythm. This is one of the reasons I feel that so many women of all different ages got such profound results with the 30-Day Fasting Reset in *Fast Like a Girl*. The change in the timing and structure of meals created a rhythm that was healing to their bodies.

What If You Should Have a Cycle but Don't?

If you are in your fertility years but don't have a cycle, my recommendation is that you follow the 30-Day Fasting Reset that I lay out in detail in Chapter 10. Start on Day 1 and go all the way to Day 30. This will allow you to experience different lengths of fasts and the two different eating styles. What I have often seen is that 30 to 90 days of this 30-Day Fasting Reset will bring your cycle back.

One important note to consider during your fertility years: Many women lose their cycles because of imbalances in their thyroid. There are many reasons why the thyroid malfunctions, so if you suspect this to be your situation, please reach out to an integrative doctor who can correctly look at all aspects of your thyroid health. The one destroyer of the thyroid that I want to touch on here is an insufficient intake of calories. You need at least 1,200 calories a day for good thyroid health.[1] If you are keeping your calories below that, there is a good chance you will adversely affect your thyroid and lose your menstrual cycle.

Perimenopause and Menopause: What If Your Cycle Is Winding Down or Done?

Perhaps the most misunderstood hormonal time a woman will experience comes during the years in which her hormonal system is winding down. Our closing hormonal act is beautiful, turbulent, complicated, and mysterious all at the same time. It's a time that should be celebrated, yet too many of us are suffering through these years. Understanding the healing power that food can have on your menopausal years will greatly improve how you feel during this time.

Menopause happens when your ovaries slow down their hormonal production. Many experts believe that this process starts as early as age 35. It takes about 10 years for this hormonal wind-down to occur, making it a long and bumpy road for many women. As your hormones shift, so do your moods, energy, focus, cognition, and metabolism. Many of the old dieting and exercise tricks that kept you feeling at your best stop working. This is disturbing to so many of us. Fat accumulates in new areas, a good night's sleep feels like a luxury of the past, moods are all over the place, and hot flashes are now a

frequent visitor. As troubling as this can be, knowing what and when to eat during this time will greatly ease the ride. Before I dive into what that looks like, let's talk about the three phases of menopause that affect us so deeply.

PHASE 1: THE PERIMENOPAUSE YEARS

Perimenopause can begin as early as age 35, and some doctors report seeing signs as early as the late 20s. The first hormone to decline during this phase is progesterone. Here are the early signs of progesterone decline:

- Increased anxiety
- Trouble sleeping
- Irregular cycles
- Spotting
- Heavy periods with clotting
- Increased hunger
- Strong cravings for carbohydrates

As challenging as these symptoms are, let's stop and think about why some of these new symptoms happen. As your progesterone stores diminish, your body wants you to increase glucose so that you can make as much age-appropriate progesterone as possible. That makes knowing how to read progesterone's clues pivotal. When anxiety is through the roof or you start spotting for days, you are going to want to lean into more hormone feasting days to best support progesterone's needs.

Soon after progesterone starts to make her slow exit, estradiol begins to follow. Remember that you have three types of estrogen, and estradiol is the version needed to release an egg and start ovulation. As you move deeper and deeper into menopause, your estradiol production declines. With the loss of estradiol also comes a whole host of new symptoms:

- Weight gain
- Brain fog
- Depression
- Memory loss
- Inability to handle stress
- Inability to handle large amounts of work
- Inability to hold on to new information

When you put all these symptoms together, you have yourself some serious menopausal madness. Understanding that our lifestyle choices greatly influence our perimenopausal ride is important. The diet you ate at age 25 may no longer work for you at 55. Getting to know the signs of these diminishing hormones and changing your food choices to support their decline are key.

PHASE 2: THE MENOPAUSAL TRANSITION YEAR

You are not fully in menopause until you have gone a year without a period. I refer to the year between an erratic cycle and no cycle as your transition year. Although every woman experiences this year differently, for many, the symptoms that may have been on and off for the past few years stick around and intensify. This intensifying of symptoms often sends even the most medication-reluctant woman toward hormone replacement therapy, and this can be the most symptomatic time for some women. But your symptoms are temporary as your body learns to live with these new lows of estradiol and progesterone, and you can help smooth them out with food and fasting.

NAVIGATING HORMONE REPLACEMENT THERAPY

As the conversation of hormone replacement therapy has come back in vogue, more women and doctors are opening their minds to supplementing with hormones as a woman transitions into her post-menopausal years. Experience has taught me that every doctor and every woman has a different comfort level with this choice. I have also witnessed that every woman has a different experience with hormone replacement therapy. For some, it's the hormonal miracle they have been looking for. Yet for many women, it's not as simple as slapping on a patch and all their hormonal problems go away. Working very closely with your doctor to find the right hormone replacement rhythm for you is key. Whatever path you choose, keep in mind you still need to make some lifestyle changes to assist your body in learning how to live with fewer hormones, especially when it comes to food.

PHASE 3: THE POST-MENOPAUSAL YEARS

The wild ride of perimenopause often comes to a very welcome halt once you hit your post-menopausal years. Even though hormones are still at a lifetime low, for many women, their bodies and brains have adapted to the new hormonal landscape. However, some women struggle with menopausal symptoms years after their last period.

When *The Menopause Reset* was first released, I heard from thousands of post-menopausal women like this—women who had not had a period in years but were still struggling with menopausal symptoms. Symptoms like belly fat, hot flashes, memory loss, and trouble focusing persisted. When I put these women through my five menopausal lifestyle changes, their symptoms finally went away. That's because they'd matched their lifestyle to their new hormonal profile.

The five menopausal lifestyle changes:

- Change when you eat.
- Vary what you eat.
- Replenish your microbiome.
- Practice daily detox strategies.
- Slow the rushing woman.

For the sake of this book, I want to dive deeper into three of those changes: changing when you eat, varying what you eat, and replenishing your microbiome. These are deeply important at all stages of the menopausal journey, but especially if you are post-menopausal and are still experiencing strong symptoms.

Changing When You Eat

One of the greatest lifestyle tools a menopausal woman can have in her toolbox is fasting. Let me explain why. First, fasting is one of the best lifestyle hacks for moving you out of insulin resistance. For menopausal women, insulin resistance is real. This is why you start gaining weight for no reason. As estradiol diminishes, your cells become more insulin-resistant. The food you ate in your 20s no longer works for you—the menopausal version of you is more insulin-resistant. Watch your hemoglobin A1c numbers; despite very little change in diet, many women see that number go up during their menopausal years.

This is the moment you want to make sure you have an eating and fasting window every day. When you practice pulsing in different-length fasting windows, you will find not only

FASTING GUIDELINES FOR MENOPAUSAL WOMEN

- **Perimenopausal women with regular cycles:** Vary fasts to sync your cycle.
- **Perimenopausal women with irregular cycles:** Vary fasts until signs of low progesterone show up, then stop fasting until bleed.
- **Menopausal women with no cycles:** Fast according to symptoms or choose a weekly variation.

that your HbA1c numbers (an indicator of your insulin sensitivity) change, but also symptoms like hot flashes and weight gain go away. Remember how estrogen likes an insulin-sensitive environment? The more insulin-sensitive you make yourself, the more you support your age-appropriate estrogen production.

Now, here's the trick: The three phases of menopause all will require a little different fasting approach. In the box above, I have listed some general guidelines you can follow. Remember to always be your *n* of 1 and see what works best for you.

Varying What You Eat

Switching between ketobiotic and hormone feasting foods works like a charm for most menopausal women. One of my biggest pet peeves in the health world is that we are always looking for absolutes. It would be so much easier if there was one diet to follow through your menopausal years. But estrogen and progesterone demand different environments. Knowing how to switch in and out of these two styles of eating will help you use food to ease your symptoms. At the end of the chapter, you

MENOPAUSAL WEEKLY VARIATIONS

Maintenance Protocol: 5-1-1

- 5 days of intermittent fasting (13–15 hours)
- 1 day of stretching your fast (>17 hours)
- 1 day of no fasting

Weight-Loss Protocol: 4-2-1

- 4 days of intermittent fasting (13–15 hours)
- 2 days of stretching your fast (>17 hours)
- 1 day of no fasting

Anxiety-Depression Protocol: 4-2-1

- 4 days of a comfortable fasting length for you
- 2 days of no fasting
- 1 day of stretching your fast longer than comfortable

will see an overview of how to use these two food styles throughout your menopausal years.

Replenishing Your Microbiome

Throughout your entire menopause journey, you need your microbiome more than ever. Metabolizing the smaller quantity of hormones your body is providing you is imperative. A depleted microbiome can also be why some women who take oral hormone replacement therapy struggle to get good results. Your microbes break down hormones and make them usable for your cells.

Unfortunately, many women come roaring into their menopausal years after decades of being on birth control or having been exposed to multiple rounds of antibiotics—both of which destroy the health of their microbiome. Combine that past health history with this new diminished hormone state and you've got yourself one symptomatic menopausal woman. If this is your history, the good news is that with fasting and food, you can quickly repair your microbiome and get those good bacteria breaking down hormones for you again.

Fasting changes the terrain of your gut. Research shows that a 24-hour fast stimulates the production of intestinal stem cells.[2] Those are cells that repair the inner terrain of your gut. If you break that fast with foods of the three Ps—probiotics, prebiotics, and polyphenols—your microbiome will be back in the hormone game quickly. Depending on where you are in your menopausal journey, there are two ways you can approach this: weekly or monthly (see next page).

WHAT ABOUT MENOPAUSAL BELLY FAT?

Can we get real for a moment? The fat that accumulates around our midsections during our menopausal years is real. It's so frustrating because it's not developing in this area because we are eating too much. Your belly fat is where your body stores excess hormones—specifically cortisol and estrogen. Take that in for a moment. I watch so many women beat themselves up for this midsection fat. But all it consists of is excess hormones that you can

WEEKLY MICROBIOME REPAIR PROTOCOL (POST-MENOPAUSAL)

Weekly Microbiome Repair Protocol (post-menopausal): 4-2-1

- 4 days of intermittent fasting (<17 hours)
- 2 days of gut reset fast (24 hours)
- 1 day of no fasting

Break all fasts with bone broth or foods of the three Ps: probiotics, prebiotics, and polyphenols.

MONTHLY MICROBIOME REPAIR PROTOCOL (PERIMENOPAUSAL)

- Follow the 30-Day Fasting Reset (covered in Chapter 10) timed to your cycle.
- Break all fasts with broth or the three Ps: probiotic, prebiotic, polyphenol foods.

learn to mobilize and detox out of your body. With that in mind, there are five steps to getting rid of this belly fat:

1. **Eat a fiber-forward diet:** Fiber is a menopausal girl's best friend. If you start randomly gaining weight around your midsection, go all in on vegetables. Make sure you have a big green salad with every meal. What fiber does is fuel the microbes that break down both estrogen and cortisol. Once estrogen gets broken down, your cells can use it, which avoids the excess storage trap. Try it for a week and see for yourself how powerful this tool can be for that excess belly weight.

2. **Stop the liver agitators:** Since your liver also contributes to the breakdown of hormones, make sure you are avoiding all the liver agitators that I mentioned earlier in this book. Unfortunately, alcohol is a menopausal woman's worst enemy. Although it can relax you, pinch-hitting for the loss of progesterone, it's a temporary calm that leads to extra weight gain. When

your liver is processing alcohol, it is not metabolizing hormones. Your nightly glass of wine may be that subtle habit that is the source of your belly fat. Try 30 days without it and see what happens. You have nothing to lose but extra belly weight.

3. **Lower cortisol:** High-stress living is fuel for the menopausal fire. The more cortisol your body makes in response to stress, the more it stores it in your belly. There are two ways you can approach this situation. First, lower your stress loads. This may look like learning to say no more often, setting better boundaries, or maybe just building more downtime into your schedule. I know that I had to learn all three of those as I moved into my menopausal years.

Second, learn how to use cortisol instead of storing it. This is fairly easy. Cortisol is meant to make you move. It winds you up for a reason. You are meant to run from a tiger when cortisol is around. If you sit and don't move when a stressful event hits you, cortisol will be stored as fat, right in the middle of your belly. Make it a golden rule that anytime a stressful moment happens, go for a walk. If it's a low-level chronic stress, then build into your weekly routine

MAPPING YOUR FOOD AND FAST TO THE MOON CYCLE

When you stop and look at many of nature's patterns, you start to realize how synced our feminine bodies are with the earth. One of those magical ways is with the moon. A woman's menstrual cycle is on average 28 to 29 days. The average lunar cycle is 29 days. Human biology operates in cycles; for all humans, our 24-hour circadian rhythm controls our appetite, energy, and even moods, and it signals hormonal changes based on the sunlight in the sky. And we observe that the menstrual-cycle rhythm also sees fluctuations in hormones. Ever wondered what controls that? Well, many experts hypothesize it's the monthly changes in the moon. If the moon is powerful enough to control the ocean tides, surely it has the power to affect our menstrual cycles, especially considering that the body is more than 70 percent water.

Whatever the reason your cycle is nonexistent or unpredictable, you can map your fasts and foods to the four phases I've set out in previous chapters, or you can choose to align them with the moon cycle. One question I get when I speak of the moon cycle: "Why then don't all women menstruate together?" Welcome to synthetic blue light. We are bombarded by it. The light from our LED light bulbs, laptop computers, and cell phones has thrown off many of our natural rhythms, including our menstrual cycle.

If you do choose to map your fasts and food to the moon, here's how that would look: Day 1 of your menstrual cycle is the new moon. The full moon would hit mid-ovulation, around Day 14. Go to either the Fasting Cycle or the 30-Day Fasting Reset, look at the day of the moon (you can find that online), and sync up the day of the moon with the days of food and fasts I have mapped out for cycling women. The moon then becomes your cycle.

some walks in nature. Nature does an incredible job of bringing down your cortisol levels. Research even shows that looking at pictures or hearing nature sounds can bring cortisol down.[3] So if life is crazy-stressful and the belly fat is accumulating around your midsection, let nature be your doctor and surround yourself with as much natural beauty as possible.

4. **Open up detox pathways:** To properly detox your hormones, your pathways need to be open. In Chapter 3, I spoke about how important your detox organs are for getting rid of hormones. Let's revisit them. These are your primary detox pathways:

 - Liver
 - Gut
 - Kidneys
 - Lungs
 - Lymphatic system
 - Skin

There are many ways you can support these pathways. Castor oil packs and coffee enemas can help open up the liver. Lots of fiber will get your bowels moving. Hydrating with a large amount of water supports your kidneys. Deep

MATCHING YOUR SYMPTOMS TO YOUR FOOD STYLE

Ketobiotic Food Style

Ketobiotic is your food style to level out age-appropriate estrogen levels.

- Hot flashes
- Night sweats
- Vaginal dryness
- Inability to handle stress
- Dry skin
- Cognitive changes
- Memory loss
- Bone density loss
- Chronic musculoskeletal injuries
- Increased urgency and frequency of urination
- Weight gain

Hormone Feasting Food Style

Hormone feasting foods help elevate age-appropriate progesterone levels.

- Insomnia
- Chronic pain
- Trouble relaxing your body
- Brain anxiety
- Feelings of impending doom
- Spotting and irregular periods
- Increased hunger
- Trouble fasting
- Migraines and headaches
- Breast tenderness
- Increased belly fat

breathing exercises help your lungs. And a good lymph massage will get your lymph flowing again. Once your body has open detox pathways, it will no longer store your hormones in fat.

5. **Try longer fasts:** When in doubt, fast it out. I can't tell you the amount of weight that has been lost, especially around the midsection, by post-menopausal women in my community. Fasts longer than 24 hours lovingly encourage the body to mobilize fat. If you have tried all the above and still aren't dropping that midsection weight, I highly recommend you try some longer fasts. Anything from 24 to 70 hours will do the trick. The beautiful part of these longer fasts is they tend to not only encourage your body to burn that weight now, but it seems to flip a switch that allows the body to keep burning belly fat long after the fast is over.

FOOD AND MENOPAUSE SYMPTOMS

To help you match your symptoms to a food style, I am including a key here where you can see the recurring symptoms and know which food style to move into. This should be especially helpful for my post-menopausal friends who don't have a cycle to which to map their food and fasts.

Keep in mind that in the next chapter, I have outlined a 30-Day Fasting Reset that will move you in and out of both eating styles along with several different-length fasts. Many menopausal women like following that to get the hang of what this food rhythm looks like.

If you don't have a cycle to time this 30-Day Fasting Reset to, on the previous page, I shared instructions on how to time the Fasting Reset to the moon cycle—a popular tool used in my Reset Academy for post-menopausal women.

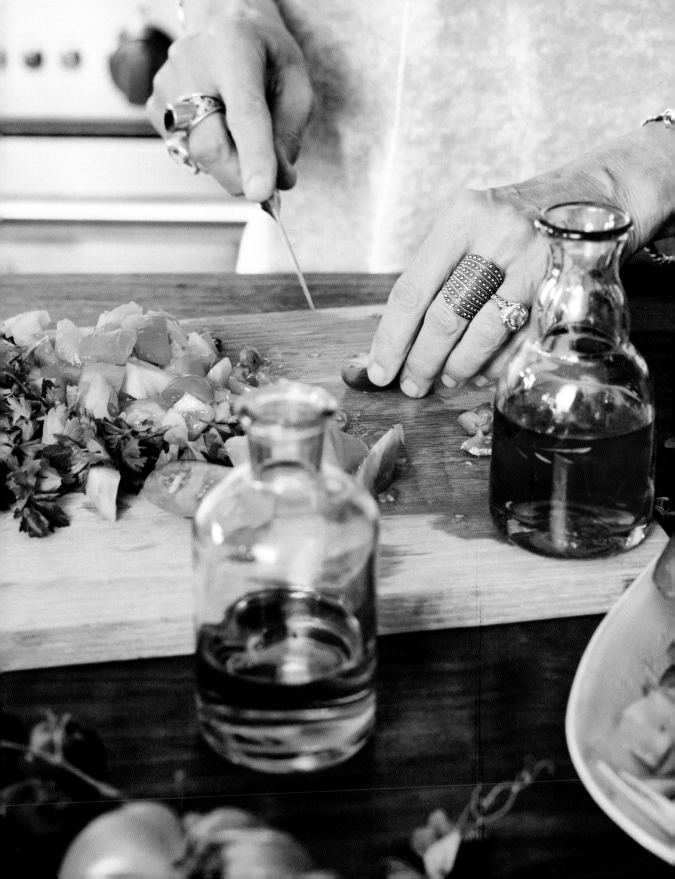

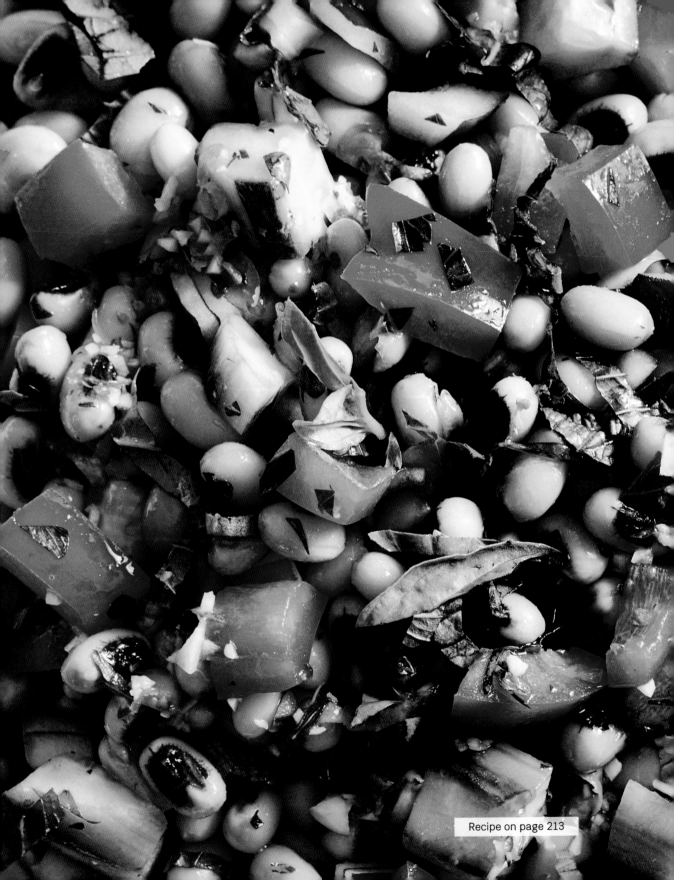

Recipe on page 213

10

The 30-Day
Fasting Reset

YEARS AGO, I HEARD A STATISTIC that blew my mind: We may retain only about 10 percent of the information we hear. As a lover of new information, this bummed me out. I am obsessed with elevating my thoughts through new perspectives. I have stacks of books all over my home, love listening to insightful podcasts, and a good old-fashioned deep conversation with a growth-minded human is my jam! To think that I am retaining only 10 percent of the information these resources provide me is frustrating. Although some experts say this 10 percent stat is an urban myth, I think it leads us to an interesting question: How can we get our brains to retain more of the content we are exposed to? This is how I came up with the idea that we needed to *experience* the new information so it sticks in our brains better.

Neuroplasticity is a term used to explain the brain's ability to change and adapt as a result of an experience. Our brains have a remarkable capacity to reorganize information by creating new neuronal connections. A neuron is the brain highway that carries information. The fact that our brains can reorganize these information highways is critical

for sticking to a new health habit. When I learn something new, I liken it to the birth of a new neuron—a baby neuron that needs love, care, and lots of positive experiences to grow into a healthy, mature neuron. It takes time, repetition, and energy to integrate that baby neuron into the neuronal highways already existing in my brain. I have come to realize that if I can have an experience with that new information, the more baby neurons mature.

My hope is that this book has birthed a whole nursery full of baby neurons. Now it's time to grow them. How do you best do that? Well, it turns out that you can facilitate neuroplasticity with novel experiences. Your brain becomes curious when a new adventure is before it. If it's a novel adventure, meaning that you never did it before, you also stimulate dopamine, firing up your motivation to explore the depths of that new experience. Mix a good shot of dopamine with amplified neuroplasticity, and you will find it becomes effortless to establish a new habit.

For years, I taught lifestyle tools in my practice. Once a month, I would hold workshops teaching different health topics, and then

I'd lead my patients through an experience together. I called them *resets*. Some resets were only a week long, while others lasted a month. These resets became the glue that helped the new information stick in my patients' brains, and they became a critical component in their healing journeys.

Now it's time to help your baby neurons grow into mature neurons that will keep you healthy for years to come. Welcome to my 30-Day Fasting Reset! I'm just going to introduce it to you in this chapter, and then there is a detailed plan for you to follow on pages 296 to 305. Hundreds of thousands of people have already gotten incredible results from this reset, and I am thrilled that I can now add some ridiculously yummy recipes to ensure even greater success.

Before I dive into the reset's logistics, I want to introduce you to four key principles that will help you get the best result.

Principle #1: Choose a Track

My general rule on nutrition is to pick a food style that works for both your ethos and your body. What I mean by that is if your belief system is to be plant-based and you love how your body feels and functions on a plant-based diet, then you will want to do our plant-based track. I can tell you firsthand that Chef Leslie's passion for plant foods is infectious! As it does for many of you, plant-based eating works incredibly well for her. That's why I wanted her to build out plant-based recipes for you all—she's a plant-based zealot in all the right ways!

On the flip side of that, I have seen people try a new food style because it's trendy. Whole food cultures are often stimulated by new books, popular documentaries, or viral social media. But just because a food style is popular doesn't mean it's right for you. We always need to keep the *n* of 1 in mind. There is no perfect diet for everyone. There is only the perfect diet for you! This is why I have both plant-based and omnivore tracks for the 30-Day Fasting Reset.

You will also see these two different tracks reflected in the menu plans. You get to choose which fits best for you. If you already know you are committed to one of these eating styles, then it should be easy to navigate which reset you will do. If you are still trying to figure out which way of eating is optimal for you, I recommend that for one month you try the plant-based track, and then try the omnivore track the following month. See how you feel on both, and then make a choice for yourself.

Principle #2: Choose Your Healing Intensity

Within each track, I created a beginner version and an advanced version. The differences between these two are the length of fasts. If you have never fasted before, I highly recommend that you start with the beginner. Start off slow and get used to the eating and fasting windows; then once you get the hang of it, you can move on to the advanced track. The longer fasts will deepen your healing experience. This may mean more weight loss, gut repair, or improved moods.

You may choose to look at the beginner track as one you can effortlessly lean into to maintain your health and the advanced track as one you dip in and out of when you need a deeper healing moment for your body. Find the rhythm that works best for you!

Principle #3: Choose How to Cycle Your Reset

The whole idea behind eating and fasting like a girl is rhythm. The 30-Day Fasting Reset has a rhythm already built into it—one that has proved to work for millions of women. How you enter this reset is based on two different cycles: your menstrual cycle or the moon cycle.

If you have a menstrual cycle, you will start your reset on the day of the cycle you are on. For example, if you are on Day 3 of your cycle, then your 30 days start on Day 3 of the reset. You will then follow the reset for 30 days total. It's that simple.

If you don't have a menstrual cycle, you have two choices. You can either start on Day 1 of the reset and follow it 30 days through, or you can follow the moon cycle. It is no coincidence that the lunar cycle is around 30 days and so is a woman's menstrual cycle. If you want to follow the lunar cycle, Day 1 of your reset will be synced up with the new moon.

Principle #4: Choose an Accountability Buddy

Any worthy health endeavor is best done in community. For years, I had a friend who was my health challenge go-to. If I wanted to test out a new health habit, I asked her to join me in that experience. She was always game! Not only did this add oxytocin to the mix of neurochemicals I was stimulating, but it gave me someone to be accountable to on the days I wanted to give up. I cannot emphasize enough how much easier this reset will be if you have an accountability buddy.

If you are struggling to find that buddy, please know we have lots of ways you can practice these principles with me and my team. First, I have a free Facebook group called the Resetter Collaborative. This is a passionate group that knows fasting well! You will get lots of support there. Just announce that you are doing the 30-Day Fasting Reset, and you will find many kindred spirits who will happily join you in that journey. I also have a low-cost membership group called the Reset Academy. This is where you will find me, my health coaches, and my incredible team. We do fat-burning experiences together, dive deep into hormonal concepts together, and we even work out together on Saturday mornings. So if you need more support, please join us in my Reset Academy.

Your 30-Day Fasting Reset

Here's how the 30-Day Fasting Reset works: In a 30-day period you will cycle in and out of two food styles and three different-length fasts. This is all built to help you metabolically flex in and out of your sugar burner and fat burner systems. There are three major components to this reset: what to avoid, what food style to eat, and how long to fast.

WHAT TO AVOID

Remember the Foundational Five I mapped out in Chapter 1? Here's where we put it into action. Throughout your 30 days, you will avoid four things:

- Bad inflammatory fats
- Highly processed flours and sugars
- Toxic fat-stimulating ingredients
- Alcohol

YOUR TWO DIFFERENT EATING STYLES

Ketobiotic Eating Style

- Consume 50 grams net carbohydrates (nature's carbs only)
- Avoid humanmade carbohydrates (breads, pastas, desserts, crackers, etc.)
- Consume 1 gram of protein for every pound of ideal body weight per day
- Good fat with every meal

Hormone Feasting Eating Style

- Consume more than 150 grams of net carbs per day
- Focus on fiber-rich nature's carbs (vegetables, fruits, squashes, and potatoes)
- Consume 1 gram of protein for every pound of ideal body weight per day
- Good fat with every meal

Go back to Chapter 1 if you need to remind yourself what constitutes a bad inflammatory fat (there is also a list of endocrine-disrupting obesogens to avoid in Appendix A). Taking these ingredients out of your diet is a huge step forward if you are looking to lose weight or balance your hormones.

WHAT FOOD STYLE YOU WILL EAT

I have mapped out two food styles here in this book: ketobiotic and hormone feasting. Throughout these 30 days, you will move in between these two. Keep in mind that keto-biotic will be your lower-carbohydrate days, while on hormone feasting days, you bring your carbohydrate load up.

You will also be choosing your protein amount based on how much muscle you are looking to build. For both eating styles, to build muscle, consume 1 gram of protein for every pound of ideal body weight. I have listed summaries of both eating styles in the box above.

TOOLS YOU NEED FOR THIS RESET

Remember how the first principle of the Foundational Five is to focus on blood sugar, not calories? To best understand how these two styles affect your blood sugar, you might find it helpful to put on a continuous glucose monitor.

When I coach a patient, this is the very first step we take together. When you can see in real time how your blood sugar responds to different foods, your mastery over your food choices accelerates. This is where you can take a baby neuron and turn it into a mature neuron in a matter of days. It's one of the most profound teaching tools I have ever seen when it comes to food. Nothing will motivate you more than seeing your food in action!

On the *Eat Like a Girl* resource page on my website (https://drmindypelz.com), you will find my favorite brands of continuous glucose monitors.

HOW TO BE A MASTER FAT BURNER

Knowing that many of you are using this reset as a weight-loss tool, I want to chat for a moment about some proven strategies for

EATING STYLES AND FASTING TIMES

Day 5
15hr fasting
Ketobiotic

BEGINNER

Days 1–4 13hr fasting Ketobiotic	**Days 6–10** 17hr fasting Ketobiotic	**Days 11–15** 13hr fasting Hormone feasting	**Days 16–19** 15hr fasting Ketobiotic	**Days 20–bleed** No fasting Hormone feasting

| 1 | | 4 | | | 8 | | | 12 | | | 16 | | 20 | | | 24 | | | 28 | 30 |

ADVANCED

Days 1–5 15hr fasting Ketobiotic	**Days 7–10** 17hr fasting Ketobiotic	**Days 11–15** 15hr fasting Hormone feasting	**Days 17–19** 17hr fasting Ketobiotic	**Days 20–bleed** 13hr fasting Hormone feasting

Day 6
24hr fasting
Ketobiotic

Day 16
24hr fasting
Ketobiotic

Avoid: bad oils, refined flours/sugars, toxic chemical ingredients, alcohol; **Food Styles**: ketobiotic, hormone feasting; **Fasting Lengths**: *Beginner*, 13hrs to 17hrs; *Advanced*, 13hrs to 24hrs.

losing weight. Releasing weight is not as easy as it used to be. This is largely because of all the toxins in food mixed with the dysregulation that has occurred in our feminine bodies from the high amounts of stress we are under. This doesn't mean that you can't release weight; it just means that you may have to play with several principles to get your body to let go of the excess accumulated years ago.

To best help you figure out where your metabolism may be stuck, I have created a master checklist for you, which is on the next page. As you progress through your 30-Day Fasting Reset, if you are not releasing the amount of weight you desire, please make sure that you go through this checklist and see if anything extra needs to be added. Many women drop large amounts of weight just by doing a couple of months of this 30-Day Fasting Reset. I always say that repeating this reset three times for a total of 90 days will give you the best fat-loss results. Typically, after 90 days, you will have found your own personal rhythm.

MINDING YOUR MELATONIN

Melatonin is a hormone that your body secretes in reaction to light. At the end of the day as the sun sets, your body responds to the red light that fills the sky by ramping up your melatonin production. Two to three hours after the sun sets, melatonin is in her full glory. She is surging through you, slowing you down and preparing you for sleep. Melatonin will hit her peak somewhere between two and four in the morning and then will decline after that. When you wake up and your eyes see light, that signals melatonin to turn off. Within 30 minutes after you wake up, melatonin abruptly turns off so that you can be awake and alert for the day.

Knowing melatonin's rhythm is important because, when she increases at night, she brings with her a decrease in insulin sensitivity. Insulin sensitivity does have a circadian pattern. This reduced insulin sensitivity at night is a normal physiological response, because the body's metabolic processes slow down during sleep. What this means is that, if you want to

CHECKLIST FOR ACCELERATED FAT BURNING

It's so frustrating when you feel like you've tried everything to drop weight and nothing is working. The reason your body holds on to weight is different for each of us. This is why following the weight-loss strategies that worked for a friend may not work for you. The following is a general checklist I used with my patients for years to make sure we didn't miss a weight-loss step. This checklist is in no particular order; think of it as a guide to ensure you have addressed all the reasons your body would hold on to weight.

- Make sure you are metabolically switching according to your hormonal cycle.
- Try some longer fasts (more than 24 hours) to train your body to retrieve the excess it has stored in fat.
- Eat fiber and good fat with every meal.
- Be sure you are eating enough protein.
- Avoid liver agitators like alcohol.
- Create an exercise variation plan that involves both strength training and high-intensity workouts.
- Go for a 20-minute walk after large meals.
- Evaluate your toxin load and minimize your obesogen exposure.
- Go on a thorough detox (preferably one that pulls heavy metals out).
- Prioritize sleep (you burn fat when you sleep).
- Eat only during daylight hours.
- Evaluate your stress levels (you can't drop weight in a chronically stressed body).

release weight, the meal you eat at 9 P.M. will more likely be stored as fat as compared to if you eat that meal at 5 P.M., when melatonin levels are lower. The same thing is true for the morning hours. Circadian rhythm expert Dr. Satchin Panda highly advises "avoiding food for at least one hour after waking up."[1] This allows melatonin levels to decline, restoring insulin sensitivity. If you want to drop weight, a guiding principle to follow is to always eat when it's light outside.

Another hormone that is affected by melatonin is cortisol. When melatonin turns off in your morning hours, it stimulates cortisol production. Within 30 to 60 minutes, your cortisol levels will be at their daily peak. Remember that cortisol's job is to make you move. Like all the other hormones, if you don't use cortisol, you will store cortisol. And the pantry for cortisol is your belly. A guiding principle for avoiding belly fat then becomes to move your body at cortisol-rich moments. This might mean working out or going for a walk an hour after rising or moving your body whenever a stressful moment hits you hard. For many rushing women who want to release weight around their midsection, they do both.

One of my goals with this book is to take the mystery out of weight loss and balancing hormones. Because of that, I have taken the nutritional counting out of the recipes. Instead, I have placed the recipes according to their effect on your blood sugar. Ketobiotic recipes will have a lower blood-sugar response, whereas the recipes that are in the hormone feasting section will elevate your blood sugar more. My other goal is to help you see that you don't have to deprive your body on your path back to health. With the fundamentals out of the way, let's dive into the beautiful recipes my chefs have provided you.

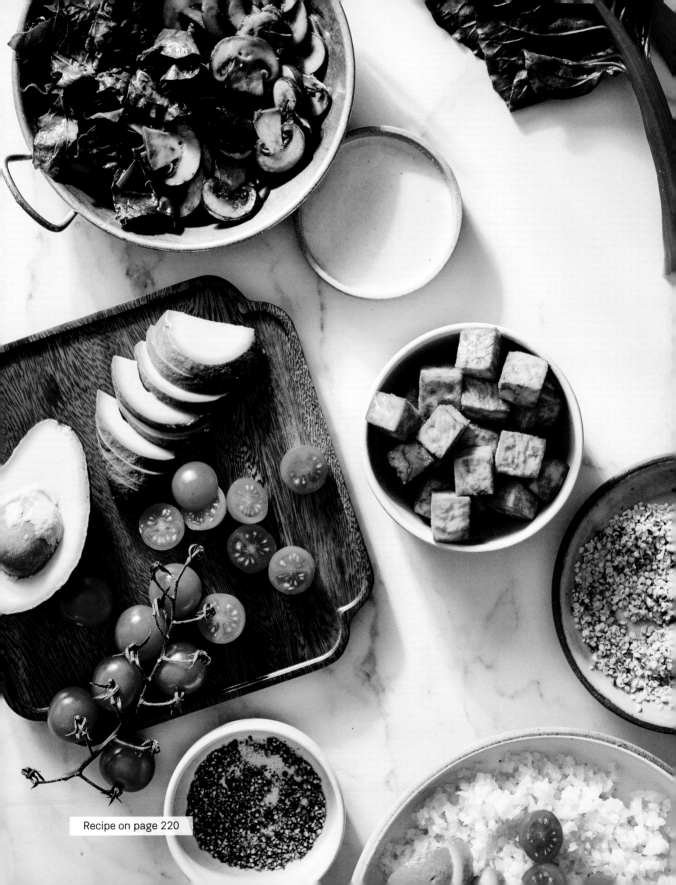

Recipe on page 220

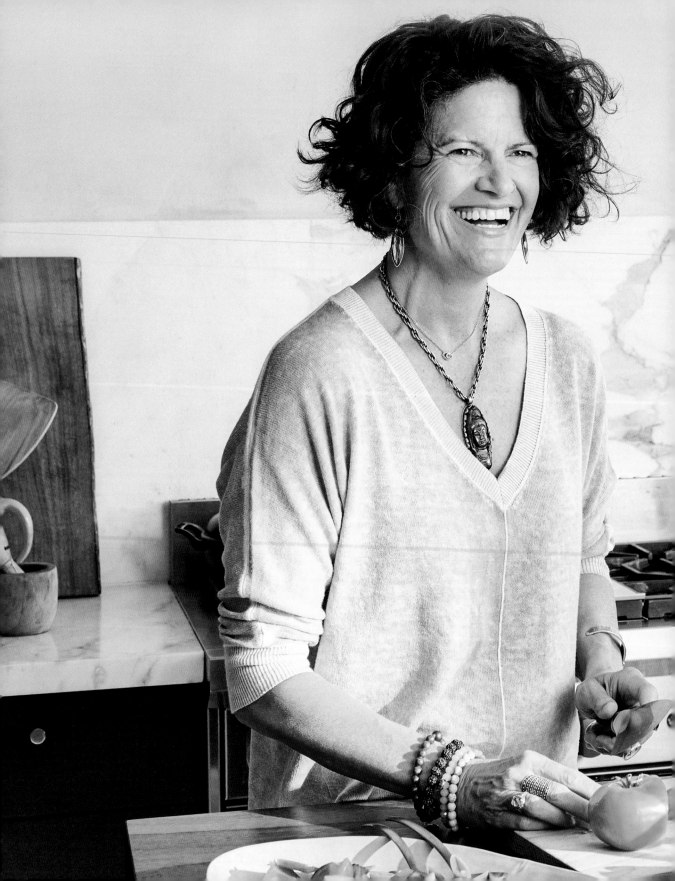

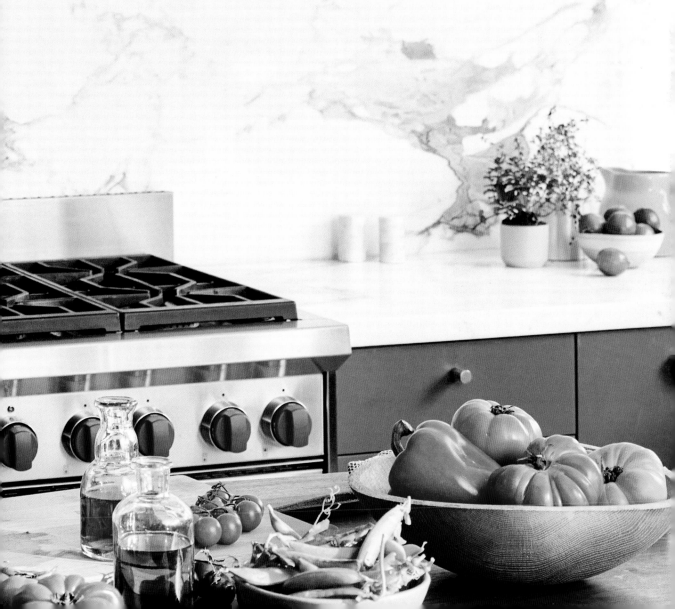

PART IV

Recipes

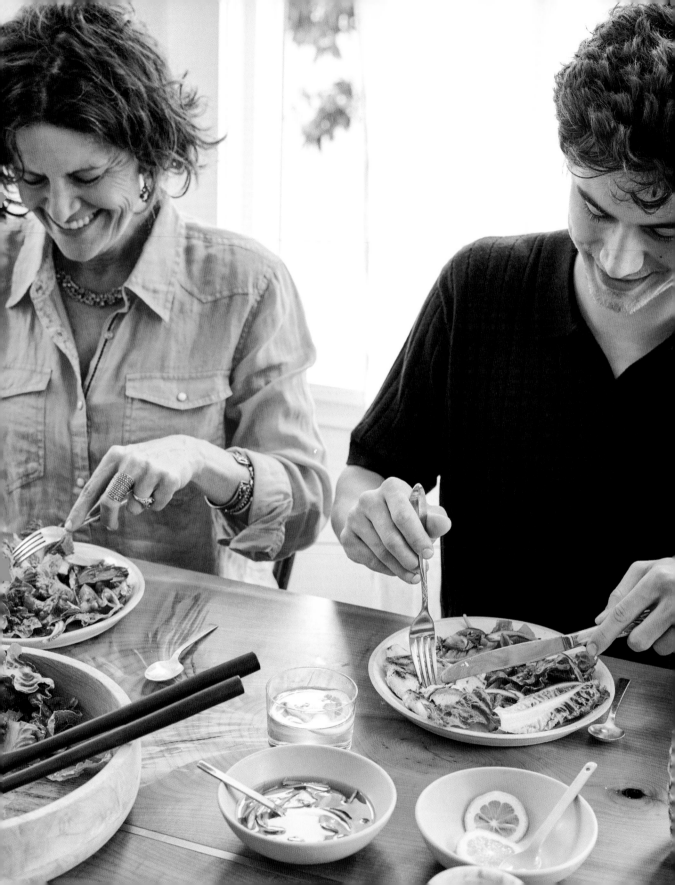

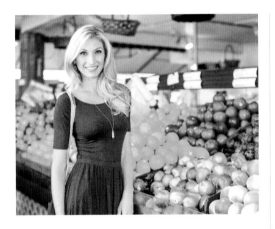

Meet Chef Leslie Durso

I first met Leslie at a retreat where she was hired to provide all the meals for us. I'm not going to lie: When I first heard we were going plant-based for three days, my omnivore brain was disappointed. Then I tasted Chef Leslie's food, and my taste buds were elated! Not to mention I had my continuous glucose reader on and was shocked at how many of Leslie's recipes didn't spike my blood sugar. I knew in that moment that there was something special about the culinary dishes she so passionately made.

When we first started to conceptualize *Eat Like a Girl*, I knew that we had to have a plant-based track for those of you who are dedicated to that style of eating. And I definitely knew

I wanted Chef Leslie to be the one to create the plant-based recipes. What I didn't know at that moment was the depth of knowledge and passion that she has for the medicinal qualities of plants.

Throughout the creation of *Eat Like a Girl*, the collaboration with Chef Leslie has been a dream. We have geeked out on hormones, the healing properties of plants, and our love of exceptional-tasting food. As I reflect on the path where both science and food intertwine to heal and uplift, Leslie's profound dedication and passion for plant-based cuisine emerge as a beacon of inspiration, infusing each carefully curated dish in this book with love and nourishment.

The decision to invite Chef Leslie to infuse her gastronomic brilliance onto the pages of *Eat Like a Girl* was born from a shared belief in the healing power of wholesome, nutrient-dense foods, and because her expertise in the culinary arts is bar none. With a culinary career spanning more than 10 years, Leslie has achieved recognition and acclaim for her innovative approach to plant-based cuisine. She works as a consulting chef for hotels, resorts, and restaurants around the world and is currently the plant-based chef at Four Seasons Resort Punta Mita, Mexico and Naviva, A Four Seasons Resort, Punta Mita, Mexico. If that is not impressive enough, the

Four Seasons named Leslie "Master Chef" in 2019.

Leslie's earliest memories of food are steeped in the tantalizing sights and scents of homemade pizzas and pastas, with her great-grandmother's treasured ravioli recipe holding a special place in her heart. Leslie's culinary artistry not only celebrates the flavors of her past, but also embodies the enduring power of women in shaping her relationships with food. Each dish she creates today is a reminder of her family's traditions, nourishment, and the indomitable spirit of women.

Some of you may recognize Chef Leslie from *Bill Nye the Science Guy*, where she was "Leslie the Lab Girl." Her experience as the Science Guy's sidekick brings a whole level of nerdiness to her culinary artistry. All you have to do is talk with her to get a glimpse of the depths of her food-science knowledge.

You can find Chef Leslie on her socials (Instagram and YouTube), at one of the aforementioned Four Seasons Resorts, or through her multiple appearances on esteemed platforms and in prestigious publications.

As we unveil the fruits (and veggies!) of our collaboration within the pages of *Eat Like a Girl*, I am filled with gratitude for the opportunity to share Leslie's culinary passion with you through these recipes. May you find not just nourishment for your body, but a reminder that every meal is an opportunity to nourish, heal, and thrive.

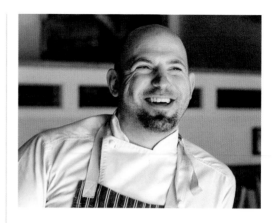

Meet Chef Jeff Weiss

Chef Jeff Weiss was an obvious choice for the omnivore track of *Eat Like a Girl* for a variety of reasons. First, nearly two decades ago, he embarked on a culinary career that has focused on seasonal, sustainable, and simple recipes. Recipes that stay true to their roots and, most importantly, taste fantastic. He also has incredible experience cooking in the kitchens of James Beard– and Michelin award–winning chefs José Andrés and April Bloomfield, as well as in the Spanish kitchens of chefs Adolfo Muñoz and Dani García. His distinguished international experience originated with being awarded the prestigious ICEX culinary scholarship in 2009—allowing him to live in Spain, learn the regional cuisines, and cook in the kitchens of top Spanish chefs. His book, *Charcutería: The Soul of Spain*, a nominee for both the James Beard Award and the Gourmand World Cookbook Award, chronicles his time working in Spain and learning the various culinary and charcuterie styles of the Iberian Peninsula.

What I love about his international experience is that many of the culinary skills he learned in Spain came from elder women in a small town—women who had passed down food wisdom through recipes that reach back through the generations. Chef Jeff has since held executive chef positions for multiple restaurants, hotels, and resorts across the country, alongside settling into the Las Vegas area to create Valencian Gold, where he showcased his passion for making "paella for the people" and introduced a fun, exciting Spanish experience outside the world of fine dining. Valencian Gold quickly soared to become one of Las Vegas's most talked-about and awarded dining experiences—a remarkable feat for an off-the-Strip restaurant.

Chef Jeff also brings a unique twist to his culinary passion. Prior to launching his career as a chef, he was a former pairs figure skater at a highly competitive level. When I asked him about his knowledge of the female body and how we can best nourish ourselves, he enthusiastically responded by sharing with me what he had learned through the years training with his partners. He knew all about how the training demands needed to change to match his partner's cycle. He also reiterated to me that his job as partner was not only to compete but to be a protector, safeguarding and showcasing his partner's talents. This fierce dedication to uplifting women touched me deeply.

Between his extensive culinary experience learning from the grandmas in Spain and his robust résumé as head chef in one of the world's most sought-after restaurants as well as his in-depth awareness of how food influences the overall well-being and performance of the female body, Chef Jeff was an incredible choice to bring you *Eat Like a Girl*'s omnivore-track recipes.

It is both an honor and a privilege to have Chef Jeff Weiss as a collaborator, a visionary whose culinary creations and philanthropic endeavors have inspired me and now all of you to embrace a future where healing and nurturing go hand in hand with the power of food.

The Recipes

Both Chef Leslie and Chef Jeff have gone to great lengths to provide you with more than 100 recipes that not only fit with the eat-like-a-girl principles, but also are unique and tasty and will act as hormonal medicine for your beautiful body.

This section is divided into four categories: Fasted Snacks, Breaking the Fast, Hormone Feasting, and Ketobiotic. Although most of the recipes fall into more than one category, I have sectioned them to help you better understand how to use these recipes in both your eating and fasting windows. To allow you to decide how to use the recipes, we have provided icons indicating all of the categories they fall into. Also, keep in mind that the two food styles that help support a healthy female body are ketobiotic and hormone feasting. The recipes that keep your blood sugar on the lower side are in the keto-biotic section, whereas the recipes that spark a higher glucose response are in the hormone-feasting section. All recipes are gluten-free, and many are vegetarian or vegan. You can substitute nonalcoholic wine or beer, water, or stock in any recipe that calls for alcohol. You'll note that the chefs treat dressings a little differently, with Chef Leslie's dressings found within her recipes, and Chef Jeff's found in Pantry.

I have mapped out guidelines for the different macronutrients of these food styles, but I purposefully did not put the macronutrient amounts in each recipe. The fasting lifestyle I'm teaching you is built around your finding your rhythm with *when* and *what* you eat—a rhythm that is unique to you and hopefully becomes effortless the more you practice it. Enjoy!

LEGEND: GF = Gluten-Free V = Vegetarian VG = Vegan
BF = Break Fast FS = Fasted Snacks HF = Hormone Feasting K = Ketobiotic

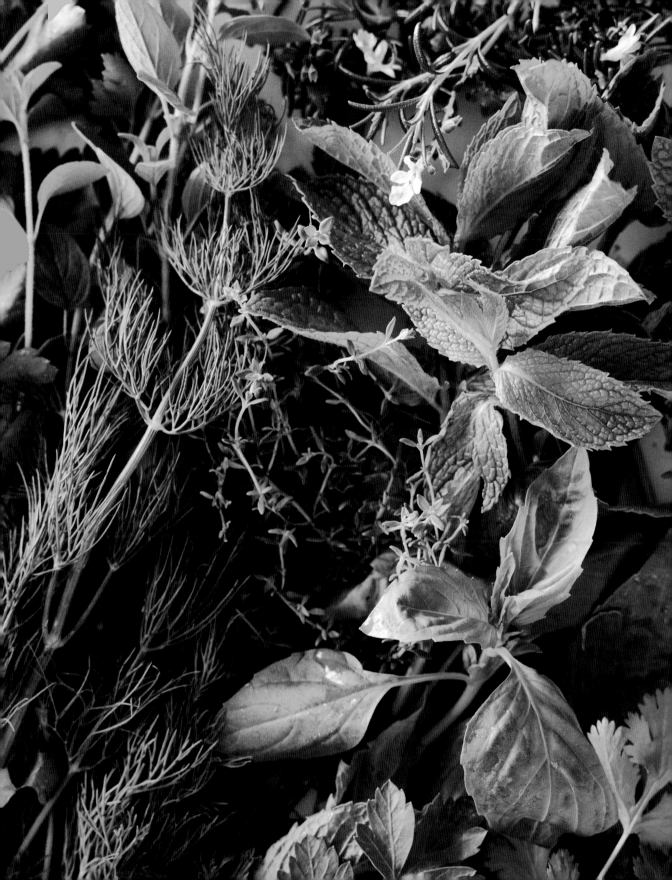

11

Fasted Snacks

WHEN I SET OUT TO WRITE THIS BOOK, my first thought was *We need recipes that showcase foods and drinks that are acceptable in the fasting window*. I am so thrilled to present those recipes to you now. Using the guidelines that fasting researchers have discovered along with the insights that studies have given us about the metabolic power of a fasted snack, my chefs offer you delicious recipes that won't pull you out of a fasted state.

Think of these recipes as a tool you use when you're first learning to fast, when you're experimenting with a longer fast, or when your brain starts chattering at you to eat while in your fasting window. As you learn the art of moving in and out of fasting and eating windows, you may notice that you need these fasted snacks less. Also, keep in mind that it's always best to test these recipes with a blood-sugar reader to ensure they don't elevate your blood-sugar levels. Since it's the microbiome that determines your blood-sugar response to food, and we all have a unique microbiome makeup, testing your blood-sugar response to these snacks can be helpful.

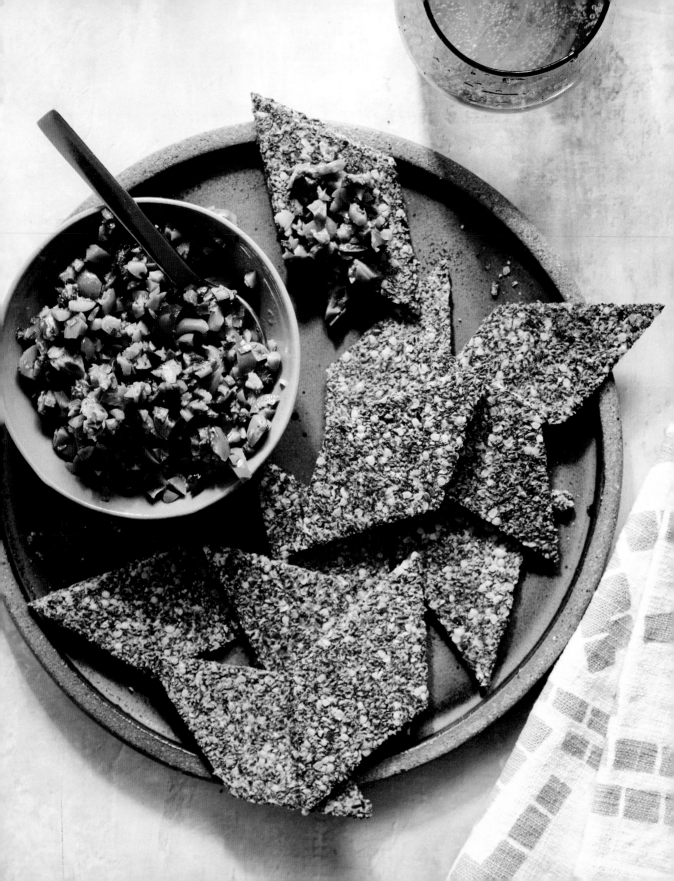

Fasting Crackers and Olive Tapenade

MAKES THIRTY 1½-INCH CRACKERS
AND ABOUT 1½ CUPS TAPENADE   CHEF LESLIE

One question I hear again and again: "Is there anything acceptable to eat during a fast?" The answer is yes—if you follow the rules of a fasted snack. These crackers do exactly that! They also provide a satisfying crunch. Make a batch of these crackers ahead of time, and they can be a go-to snack anytime. If you want to stay within a fasted state, don't eat more than five crackers within your fasting window. You can mix almost any herb into the olive tapenade, but Chef Leslie prefers basil, dill, parsley, oregano, or a combination of any of them.

FASTING CRACKERS

1 cup ground flaxseed
¼ cup hemp seeds
¼ cup chia seeds

OLIVE TAPENADE

2 cups mixed olives in a water brine, drained, pitted, and chopped
1 tablespoon chopped mixed fresh herbs, such as basil, dill, parsley, oregano, or cilantro

TO MAKE THE CRACKERS Preheat the oven to 400°F. Line a large baking sheet with parchment paper.

Combine the flaxseed, hemp seeds, and chia seeds in a bowl and mix well. Pour in ½ cup of warm water, mix well, and let sit for 10 minutes.

Lay a sheet of parchment paper on your work surface and pour the cracker mixture into the center. Place another sheet of parchment paper over it.

Using a rolling pin or your hands, roll out the mixture until it's about ¼ inch thick.

Remove the top sheet of parchment paper and use a knife or a cookie cutter to cut the dough into cracker-size shapes.

Arrange the crackers on the prepared baking sheet and bake for 10 minutes. Flip over the crackers and bake for another 10 minutes, or until they're golden brown. Remove from the oven. Let the crackers cool completely in the pan.

These crackers can be stored in an airtight container at room temperature for up to 3 weeks.

TO MAKE THE TAPENADE While the crackers are baking, mix the olives and herbs in a medium bowl.

To serve, place the tapenade and crackers in separate bowls. Top each cracker with a little of the tapenade and enjoy.

Fasting Herb Salad

MAKES 1 SERVING | CHEF LESLIE

Sometimes when we're in a fasted state, it's our microbiome that is sending us hunger signals. This recipe has a nice dose of fiber to satisfy your gut microbes while using MCT oil to turn off the hunger hormone in your brain. One serving of this delicious herb salad would make a great fasted snack.

DRESSING
¼ cup MCT oil
1½ tablespoons lemon juice
1 pinch kosher salt
1 pinch freshly ground black pepper

SALAD
1 cup arugula
½ cup whole fresh parsley leaves
½ cup whole fresh basil leaves
¼ cup whole fresh mint leaves
¼ cup olives in olive oil

TO MAKE THE DRESSING Whisk together the MCT oil, lemon juice, salt, and pepper in a small bowl until thoroughly combined.

TO MAKE THE SALAD Combine the arugula, parsley, basil, mint, and olives in a serving bowl and mix well.

Drizzle with the dressing to taste and serve.

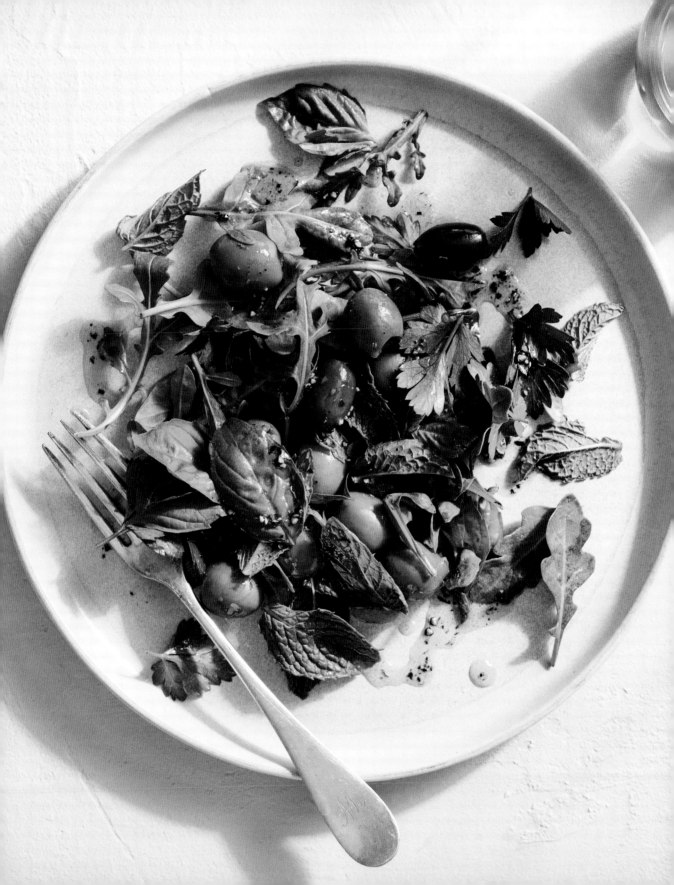

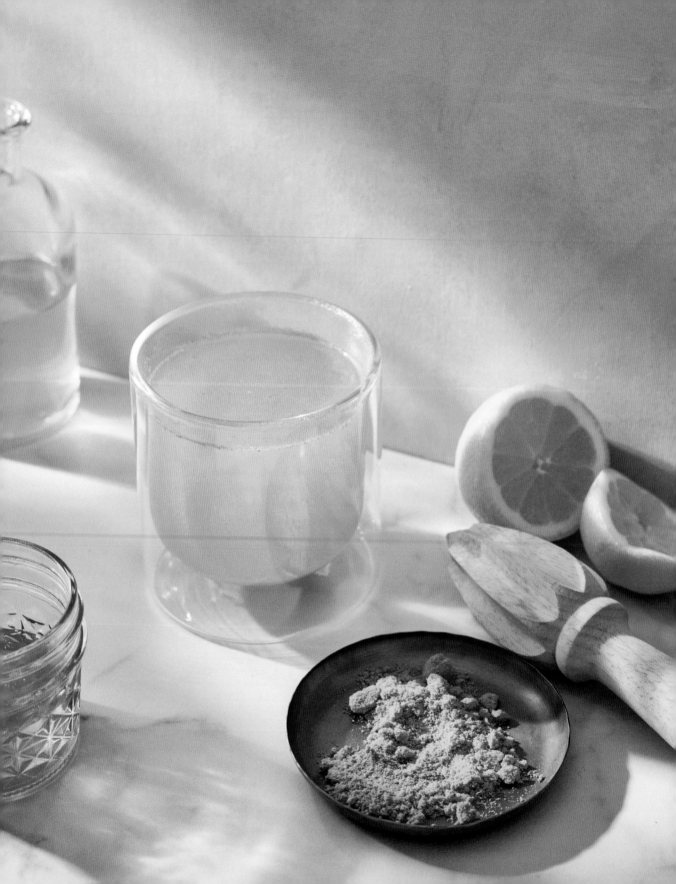

ACV Turmeric Tea

MAKES 1 SERVING | | CHEF LESLIE

I absolutely love this healing tea that Chef Leslie created. If you want to keep it as a fasted snack, don't use the optional honey. The ground turmeric has an anti-inflammatory effect that can help with any joint pain and brain fog that may show up in the longer fasts. The apple cider vinegar can lower your blood sugar, allowing your body to burn more fat and create a deeper ketogenic state.

1 tablespoon apple cider vinegar
Juice of ½ lemon
1 teaspoon honey (optional)
¼ teaspoon ground turmeric

Combine 1 cup of hot water, the apple cider vinegar, lemon juice, honey (if using), and turmeric in a mug and stir well. Serve immediately.

Lemon Basil Chia Seed Drink

MAKES 1 SERVING   CHEF LESLIE

So many people have asked me "What can I drink in my fasted state?" Oftentimes, our mind needs more flavor than what's in just a plain cup of water. This recipe gives you not only a burst of flavor to satisfy your taste buds, but also the chia seeds and lemon to support a deeper detox effect. I'd especially recommend this drink during a longer fast.

2 fresh basil leaves
Juice of ½ lemon
2 tablespoons chia seeds

Muddle the basil leaves in a tall glass. Add 1 cup of water, the lemon juice, and chia seeds and stir well.

Refrigerate for at least 20 minutes and up to overnight. Serve cold.

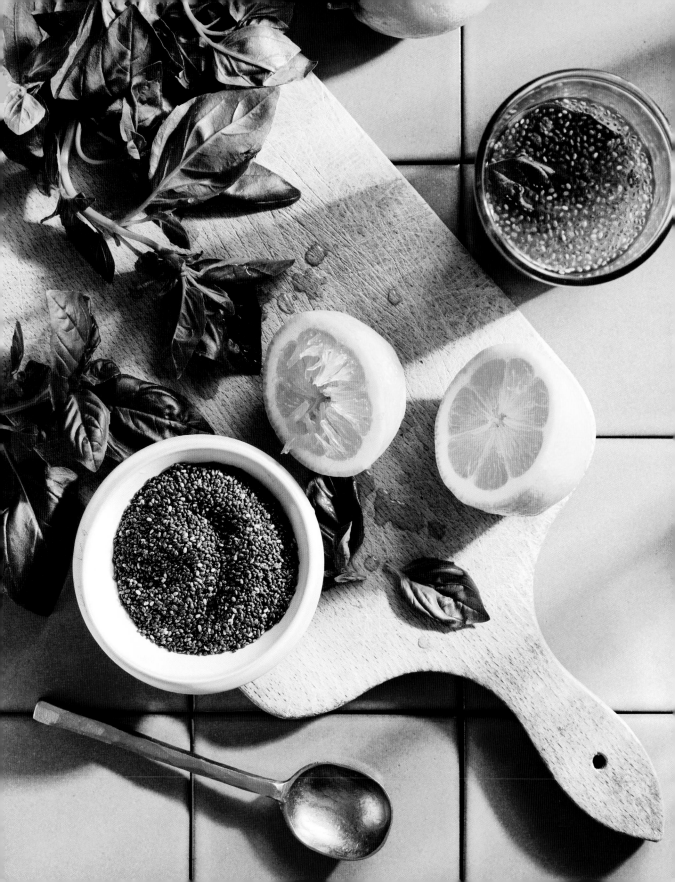

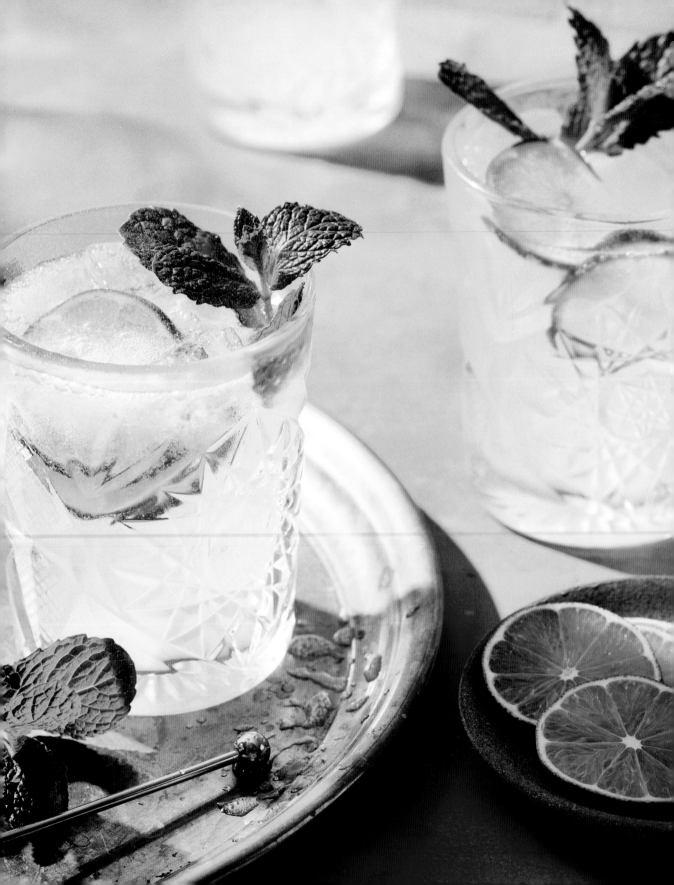

Lime Ginger Mint Mocktail

MAKES 1 SERVING | CHEF LESLIE

When we fast, we often experience waves of nausea and other gastrointestinal symptoms. If you find yourself with an upset tummy while fasting, this is your go-to drink. It keeps you in a fasted state while the ginger and mint calm your stomach.

1 sprig mint
¼ teaspoon grated fresh ginger
1 teaspoon lime juice
8 ounces sparkling water
1 sprig mint (optional)
1 to 2 slices lime (optional)

Muddle the mint and ginger in a tall glass. Pour in the lime juice.

Fill the glass with ice, then fill the rest of the glass with sparkling water and garnish with mint and lime slices.

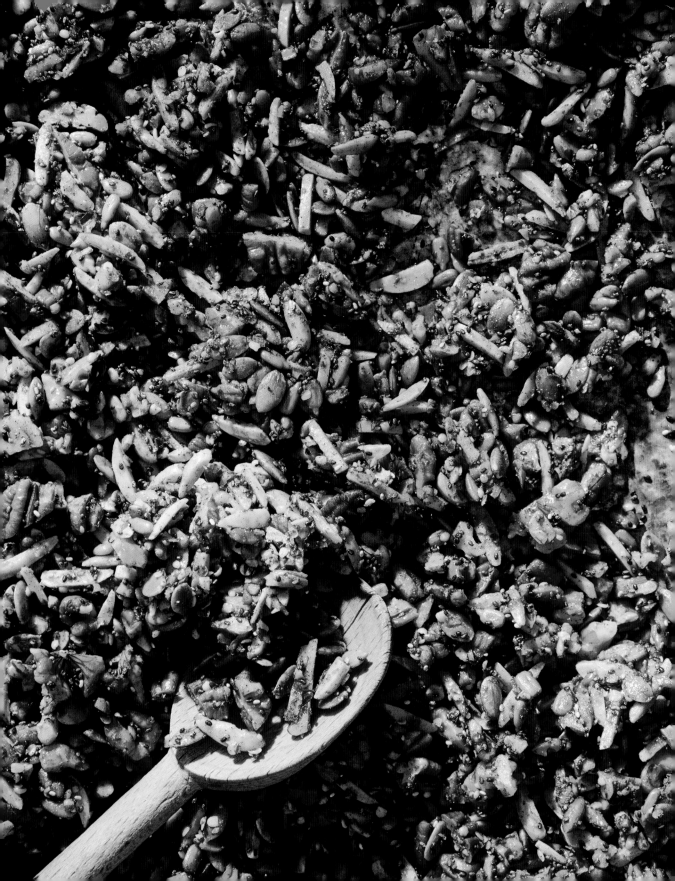

12

Breaking the Fast

YOUR FIRST MEAL MATTERS! It's so important that I guarantee you'll hear me saying this again and again. When you open up your eating window, that first meal sets the tone for healing. Fasting is a healing state, but food heals too.

Although most of the recipes in this book would be appropriate to break your fast with, I have specially categorized these recipes because they accomplish one or more of the following: They are fast and easy to make, they will curb your hunger quickly, or they can act as hormonal medicine for you. Be sure to look at the headnotes I left for you with each recipe, along with which eating style they fit in. Some recipes are perfect for your ketobiotic days, for example, while others have that added carbohydrate load that is just what your body needs on hormone feasting days.

An interesting added note here—you will know that a break-your-fast meal has worked well for you if you feel satisfied and energized and have a clear mind after you eat that meal.

If one of these recipes makes you sleepy or gives you brain fog, you may try adding more protein or fat next time for a more stable blood-sugar response.

The most important question to ask yourself when you break your fast is "What healing effect am I trying to achieve with this food?" If you want to build muscle, be sure to pick recipes that are packed with protein. If you want to repair your gut microbiome, break your fast with a plant-rich recipe. And if you want to stop your hunger, be sure that you eat a meal that is rich in good fats. In this section, I have chosen some of my favorite recipes to break a fast. Please note you are not limited to only these recipes for that first meal. Any recipe in this book with a BF icon can be used to break your fast. I encourage you to experiment with many different recipes and see how you feel after each one. Keep in mind that the best break-fast meal is one that energizes you and kills your hunger.

Pumpkin Protein Pancakes

MAKES 8 PANCAKES | | CHEF LESLIE

This is a great recipe to break your fast on your hormone feasting days. The beautiful part about this dish is that it contains a nice combination of ingredients that stabilizes your blood sugar and kills hunger. Apple cider vinegar can lower your blood sugar after a carb-rich meal, and the coconut oil turns off the hunger hormone in your brain. To facilitate muscle building, make sure the protein powder you use provides 30 grams of protein. Chef Leslie calls for refined coconut oil here; unrefined is fine, but it will add a coconut flavor to the pancakes.

1 cup unsweetened nondairy milk
1 tablespoon apple cider vinegar
⅓ cup pumpkin puree
2 tablespoons maple syrup
½ tablespoon vanilla extract
1 tablespoon melted refined coconut oil
¾ cup all-purpose gluten-free flour
¼ cup vegan protein powder
1 teaspoon baking powder
½ teaspoon baking soda
¼ teaspoon ground cinnamon
⅛ teaspoon kosher salt
1 pinch ground ginger
1 pinch ground nutmeg
¼ cup pepitas, toasted in a frying pan

Combine the milk and apple cider vinegar in a large bowl and let rest until the milk curdles slightly, about 5 minutes. Add the pumpkin, maple syrup, and vanilla and whisk to combine. Add the melted coconut oil while mixing to incorporate.

Add the flour, protein powder, baking powder, baking soda, cinnamon, salt, ginger, and nutmeg to a small bowl and combine. Add to the milk mixture and whisk.

Let the batter rest for 5 to 10 minutes.

Heat a griddle on medium heat and spritz with avocado oil cooking spray. Pour ¼-cup amounts of the batter onto the griddle, keeping them spaced apart. Cook until bubbles appear in the middle and the edges turn slightly dry, 2 to 3 minutes. Flip over and cook for 1 to 3 minutes more, or until the pancakes are set on both sides and golden brown. Transfer the pancakes to a plate and repeat with the rest of the batter. Sprinkle the pancakes with toasted pepitas and serve.

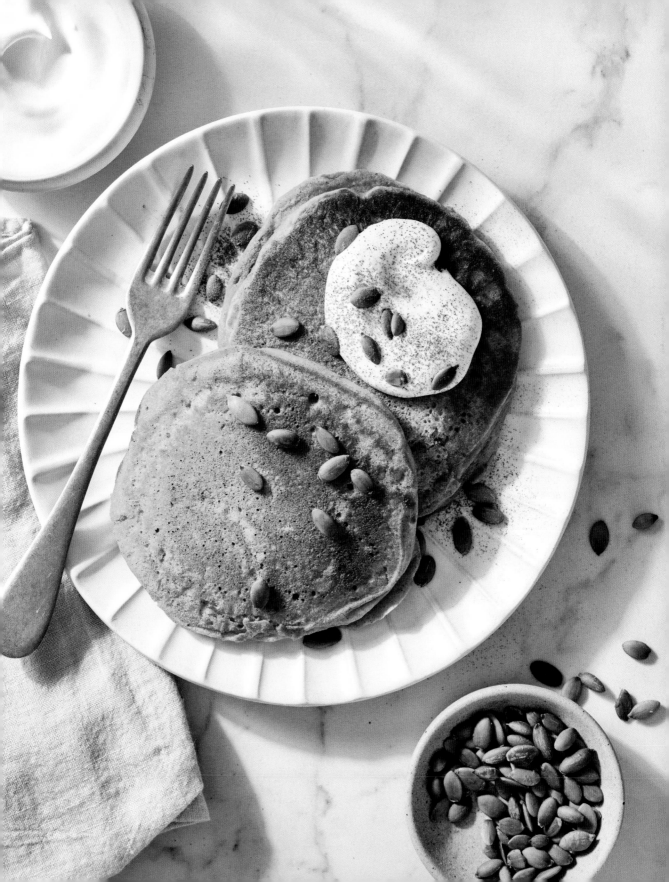

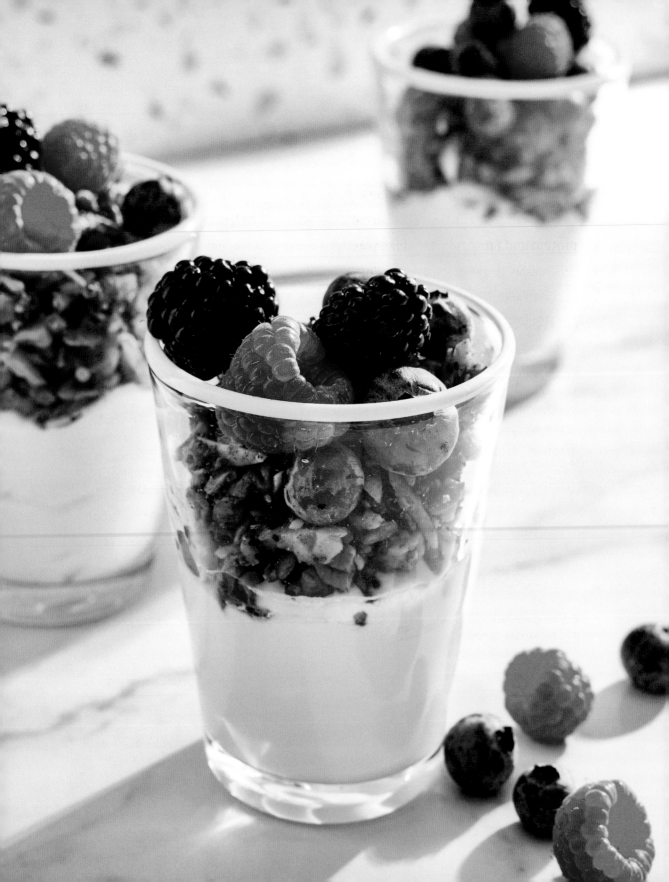

Nutty Granola Parfait

MAKES 6 SERVINGS | CHEF LESLIE

If you are opening up your eating window in the morning, this is a perfect breakfast recipe. For those of you who eat dairy, add some Greek yogurt for extra protein and fat to help stabilize your blood sugar. If you use keto maple syrup, this recipe becomes ketobiotic. The added flaxseed in this recipe makes it ideal for your manifestation stage, since flaxseed is fabulous for estrogen production. (It's also delicious—when we tested this recipe, we couldn't stop eating it!)

GRANOLA

1 cup slivered almonds
1 cup pecans, coarsely chopped
1 cup walnuts, coarsely chopped
½ cup pepitas
¼ cup sunflower seeds
¼ cup chia seeds
¼ cup melted coconut oil
¼ cup maple syrup
3 tablespoons hemp seeds
1 tablespoon ground flaxseed
1½ teaspoons ground cinnamon
1 teaspoon vanilla extract
½ teaspoon kosher salt

PARFAIT

6 cups unsweetened coconut milk yogurt
6 cups berries, such as blueberries, blackberries, and raspberries

TO MAKE THE GRANOLA Preheat the oven to 300°F. Line a baking sheet with parchment paper.

Combine the almonds, pecans, walnuts, pepitas, sunflower seeds, chia seeds, coconut oil, maple syrup, hemp seeds, flaxseed, cinnamon, vanilla, and salt in a large bowl and mix everything together thoroughly.

Pour the mixture onto the prepared baking sheet and spread it out evenly.

Bake for 15 to 20 minutes. Stir the mixture and bake for another 15 to 20 minutes, until lightly browned.

Let cool completely. Break up the granola into pieces.

The granola can be stored in an airtight container at room temperature for up to 3 weeks.

TO MAKE THE PARFAIT To serve, spoon layers of yogurt, granola, and berries into bowls or parfait glasses.

Chia Protein Bars

MAKES 12 BARS | CHEF LESLIE

I love how Chef Leslie added so many seeds to this recipe! Hemp seeds are a powerful prebiotic that also supports your gut microbiome, while chia seeds are incredible for not only feeding your gut microbiome but also having a gentle detox effect. Because of this recipe's power on your microbiome, this is a fabulous break-fast dish during your manifestation phase. Keep in mind that one of this phase's health goals is to eat foods that help your gut break down hormones. A prebiotic-rich meal like this will absolutely help your body accomplish that.

1½ cups packed pitted dates
½ cup almond butter
1 teaspoon vanilla extract
¼ teaspoon kosher salt
1 cup raw walnut pieces
½ cup chia seeds
½ cup hemp seeds
½ cup unsweetened shredded coconut
½ cup chopped nondairy dark chocolate
⅓ cup cacao powder

Line a 9 x 9-inch baking pan with parchment paper.

In a food processor, pulse the dates until a thick paste forms. Add the almond butter, vanilla, and salt and pulse again until thoroughly combined.

Add the walnuts, chia seeds, hemp seeds, coconut, chocolate, and cacao powder and pulse until thoroughly incorporated.

Using a spatula, press the mixture evenly into the prepared baking pan and freeze overnight.

Remove the pan from the freezer and cut the mixture into 12 bars. Place the bars in an airtight container and refrigerate for up to a week or freeze for up to 3 months.

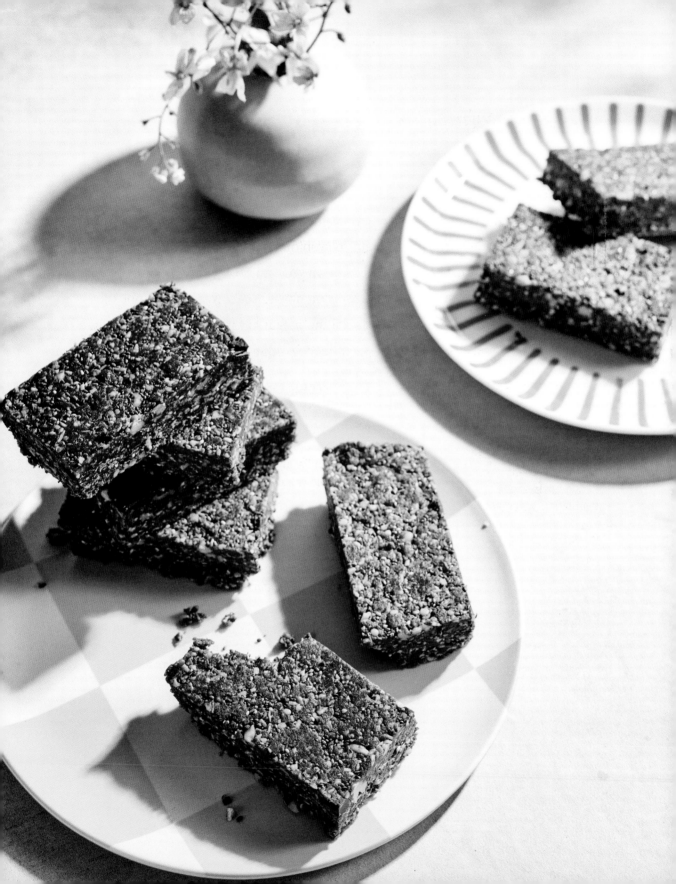

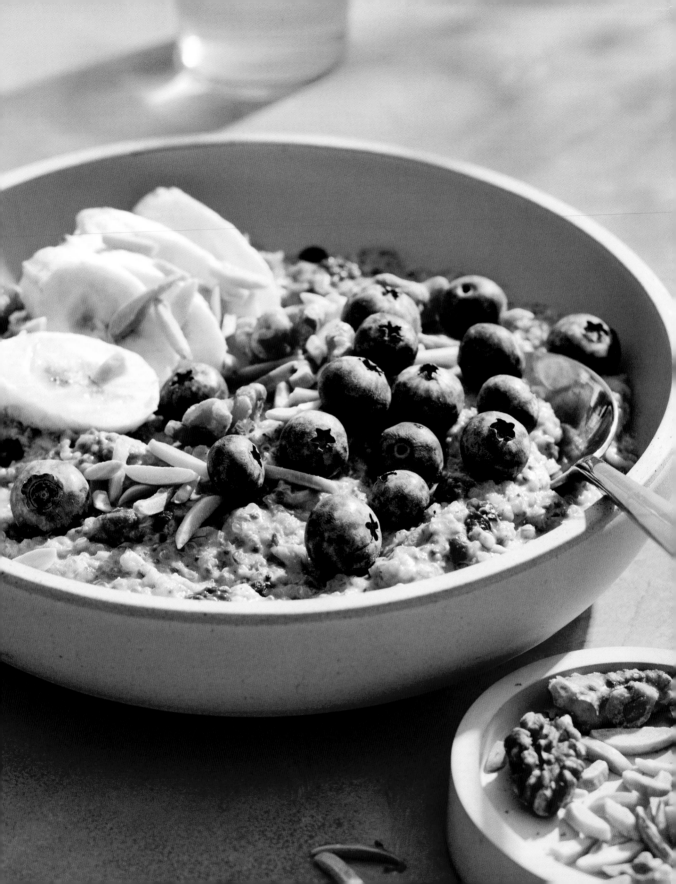

Purple Quinoa Porridge

MAKES 4 TO 6 SERVINGS | CHEF LESLIE

I love this porridge as a break-fast meal in your nurture phase. Not only is quinoa a powerful food for supporting healthy progesterone production, but it also offers a gentle blood-sugar spike and more protein than other starches like rice. Chef Leslie brilliantly added cinnamon, which is delicious but also ensures your blood sugar does not spike too high with this carb-rich meal. I love the combination of chia seeds and flaxseed for feeding the gut microbiome and gently assisting your body in detoxing.

PORRIDGE

3 cups unsweetened nondairy milk
1 cup rolled oats
½ cup dry quinoa, rinsed
½ cup frozen blueberries, preferably wild
2 tablespoons chia seeds
2 tablespoons ground flaxseed
1 tablespoon coconut oil
1 teaspoon ground cinnamon
½ teaspoon kosher salt

OPTIONAL TOPPINGS

Slivered toasted almonds
Pecans
Walnuts
Almond butter
Hemp seeds
Sliced banana
Fresh blueberries
Granola (see page 121)

TO MAKE THE PORRIDGE Combine the nondairy milk, 2 cups water, oats, quinoa, blueberries, chia seeds, flaxseed, coconut oil, cinnamon, and salt in a medium saucepan and bring to a boil over high heat.

Decrease the heat to low and let simmer until the porridge reaches your desired consistency, 10 to 15 minutes.

TO ASSEMBLE THE DISH Spoon the porridge into bowls and serve immediately with any of the optional toppings.

Tofu Scramble

MAKES 2 SERVINGS | | CHEF LESLIE

This delicious, savory scramble is perfect for breaking your fast during your power phases. In Power Phase 1, the goal is to help support estrogen production. Tofu is an effective phytoestrogen that can give your body the added protective estrogen needed for a healthy menstrual cycle. Turmeric is an anti-inflammatory superpower, making this dish helpful for menopausal symptoms like hot flashes or brain fog.

2 tablespoons extra-virgin olive oil
½ medium yellow onion, diced
1 cup sliced mushrooms
¼ cup diced bell pepper of any color
1 garlic clove, minced
¼ cup diced tomato
2 tablespoons nutritional yeast
1 tablespoon smoked paprika
1 tablespoon ground turmeric
1 teaspoon ground cumin
Kosher salt
One 14- to 16-ounce package firm tofu, drained
1 cup coarsely chopped spinach or baby kale

Heat the olive oil in a sauté pan over medium-high heat. Add the onion, mushrooms, bell pepper, and garlic and sauté until they start to turn a bit soft, about 5 minutes. Add the tomato, nutritional yeast, paprika, turmeric, cumin, and 1 teaspoon of salt and mix well. Crumble the tofu into the pan, add the spinach, and cook, stirring often, until heated through, about 2 minutes.

Taste and adjust the seasoning with more salt if desired. Serve warm.

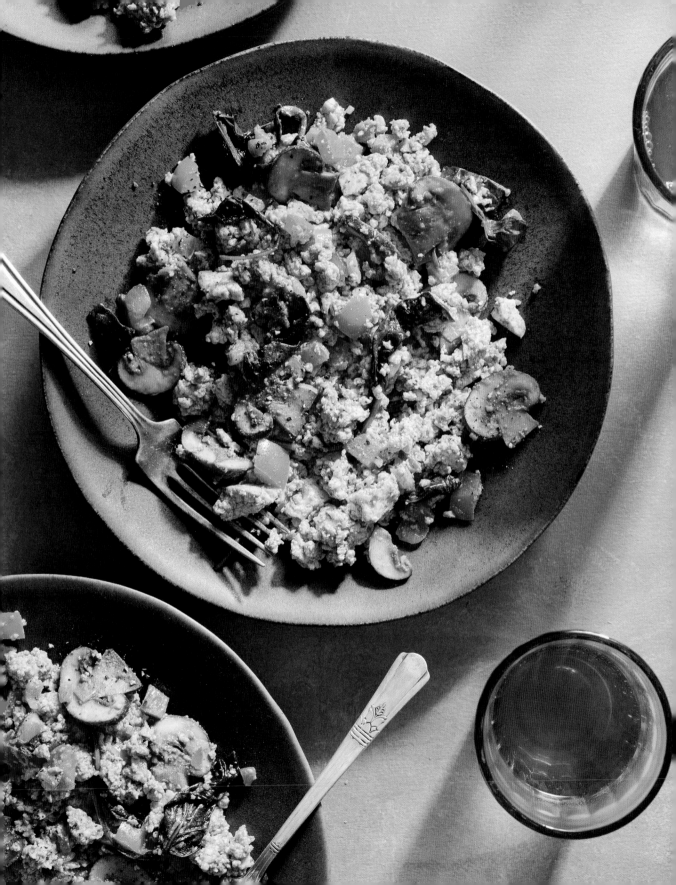

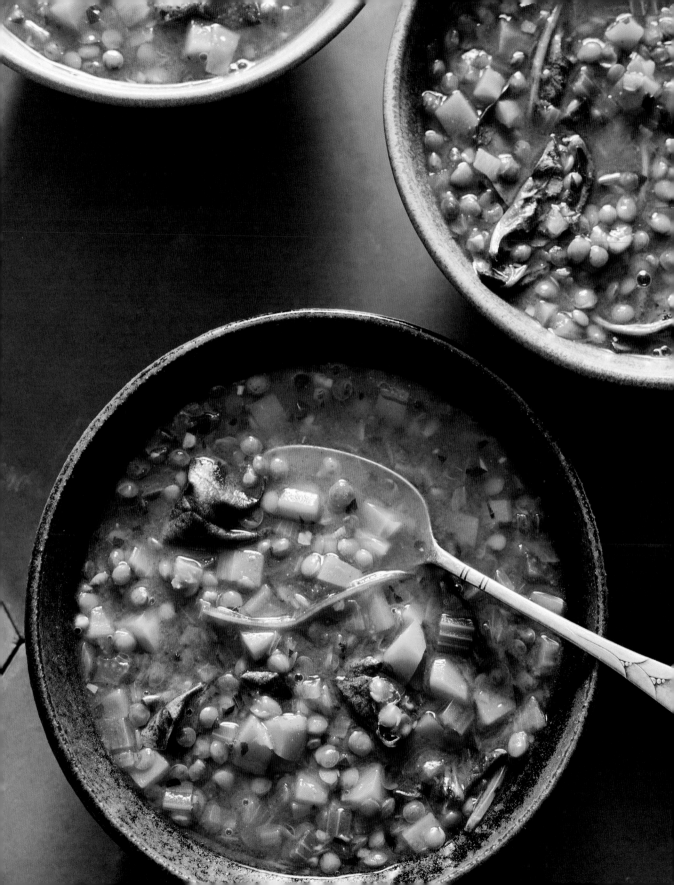

Lentil Soup

MAKES 2 TO 3 SERVINGS | | CHEF LESLIE

Break your fast with this hearty soup during your nurture phase. Lentils are one of my favorite progesterone-building foods, and I use them often, even sprinkling them over my salads, so an entire lentil soup is a progesterone dream. The cinnamon provides a gentler blood-sugar spike while the garlic supports a healthy immune system and is a great prebiotic to feed your gut microbiome.

3 tablespoons extra-virgin olive oil, plus more for serving
1 medium yellow onion, finely chopped
4 large celery stalks, chopped
2 large peeled carrots, chopped
4 garlic cloves, minced
1 teaspoon ground coriander
1 teaspoon ground cumin
¼ teaspoon ground allspice
¼ teaspoon ground cinnamon
8 cups Vegetable Broth (page 270)
1 cup green or yellow lentils, rinsed
1 cup fresh baby spinach
¼ cup chopped parsley, plus more for serving
Kosher salt and freshly ground black pepper

Heat the olive oil in a large pot over medium-high heat. Add the onion, celery, carrots, and garlic and sauté until the vegetables are soft and browned, 6 to 10 minutes.

Add the coriander, cumin, allspice, and cinnamon and mix well. Add the vegetable broth and lentils and bring to a boil.

Decrease the heat to low, cover, and let simmer, stirring occasionally, until the lentils are tender, 20 to 25 minutes.

Add the spinach and parsley and stir until they are wilted. Taste and season with salt and pepper as desired.

Spoon the soup into bowls, garnish with a drizzle of olive oil, and top with additional parsley. Serve warm.

Split Pea Soup with Chickpea Crunchies

MAKES 4 TO 6 SERVINGS | | CHEF LESLIE

Whenever you see any kind of legumes in a recipe, think progesterone building. I love how this recipe offers two different types of legumes along with lots of prebiotic-filled veggies and spices. A fabulous break-fast meal!

SOUP

3 tablespoons extra-virgin olive oil, plus more for serving
1 medium yellow onion, diced
4 garlic cloves, minced
4 large celery stalks, chopped
4 carrots, peeled and chopped
1 pinch kosher salt
1 pound dry split peas
6 cups Vegetable Broth (page 270)
½ tablespoon smoked paprika
½ teaspoon dried oregano
½ teaspoon dried thyme
Kosher salt and freshly ground black pepper
¼ cup chopped fresh parsley, divided

CHICKPEA CRUNCHIES

One 15½-ounce can chickpeas, drained and rinsed
3 tablespoons extra-virgin olive oil
¼ teaspoon kosher salt

TO MAKE THE SOUP Heat the olive oil in a large pot over medium-high heat. Add the onion, garlic, celery, carrots, and salt and sauté until the veggies are soft, 6 to 10 minutes.

Add the split peas, vegetable broth, paprika, oregano, and thyme to the pot. Increase the heat to high and bring to a boil. Decrease the heat to low and let simmer for 45 minutes, stirring occasionally. The split peas will break down and the soup will become thick.

Season with salt and pepper and stir in 2 tablespoons of the parsley.

TO MAKE THE CHICKPEA CRUNCHIES Meanwhile, preheat the oven to 425°F. Line a baking sheet with parchment paper. Spread the rinsed chickpeas on a clean kitchen towel and pat them dry.

Transfer the chickpeas to the baking sheet and drizzle with olive oil and salt. Shake the pan to evenly coat the chickpeas with oil.

Place the chickpeas in the oven and roast for 20 to 30 minutes or until they turn golden brown and crisp.

Remove and let cool. Store in a container lined with a paper towel to absorb extra oil until used.

TO ASSEMBLE THE SOUP Spoon the soup into bowls, garnish with a drizzle of olive oil, and top with the remaining parsley and pepper and chickpeas. Serve warm.

Portuguese Pork, Kale, and Potato Stew

MAKES 4 HEARTY SERVINGS OR 6 SMALL SERVINGS | CHEF JEFF

This recipe has a phenomenal combination of the Key 24 nutrients needed for hormonal production. It hits all Three Food Rules of eating like a girl and is delicious and warming on a cold night.

2 tablespoons extra-virgin olive oil

1 medium white, yellow, or red onion, cut into medium dice

1 medium-large leek, white and pale green parts only, halved lengthwise and thinly sliced

1 link Portuguese chouriço, linguiça, or any smoked sausage (about 6 ounces), sliced crosswise into rounds

3 garlic cloves, minced

½ teaspoon red pepper flakes, or to taste

1 dried bay leaf

1 teaspoon kosher salt

1 teaspoon freshly ground pepper

2 tablespoons white miso

12 ounces yellow potatoes, such as Yukon golds, peeled and cut into ½-inch chunks

½ cup white wine

3 cups Chicken Bone Broth (page 268) or water

4 ounces collard greens, center ribs removed, leaves chopped into small pieces

4 ounces curly green kale, center ribs removed, leaves chopped into small pieces

2 tablespoons apple cider vinegar

½ bunch chives, minced

Heat the olive oil in a medium Dutch oven or saucepan over medium heat. Add the onions, leeks, chouriço, garlic, red pepper flakes, bay leaf, salt, and black pepper. Cook until the vegetables are soft and translucent but not browned and the chouriço is cooked through, about 6 minutes. (If the vegetables are cooking too quickly and browning, reduce the heat to medium-low.)

Add the miso and potatoes and stir to combine. Add the white wine, increase the heat to medium-high, and boil until the wine has reduced by half, about 2 minutes. Add the bone broth and bring to a simmer, then reduce the heat to medium-low and simmer, stirring occasionally, until the potatoes are tender, about 12 minutes.

Add the collards and kale and continue simmering until the greens are wilted and tender, 3 to 5 more minutes.

Right before serving, whisk in the apple cider vinegar and the chives. Taste and season.

Keep in an airtight container in the fridge for up to 7 days or freeze for up to 1 month.

Gazpacho

MAKES 4 TO 6 SERVINGS | CHEF LESLIE

When you're breaking a longer fast, something cool and refreshing can be incredibly satisfying. This break-fast meal is perfect if you're trying to repair your gut microbiome. It pairs nicely with a grilled chicken breast, giving you 30 grams of protein for building muscle as you open up your eating window.

3 pounds Roma tomatoes, halved
1 large cucumber, peeled and seeded, and diced
1 red bell pepper, seeded and roughly chopped
½ large red onion, quartered
2 garlic cloves, peeled
½ cup fresh basil
¼ cup extra-virgin olive oil
2 tablespoons sherry vinegar
2 teaspoons kosher salt
½ teaspoon ground cumin
1 pinch freshly ground black pepper

In two batches, puree the tomatoes, cucumber, bell pepper, onion, and garlic in a blender on high speed until chunky or smooth, depending on your preference.

Add the basil, olive oil, sherry vinegar, salt, cumin, and black pepper to one batch and then blend again. Combine in an airtight container and refrigerate for at least 2 hours or up to overnight.

Serve chilled.

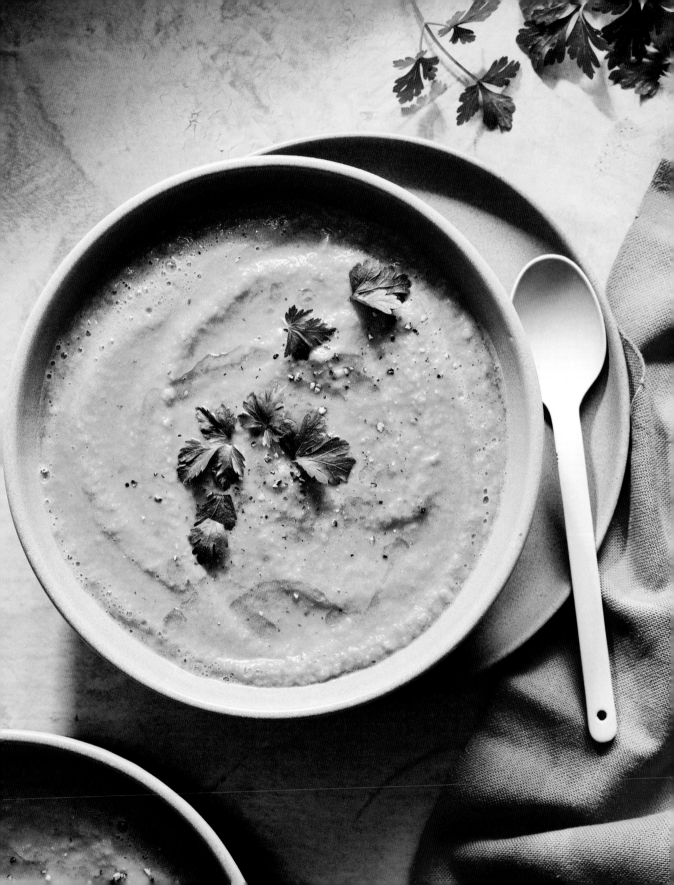

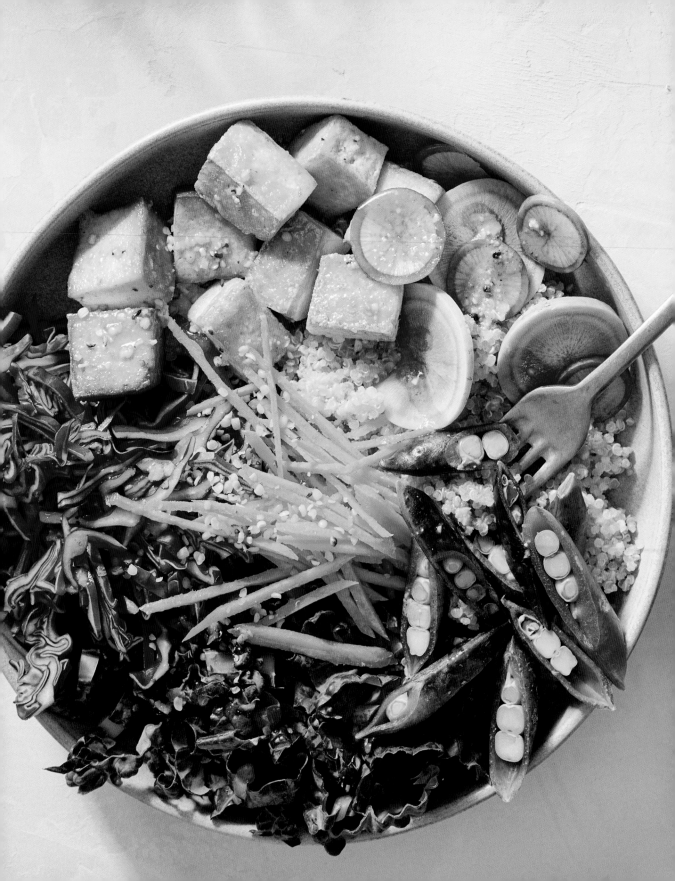

Buddha Bowl

MAKES 1 SERVING | | CHEF LESLIE

This unique recipe may work for both hormone feasting and ketobiotic days, making it a break-fast meal that would work at any time. If you want a lower blood-sugar spike (which is good for ketobiotic days), use less agave and maple syrup and add a little extra olive oil. Tofu is a fabulous phytoestrogen, so feel free to add more on the days your body needs an extra dose of estrogen.

DRESSING

3 tablespoons extra-virgin olive oil

¼ cup unseasoned rice wine vinegar

1½ tablespoons white miso paste

1½ tablespoons tamari

½ tablespoon agave or maple syrup

½ teaspoon grated fresh ginger

1 small garlic clove, minced and mashed to a paste

Kosher salt and freshly ground black pepper

BOWL

½ teaspoon olive oil

½ cup dry quinoa, rinsed

1 cup chopped Lacinato kale, center ribs removed

1 cup diced store-bought baked tofu

¼ broccoli sprouts

¼ cup shredded carrot

¼ cup sliced sugar snap peas

¼ cup shredded purple cabbage

1 tablespoon hemp seeds

1 watermelon radish, sliced (optional)

TO MAKE THE DRESSING Whisk together the olive oil, rice vinegar, miso, tamari, agave syrup, ginger, and garlic in a small bowl. Taste and season with salt and pepper.

TO MAKE THE QUINOA Bring ½ cup of water to a boil in a small pot over high heat. Add the quinoa, cover, and decrease the heat to medium-low. Let it simmer for 10 to 15 minutes, or until the quinoa has absorbed all the water. Remove from the heat and let sit for 5 minutes with the lid on. Fluff with a fork and set aside.

TO ASSEMBLE THE BOWL Drizzle the kale with olive oil and massage with your hands until the kale is softened. In a bowl, arrange separate sections of quinoa, kale, baked tofu, broccoli sprouts, carrots, sugar snap peas, and purple cabbage. Drizzle with the dressing, sprinkle with hemp seeds, garnish with radish, and enjoy.

Fettuccine "Alfredo"

MAKES 4 SERVINGS | | CHEF LESLIE

This creamy, comforting break-fast meal is ideal for your manifestation and nurture phases, with lots of spices like garlic and onion powder combined with hemp seeds that make it a healing meal to use when you want to give your microbiome some extra love. Tofu is a phenomenal phytoestrogen that supports your protective estrogen levels. When buying any tofu product, always make sure it's organic.

HEMP "PARMESAN"

½ cup hemp seeds

½ cup raw cashews

¼ cup nutritional yeast

¼ teaspoon kosher salt

¼ teaspoon dried oregano

¼ teaspoon garlic powder

¼ teaspoon onion powder

"ALFREDO" SAUCE

One 16-ounce package silken tofu

½ cup raw cashews

¼ cup nutritional yeast

¼ cup Vegetable Broth (page 270)

2 tablespoons extra-virgin olive oil

1 tablespoon lemon juice

1 teaspoon white miso paste

1 teaspoon garlic powder

1 teaspoon onion powder

1 teaspoon kosher salt

¼ teaspoon freshly ground white pepper

1 pound gluten-free fettuccine

TO MAKE THE HEMP "PARMESAN" Pulse the hemp seeds, cashews, nutritional yeast, salt, oregano, garlic powder, and onion powder in a food processor until the mixture reaches the consistency of grated Parmesan cheese. Set aside.

TO MAKE THE "ALFREDO" SAUCE Place the tofu, cashews, nutritional yeast, vegetable broth, olive oil, lemon juice, miso paste, garlic powder, onion powder, salt, and white pepper in a blender and blend on high speed until smooth and pureed. Set aside.

TO ASSEMBLE THE PASTA Bring a large pot of water over medium-high heat to a boil and cook the fettuccine according to the package instructions.

When the fettuccine is al dente, drain it in a colander and return it to the pot. Remove from the heat. Pour the "Alfredo" sauce over the fettuccine and mix thoroughly until the pasta is evenly coated.

Serve topped with the hemp "Parmesan."

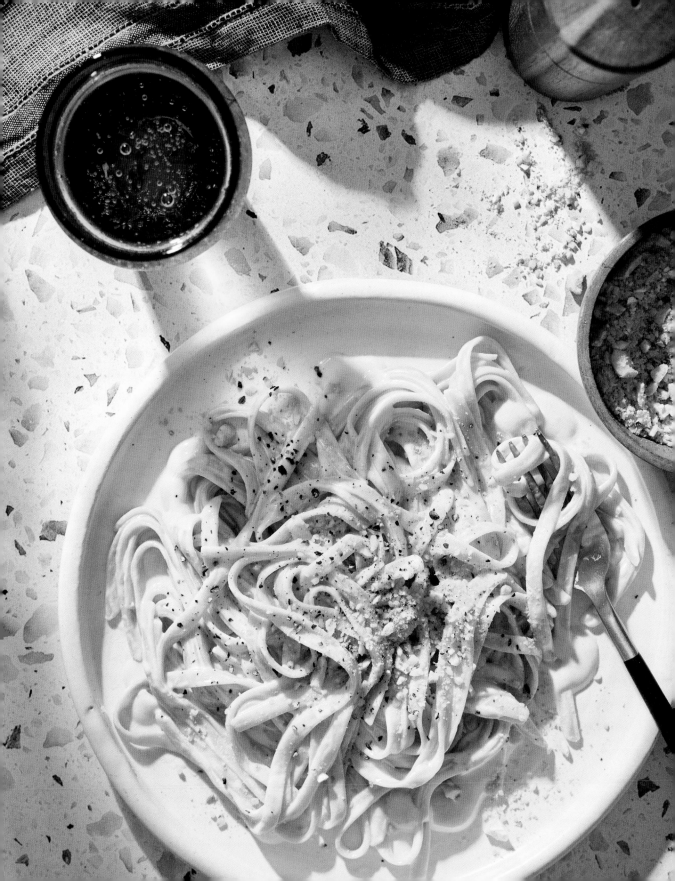

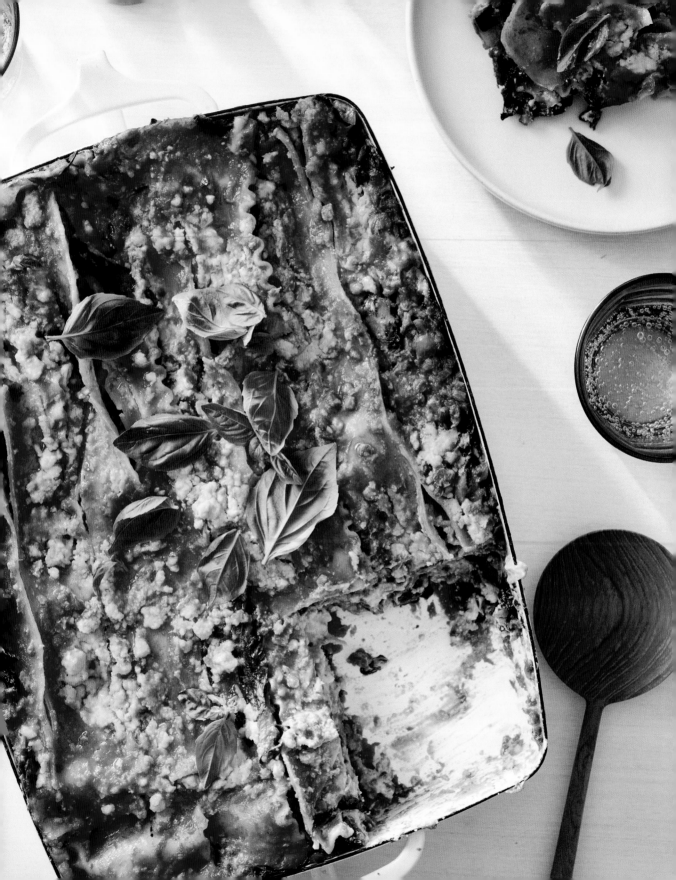

Lasagna

MAKES 6 TO 8 SERVINGS | CHEF LESLIE

This is one of my favorite recipes in this book. It makes a convenient break-fast meal because you need only a small serving to satisfy your taste buds and appease your hunger. You can also prep it ahead of time; make it on a Sunday afternoon and you'll have your break-fast meals ready to go for the week. The prebiotic ingredients in this recipe make it a suitable meal for your manifestation phase while the lentils support progesterone production in your nurture phase. A splash of organic wine in the sauce adds flavor, but it can be left out if you're avoiding alcohol.

TOMATO SAUCE

1 tablespoon extra-virgin olive oil

3 garlic cloves, minced

One 28-ounce can crushed tomatoes

1 teaspoon dried oregano

6 to 8 fresh basil leaves, chopped

BOLOGNESE SAUCE

3 tablespoons extra-virgin olive oil

1 cup diced medium yellow onion

1 large carrot, peeled and finely chopped

1 large celery stalk, finely chopped

4 to 8 garlic cloves, minced

1 teaspoon dried oregano

1 teaspoon kosher salt

1 pinch red pepper flakes (optional)

One 28-ounce can crushed tomatoes

½ cup red wine

½ cup chopped walnuts

1 cup canned or cooked lentils

VEGAN RICOTTA

¾ cup raw cashews

½ cup nutritional yeast

½ teaspoon kosher salt

One 14-ounce package firm tofu, drained and patted dry

1 tablespoon chopped fresh parsley

VEGAN BÉCHAMEL SAUCE

1 cup raw cashews

¼ cup nutritional yeast

4 teaspoons tapioca starch

1 teaspoon white miso paste

½ teaspoon garlic powder

½ teaspoon kosher salt

SPINACH AND MUSHROOMS

3 tablespoons extra-virgin olive oil

1 pound cremini or baby bella mushrooms, sliced

Kosher salt

1 pound fresh baby spinach

Two 10-ounce boxes gluten-free no-boil lasagna sheets, or 2 eggplants, cut lengthwise into thin strips and grilled

CONTINUED ▶

Lasagna
CONTINUED

TO MAKE THE TOMATO SAUCE Heat the olive oil and garlic in a medium pot over medium heat. As soon as the garlic starts to sizzle, add the crushed tomatoes and oregano and stir to combine. Decrease the heat to low and let simmer, stirring occasionally, for 15 minutes. Just before you are going to use it, stir in the fresh basil leaves. Set aside.

TO MAKE THE BOLOGNESE SAUCE Heat the olive oil in a large pot over medium heat. Add the onion, carrot, celery, and garlic and sauté until the veggies turn soft, about 10 minutes.

Add the oregano, salt, and red pepper flakes (if using) and mix well. Cook for 2 minutes. Add the tomatoes, wine, and walnuts and stir to combine. Cook until the sauce starts to simmer, and then decrease the heat to low, cover, and let simmer for 10 minutes. Stir in the lentils and cook for another 5 minutes. Set aside.

TO MAKE THE VEGAN RICOTTA Combine the cashews, ½ cup of water, nutritional yeast, and salt in a blender and blend on high speed until smooth and pureed.

In a large bowl, crumble the tofu with a fork or your hands. Pour in the cashew mixture and parsley and stir well. Set aside.

TO MAKE THE VEGAN BÉCHAMEL SAUCE Combine the cashews, 2 cups of water, nutritional yeast, tapioca starch, miso paste, garlic powder, and salt in a blender and blend on high speed until smooth and pureed.

Pour the sauce into a small saucepan over medium heat and bring to a boil. Whisk constantly until the sauce boils and thickens, about 5 minutes. Remove from the heat and set aside.

TO MAKE THE SPINACH AND MUSHROOMS Heat the olive oil in a medium pan over high heat.

Add the mushrooms and sprinkle with ½ teaspoon of salt. Cook until the mushrooms are tender, 7 or 8 minutes. Gradually add the spinach to the mushrooms in the pan, stirring and adding more spinach as it cooks down. Cook until all the spinach is wilted, then season with more salt. Set aside.

TO ASSEMBLE THE LASAGNA Preheat the oven to 375°F.

Ladle 1½ cups of the tomato sauce into a deep 9 x 13-inch baking dish until it evenly covers the bottom. Place a layer of lasagna noodles over the tomato sauce, about 4 sheets, making sure they don't overlap much.

Top with one-third of the Bolognese sauce, one-third of the spinach-mushroom mixture, one-fourth of the vegan ricotta, and one-third of the vegan béchamel sauce. Repeat the layering 2 more times, ending with the noodles. Top with the remaining tomato sauce. Dollop the final fourth of the vegan ricotta over the lasagna.

Cover with aluminum foil and bake for 45 minutes.

Remove the foil and bake for another 10 minutes. Let stand for 10 to 15 minutes before serving.

Protein Banana Donut Holes

MAKES 16 DONUT HOLES | **CHEF LESLIE**

If you crave carbohydrates when you open up your eating window, these delicious treats will satisfy your sweet tooth while keeping your blood sugar stable. If you don't consume dairy, use an organic nut milk because it contains more protein and triggers less of a blood-sugar spike than oat milk. Adding extra protein powder and MCT oil also helps stabilize your blood sugar as you open up your eating window.

DONUT HOLES

1 banana, mashed
¼ cup unsweetened nondairy milk
¼ cup almond butter
1 tablespoon melted coconut oil or MCT oil
1 teaspoon vanilla extract
½ cup all-purpose gluten-free flour
½ cup vegan vanilla protein powder
1 teaspoon baking powder
½ teaspoon baking soda
½ teaspoon ground cinnamon
½ teaspoon kosher salt
Spray coconut oil

MELTED DARK CHOCOLATE DRIZZLE

1 tablespoon coconut oil
½ cup nondairy chocolate chips

TO MAKE THE DONUT HOLES Preheat an air fryer or the oven to 350°F.

Mix together the mashed banana, nondairy milk, almond butter, melted coconut oil, and vanilla extract in a medium bowl.

Combine the flour, protein powder, baking powder, baking soda, cinnamon, and salt in another medium bowl.

Pour the wet ingredients into the dry ingredients and mix until thoroughly combined. Let sit for 5 minutes.

Using your hands, on a lightly floured surface, form the dough into sixteen 1-inch balls. Spray the balls with spray coconut oil.

If you're using an air fryer, place the balls into the basket and air-fry for 10 minutes, or until golden.

If you're using an oven, place the balls on a parchment paper–lined baking sheet and bake for 10 to 15 minutes, or until golden.

TO MAKE THE CHOCOLATE DRIZZLE Combine the chocolate chips and coconut oil in a glass bowl and microwave them in 15-second increments, stirring each time, until the chips have dissolved completely and the mixture is smooth.

Serve the donut holes as is or drizzle them with the melted dark chocolate mixture, if desired.

Leftover donut holes can be stored in an airtight container at room temperature for up to 4 or 5 days.

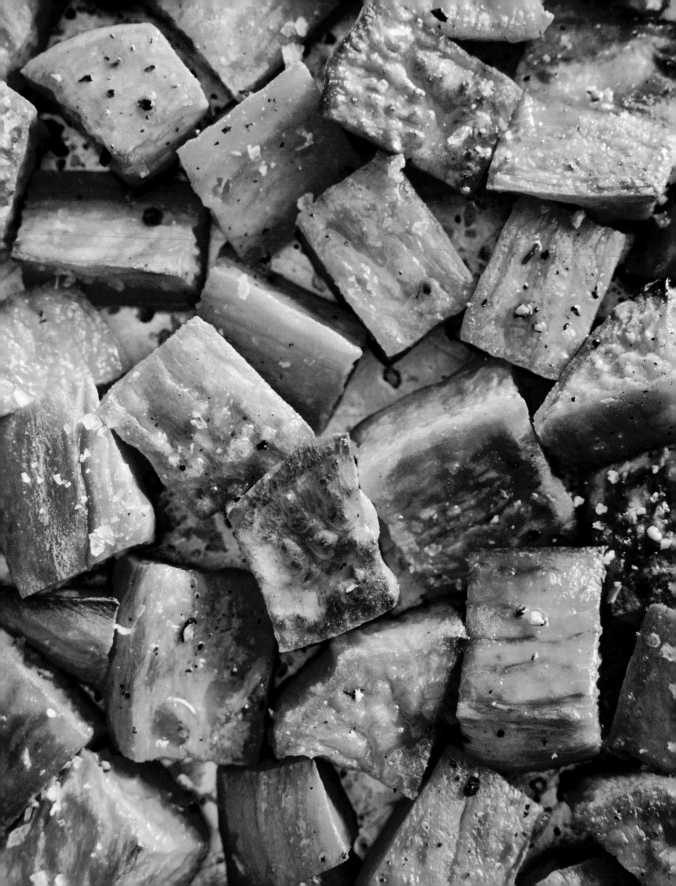

13

Hormone Feasting

YOUR FEMININE BODY has times when it needs carbohydrates. Low-carb diets failed us when they forgot to mention how important it is for women to cycle in and out of low-carb living. Hormone feasting foods bring the right carbohydrates back into your diet, giving you the fuel needed to make one of your major sex hormones: progesterone. This style of eating will benefit you most during your manifestation and nurture phases, when progesterone makes her appearance. For my perimenopausal friends, these recipes are fabulous on days when you're spotting, anxiety levels are high, or you're struggling to sleep.

What I love about many of the recipes in this section is the variety of ingredients my chefs chose. From a diverse array of fruits, vegetables, and starches to a wonderful selection of spices, these meals hit all Three Food Rules of eating like a girl. Not only will your taste buds scream *Yes!* with these recipes, but your hormones and microbiome will too!

Red, White, and Green Salad

MAKES 4 SERVINGS AS A SIDE DISH | | CHEF LESLIE

Legumes of all kinds are incredibly supportive of progesterone production in our bodies, so this is a tasty meal for your nurture phase. Avoid using artichoke hearts in canola oil; always opt for olive oil– or water-packed artichokes.

2 cups green beans, trimmed and halved

Kosher salt and freshly ground black pepper

One 15-ounce can cannellini beans, drained and rinsed

1 cup quartered artichoke hearts (jarred in olive oil or canned in water)

¼ cup sun-dried tomatoes packed in olive oil, sliced

4 tablespoons extra-virgin olive oil

2 tablespoons red wine vinegar

1 tablespoon chopped fresh parsley

6 or more fresh basil leaves, sliced

Bring a medium pot of water to a boil over medium-high heat and then add 1 teaspoon salt. Add the green beans and boil for 3 minutes. Drain the beans in a colander and immediately rinse them with cold water to stop their cooking.

In a medium bowl, combine the cannellini beans, artichoke hearts, sun-dried tomatoes, olive oil, red wine vinegar, parsley, basil, and green beans. Toss to combine. Taste and season with salt and pepper.

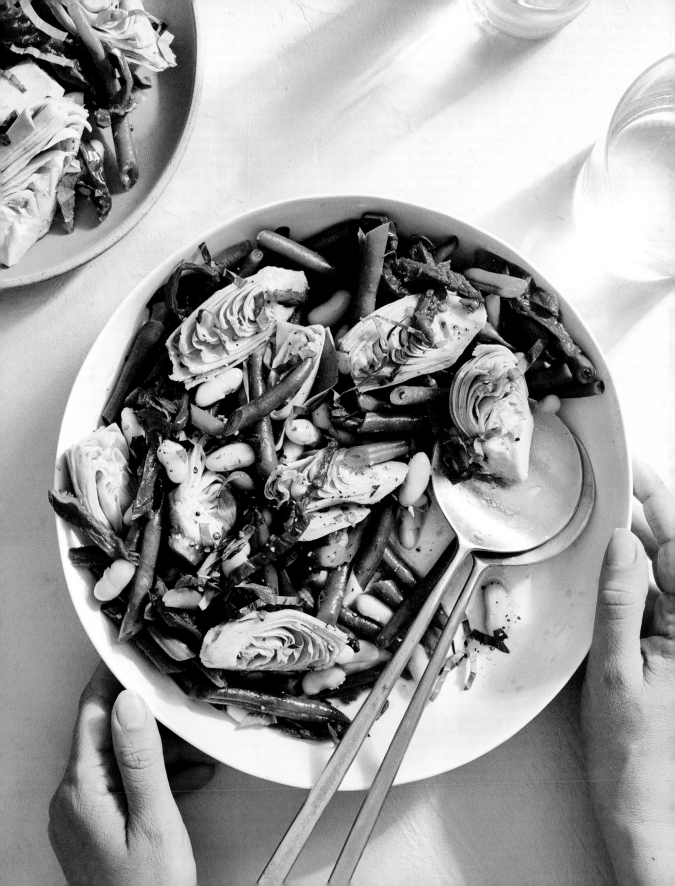

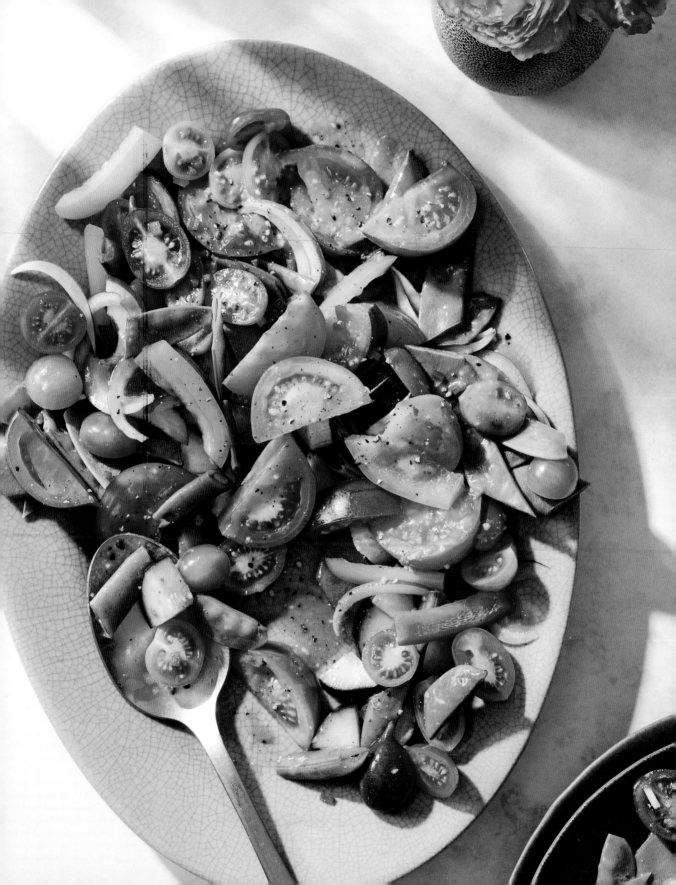

Height-of-Summer Veggie Salad

MAKES 4 TO 6 SERVINGS | | CHEF JEFF

I absolutely love the diversity of textures in this recipe, with lots of crunch for those of you who find that crunchy foods satisfy your hunger. The second rule of eating like a girl is Eat to Metabolize Hormones, making this combination of vegetables a perfect meal during your manifestation phase. If you can't find flat or romano beans, you can increase the amount of peas.

1 small red onion, cut into medium julienne

1 medium heirloom or beefsteak tomato, cored and cut into wedges

1 pint heirloom cherry, grape, Sungold, or similar small tomatoes, cut in half

1 medium orange or red bell pepper, seeded and cut into bite-size pieces

1 medium kirby cucumber, quartered lengthwise and thickly sliced crosswise into bite-size pieces

3 ounces romano or flat beans, trimmed and cut into bite-size pieces (1 scant cup)

3 ounces snow peas, trimmed and cut into bite-size pieces (1 scant cup)

3 ounces sugar snap peas, trimmed and cut into bite-size pieces (1 scant cup)

1 small Fresno or jalapeño pepper, cored, seeded, and minced (optional)

1 tablespoon coconut sugar

1 teaspoon kosher salt

2 garlic cloves, peeled

¼ cup Spain's Favorite Sherry Vinaigrette (page 287)

Flake sea salt, such as Maldon

Combine the onion, both tomatoes, bell pepper, cucumber, romano beans, snow and sugar snap peas, and Fresno or jalapeño pepper (if using) in a large bowl and mix well. Add the coconut sugar and salt, mix well, and let sit for 10 minutes to marinate.

Grate the garlic with a microplane or the small holes of a box grater, add it to the veggies, and toss to combine.

Drizzle with the vinaigrette and toss well. Taste and season the salad with more salt.

Serve on individual plates and top with the flake salt.

All the Greens Bowl

MAKES 4 SERVINGS | | CHEF LESLIE

This terrific recipe helps you detox hormones at the end of your manifestation phase (Days 13, 14, and 15). It's also excellent for menopausal women when feeling bloated or gaining belly weight; its variety of greens helps detox hormones to alleviate those symptoms. Also use this recipe during your nurture phase because quinoa and sweet potatoes support healthy progesterone production.

CHIMICHURRI DRESSING

1 cup extra-virgin olive oil

⅓ cup chopped fresh basil

¼ cup chopped fresh parsley

¼ cup chopped fresh chives

2 tablespoons chopped fresh mint

2 tablespoons chopped fresh dill

1 teaspoon red pepper flakes

Zest of 1 lemon

Kosher salt and freshly ground black pepper

BOWL

1 cup dry quinoa, rinsed

1½ pounds sweet potatoes, cut into
   ¾-inch cubes

2 tablespoons extra-virgin olive oil, divided

1 medium head Romanesco or regular cauliflower, cut into 2 x 1-inch florets

2 cups packed fresh spinach

1 bunch Lacinato kale, center ribs removed,
   coarsely chopped

1 medium avocado, cut into quarters and
   sliced

2 tablespoons hemp seeds

2 tablespoons pumpkin seeds

1 cup broccoli microgreens

TO MAKE THE CHIMICHURRI DRESSING Combine the olive oil, basil, parsley, chives, mint, dill, red pepper flakes, and lemon zest in a bowl. Season with salt and pepper. Whisk.

TO MAKE THE QUINOA Bring 2 cups of water to a boil in a small pot over high heat. Add the quinoa, cover, and decrease the heat to low. Let it simmer for 15 minutes, or until the quinoa has absorbed all the water. Remove from the heat and let sit for 5 minutes with the lid on. Fluff with a fork and set aside.

TO ASSEMBLE THE BOWL Preheat the oven to 375°F.

On a baking sheet, toss the sweet potatoes in 1 tablespoon of the olive oil. On a second baking sheet, toss the cauliflower florets with the remaining 1 tablespoon of olive oil. Roast the vegetables until they're lightly browned and tender, about 30 minutes, switching pans between the oven racks halfway through.

Combine the spinach and kale in a large bowl.

To serve, arrange the quinoa, sweet potatoes, cauliflower, spinach and kale, and avocado in each bowl. Drizzle with the dressing and sprinkle with seeds and broccoli microgreens.

Black Bean Soup

MAKES 2 SERVINGS | CHEF LESLIE

This warm, comforting soup is a great recipe for breaking your fast in either your manifestation or nurture phases. Black beans help with progesterone production. Garlic superbly supports the immune system, and hemp seeds are a prebiotic that feeds your gut microbiome. Even celery is a terrific alkalizing food that also supports a gentle detox.

SOUP

4 tablespoons extra-virgin olive oil

1 yellow onion, chopped

1 large carrot, diced

1 large celery stalk, diced

6 garlic cloves, chopped

1 jalapeño, minced (optional)

Two 15½-ounce cans black beans, with their liquid

2 cups Vegetable Broth (page 270)

1 tablespoon ground cumin

1 tablespoon smoked paprika

1 teaspoon dried oregano

1 teaspoon kosher salt

OPTIONAL TOPPINGS

Chopped fresh cilantro

Hemp seeds

Diced raw onion

Sliced or diced avocado

TO MAKE THE SOUP Heat the olive oil in a large pot over medium-high heat. Add the onion, carrot, celery, garlic, and jalapeño (if using), and sauté until the vegetables turn soft on the edges, 6 to 10 minutes.

Add the black beans and liquid, vegetable broth, cumin, smoked paprika, oregano, and salt. Mix well and increase the heat to medium-high to bring to a boil. Then decrease the heat to low and let simmer for about 10 minutes.

Transfer 1 cup of the soup to a blender and blend on high speed until smooth. Return the pureed soup to the pot and mix well. Alternatively, you can use an immersion blender or a potato masher to mash some of the beans.

TO ASSEMBLE THE SOUP Spoon the soup into bowls and serve with the optional toppings on the side.

Navy Bean Tuscan Kale Soup

MAKES 6 SERVINGS | CHEF LESLIE

Legumes of all kinds give the female body two key resources: They help with progesterone production, and they are rich in protein to promote muscle building. If you're looking for less of a blood-sugar spike, drizzle your favorite healthy oil on top of this soup. You can pair this with our recipe for Fasting Crackers (page 107) for a yummy meal that supports a healthy gut microbiome.

3 tablespoons extra-virgin olive oil
1 cup diced yellow onion
1 cup peeled, sliced carrots
1 cup sliced celery
6 garlic cloves, chopped
1 teaspoon dried oregano
1 teaspoon dried thyme
1 pinch to 1 teaspoon red pepper flakes (optional)
Three 15-ounce cans navy beans, drained and rinsed
6 cups Vegetable Broth (page 270)
3 cups chopped Lacinato kale, center ribs removed
Kosher salt and freshly ground black pepper
¼ cup pine nuts, toasted

Heat the olive oil in a large pot over medium-high heat. Add the onion, carrots, celery, and garlic and cook until the edges of the veggies are soft, about 10 minutes.

Add the oregano, thyme, and red pepper flakes (if using) and mix well. Cook for 1 minute.

Add the navy beans and vegetable broth and bring to a boil over high heat. Decrease the heat to low and let simmer until everything is soft, 15 to 20 minutes.

Transfer 2 cups of the soup to a blender and blend on high speed until smooth. Pour the pureed mixture back into the soup in the pot and mix well.

Add the kale and stir until it wilts, 2 to 3 minutes. Taste and season with salt and pepper.

Ladle the soup into bowls and sprinkle each serving with pine nuts. Serve warm.

Store in an airtight container in the fridge for up to 4 days or freeze for up to 1 month.

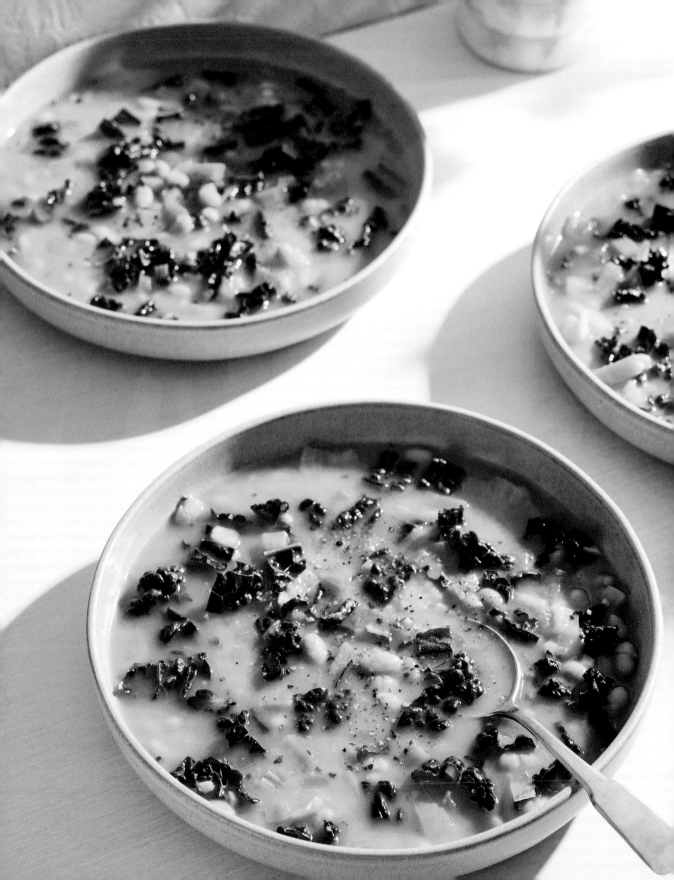

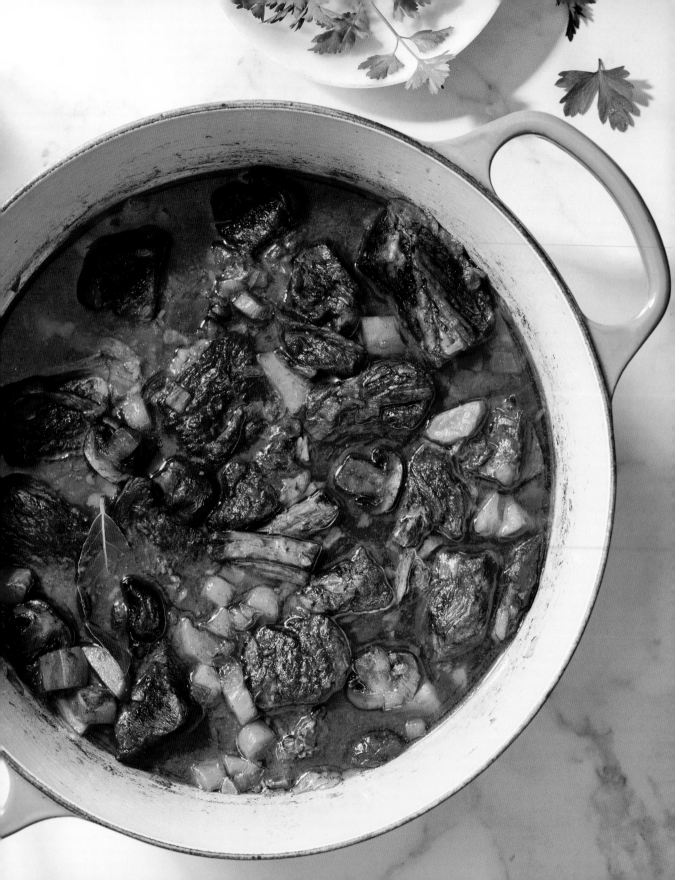

Beef Stew with Beer

MAKES 4 SERVINGS | CHEF JEFF

If you're seeking to build muscle, this is the stew for you—it is packed with protein. Chef Jeff has also ensured that all the sweeteners in this recipe are low-glycemic to avoid huge blood-sugar spikes.

2 pounds beef chuck roast, cut into 1-inch chunks
Kosher salt and freshly ground black pepper
4 tablespoons unsalted butter, cut into cubes
Extra-virgin olive oil
1 large white, yellow, or red onion, peeled, cut into medium chunks
2 tablespoons Keto Chili Sauce (page 284)
1 tablespoon coconut sugar
1 dried bay leaf
½ teaspoon ground allspice
1 cup gluten-free dark beer, such as a stout, porter, or Belgian-style dubbel
1 cup Beef Bone Broth (page 266) or water
Dijon or stone-ground mustard
2 large carrots, peeled and cut into ½-inch chunks
2 medium turnips, peeled and cut into ½-inch chunks
½ pound small cremini mushrooms, halved
½ bunch Italian parsley, coarsely chopped (about ⅓ cup, loosely packed)

Set aside a platter for holding the cooked beef. Season the beef pieces all over with salt and pepper and set aside.

Heat a large Dutch oven over medium-high heat. Combine the butter and 2 tablespoons of olive oil in the pot and add half of the beef without crowding the pot. Cook the beef without stirring until a deep brown crust forms on one side, about 5 minutes. Flip and cook on the other side for another 5 minutes, or until a deep brown crust forms. Transfer the beef to the platter. Repeat with the remaining beef and set aside.

Add more oil to the pot, if needed, then add the onion and a large pinch of salt. Cook, stirring and scraping up the browned bits from the bottom of the pot, until the onions soften and turn golden brown, about 6 minutes. Decrease the heat to medium. Add the keto chili sauce, coconut sugar, bay leaf, and allspice and continue cooking, stirring often, until well combined, about 2 minutes.

Add the reserved beef and its juices, beer, bone broth, 1 tablespoon of mustard, and 2 teaspoons salt, and stir to combine. Increase the heat to medium-high and bring the stew to a boil. Decrease the heat to low, cover, and let simmer, stirring occasionally, for about 1 hour.

Add the carrots, turnips, and mushrooms and let simmer for another hour until the liquid is reduced and the vegetables are tender.

Taste and season the stew with more salt, pepper, or mustard as desired.

Serve the stew in bowls, garnished with the chopped parsley.

Chana Masala

MAKES 4 SERVINGS | | CHEF JEFF

Not only does this recipe taste delicious, but it also looks beautiful. The diversity of spices makes this an incredible prebiotic meal to support great gut health. If you don't normally eat foods with this spice profile, remember that one of the most important principles of eating like a girl is to increase the diversity of the types of foods you eat. Try this recipe on your manifestation and nurture phase days. Serve this with greens and summer squash for even more color.

SPICE PASTE

¼ white or yellow onion, chopped

2 large garlic cloves, chopped

One 1-inch piece fresh ginger, peeled and chopped

1 jalapeño, seeds discarded, chopped

Juice of 1 lemon

CHANA MASALA

¼ cup ghee or unsalted butter or avocado oil

1 small white, yellow, or red onion, cut into medium chunks

1 tablespoon Keto Chili Sauce (page 284)

1 tablespoon dried fenugreek leaves (optional)

2 teaspoons garam masala

2 teaspoons mild curry powder

1½ teaspoons black mustard seeds

1½ teaspoons yellow mustard seeds

2 dried bay leaves

Kosher salt and freshly ground black pepper

Coconut sugar

One 28-ounce can diced tomatoes with their juices

Two 15-ounce cans chickpeas, rinsed and drained

½ bunch cilantro leaves, chopped

TO MAKE THE SPICE PASTE Combine the onion, garlic, ginger, jalapeño, and lemon juice in a mini food processor, and process until smooth. Set aside.

TO MAKE THE CHANA MASALA Melt the ghee in a medium saucepan or Dutch oven over medium heat. Once the ghee is melted and hot, add the onion and cook until it starts to turn golden brown, about 6 minutes. Add the spice paste, keto chili sauce, fenugreek, garam masala, curry powder, black and yellow mustard seeds, bay leaves, 2 teaspoons of salt, 1 teaspoon of black pepper, and 1 tablespoon of coconut sugar. Cook, stirring often, until the onions start to caramelize, 6 to 10 minutes. (Decrease the heat to medium-low if it browns too quickly.)

Add the diced tomatoes, the chickpeas, and ½ cup of water. Increase the heat to medium-high and bring to a boil. Then decrease the heat to medium-low and let simmer, partially covered, while stirring occasionally, until the sauce thickens, 15 to 20 minutes.

Stir in the cilantro. Taste and season with more salt, black pepper, and coconut sugar.

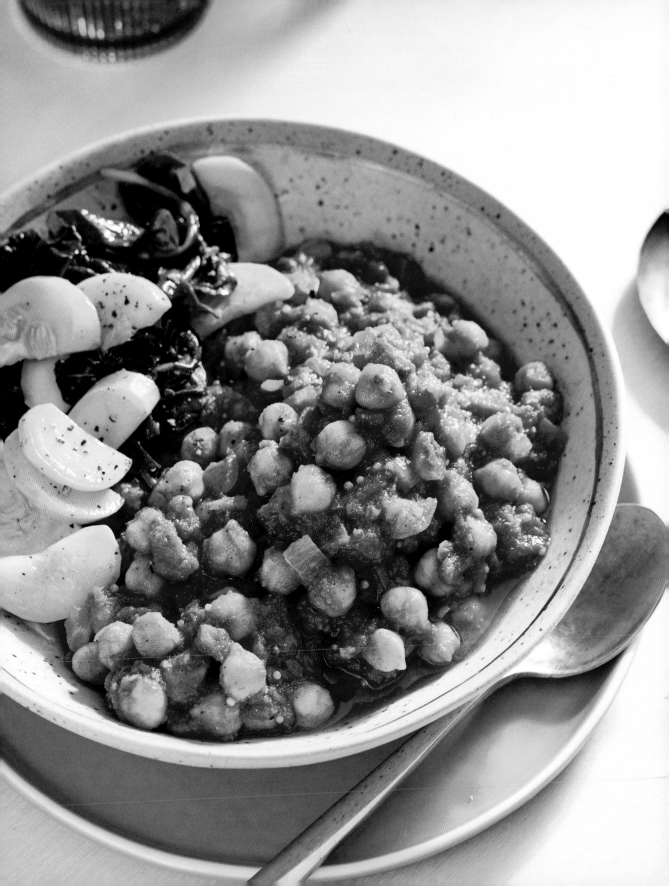

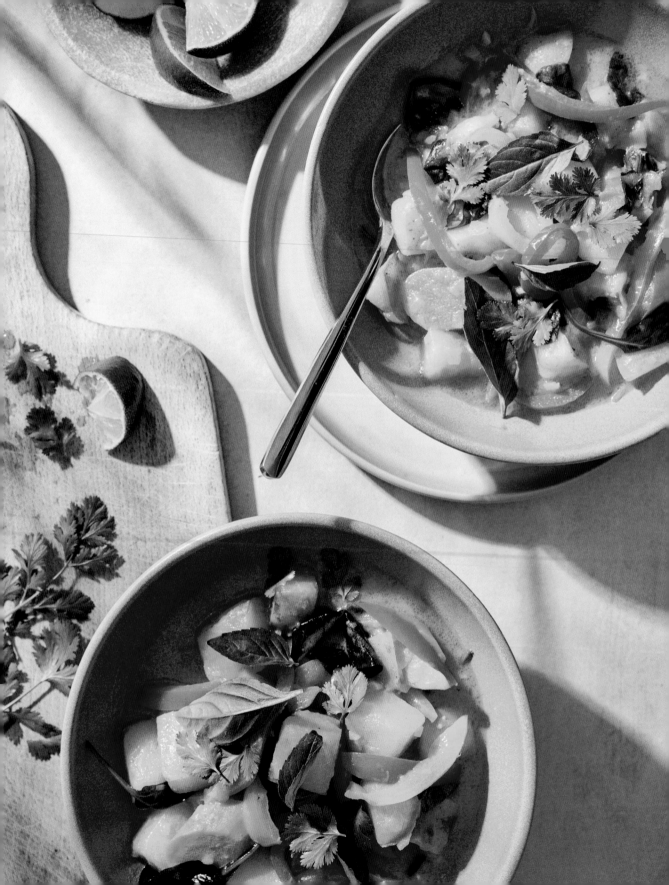

Red Thai Curry

MAKES 4 SERVINGS 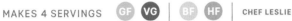 CHEF LESLIE

This is a beautiful gut microbiome–supporting meal. Between all the fibrous vegetables and a healthy dose of ginger, it is beneficial during both manifesting and nurture stages. Chef Leslie recommends serving it with rice, and I suggest using wild or forbidden rice, as they provide more stable blood-sugar responses.

1 tablespoon avocado oil

1 cup diced yellow onion

4 garlic cloves, chopped

One 2-inch piece fresh ginger, minced

4 Yukon gold potatoes, peeled and cut into 1-inch dice

2 large peeled carrots, cut into ½-inch slices on the diagonal

1 red bell pepper, seeded and julienned

1 yellow bell pepper, seeded and julienned

4 tablespoons Thai red curry paste

One and one-half 15-ounce cans full-fat coconut milk

1½ cups fresh spinach

¼ cup Thai basil leaves

¼ cup fresh cilantro leaves

1 lime, cut into 8 wedges

Heat the avocado oil in a large skillet over medium heat. Add the onion, garlic, and ginger and sauté until the onions begin to soften, 2 to 3 minutes.

Add the potatoes and ¼ cup of water and place a lid over the skillet. Let the veggies steam until the water has evaporated and the potatoes are just fork-tender, about 5 minutes. Add more water as needed.

Uncover, add the carrots and the red and yellow bell peppers, and sauté for 8 minutes until soft.

Stir in the Thai red curry paste. When it's thoroughly mixed in, add the coconut milk, stir, and decrease the heat to low. Simmer until the veggies are soft but still retain some firmness, about 5 minutes.

Remove from the heat and stir in the spinach.

Serve topped with fresh basil, cilantro, a squeeze of lime, and another wedge of lime for garnish.

Chickpea "Omelet"

MAKES 1 SERVING | CHEF LESLIE

I love how Chef Leslie uses chickpea flour in this omelet. Chickpeas supply a healthy dose of protein, so this could be a fantastic post-workout meal if you're doing a plant-based diet and trying to build more muscle. Note that while black salt has a lovely flavor, you can swap in kosher salt if you have trouble finding black salt. Chickpea flour can be a little bit sticky, so be sure to warm the olive oil in the pan before adding the batter and use a spatula to loosen.

¼ cup chickpea flour
2 tablespoons nutritional yeast
¼ teaspoon ground turmeric
¼ teaspoon baking powder
¼ teaspoon black salt or kosher salt
4 tablespoons extra-virgin olive oil, divided
1 sliced cremini or white button mushroom
½ cup chopped fresh spinach
¼ cup sliced leek, white parts only
1 garlic clove, minced

Combine the chickpea flour, nutritional yeast, turmeric, baking powder, and black salt in a large bowl and mix well. Add ⅓ cup of water and whisk until smooth. Set aside.

Heat 3 tablespoons of the olive oil in a large skillet over medium heat. Add the mushrooms, spinach, leeks, and garlic and sauté until they turn soft, about 5 minutes. Transfer this filling to a plate.

In the same skillet over medium heat, pour in the remaining 1 tablespoon of olive oil. Wait until the olive oil is warm and then pour in the chickpea batter. Tilt the skillet around until the mixture is evenly spread throughout the bottom of the pan. Cook until the center of the mixture becomes dry, about 5 minutes. Shake the skillet to loosen the omelet. If the omelet starts to stick to the sides, use a spatula to loosen.

Spoon the mushroom-spinach filling over half of the omelet, and carefully fold the other half over the filling. Serve warm.

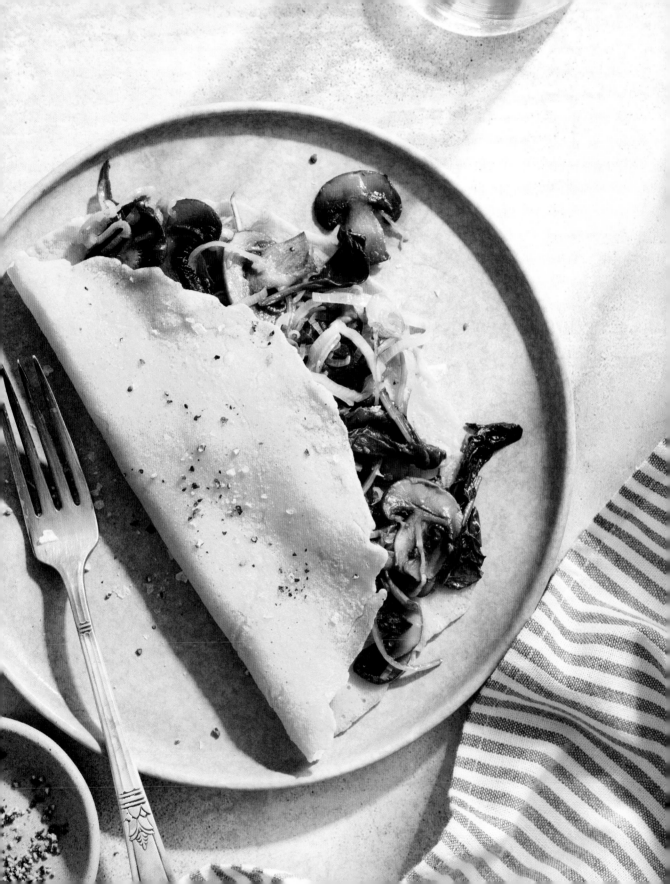

Tortilla Española

MAKES 4 SERVINGS | | CHEF JEFF

This is one of those recipes that gets better the more you make it. The eggs supply an incredible leucine punch for those of you looking to get more protein in your diet. And feel free to experiment with different types of potatoes in this recipe, since they all feed different microbes in your gut. So branch out and try varieties that you don't usually eat, and your microbes will be happy! The beauty of the Spanish tortilla is that it can be a perfect lunch or dinner with a side salad or on its own for breakfast or a snack.

1½ cups extra-virgin olive oil
1 large yellow or white onion, halved and cut into thin julienne or half-moons
3 russet potatoes (1½ pounds), peeled, halved lengthwise, and cut crosswise into thin slices
6 large eggs
2 teaspoons kosher salt

Heat the olive oil in a large skillet over medium heat. Add the onion and sauté, stirring occasionally, until it softens, about 4 minutes. Add the potatoes and continue to cook, stirring occasionally, until they become fork-tender but still hold their shape, about 10 minutes.

Place a large fine-mesh sieve over a bowl and carefully pour the potato-onion mixture into the sieve, capturing the oil in the bowl. Allow the potato-onion mixture to cool to room temperature, about 10 minutes, or refrigerate the mixture until ready to use.

Combine the eggs and salt in another large bowl and whisk well. Add the potato-onion mixture to the eggs and gently mix until the potatoes are well coated.

Heat a 10-inch nonstick skillet over medium heat. Get a round plate ready that is the same diameter as the top of the pan, as well as a serving platter.

Add 2 tablespoons of the reserved onion oil to the skillet.

Add the egg-potato mixture and begin shaking the skillet; the goal is to get the egg to cook without anything sticking to the bottom or sides of the skillet. Use a heatproof spatula to continually loosen the mixture around the edges and keep them from sticking.

Decrease the heat to medium-low as the tortilla cooks so it doesn't get overly brown. Continue to shake the skillet until the tortilla is bubbling and its edges have set, about 5 minutes.

Here's the fun part: Using oven mitts, remove the skillet from the heat and invert the round plate over the top of the skillet. With one hand on the plate and the other holding the skillet, flip the tortilla in one motion onto the plate. Return the skillet to medium-low heat and add 1 tablespoon of the reserved onion oil. Slide the tortilla back into the skillet to cook the other side. Continue to shake the skillet to keep the tortilla from sticking, until it is cooked all the way through in the middle, about 6 to 10 minutes.

Flip the tortilla one more time onto the serving platter and allow it to rest for at least 5 minutes before cutting into slices.

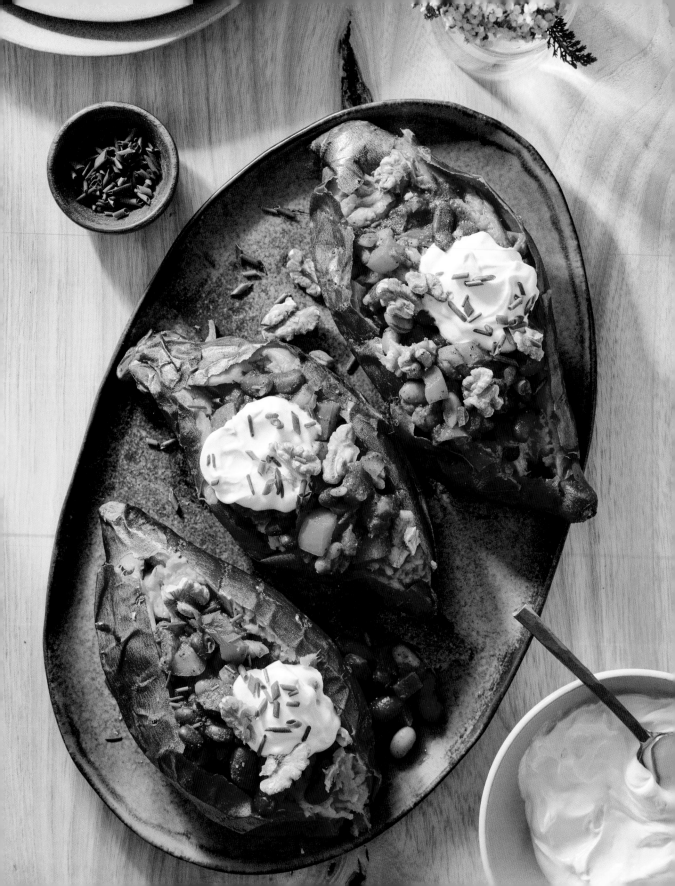

Chili-Loaded Sweet Potato

MAKES 6 SERVINGS (7½ CUPS OF CHILI)   CHEF LESLIE

Sweet potatoes and legumes are my favorite hormone feasting foods. This recipe could have been named Progesterone-Loaded Sweet Potato, as it has the perfect combination of foods to support your body's progesterone production. Enjoy this one in your nurture phase.

POTATOES

6 large sweet potatoes
1 tablespoon extra-virgin olive oil
Kosher salt

CHILI

3 tablespoons extra-virgin olive oil
Kosher salt
1 cup diced yellow onion
1 red bell pepper, seeded and diced
¼ cup chili powder
1 tablespoon cacao powder
1½ teaspoons ground cumin
1 teaspoon dried oregano
1 teaspoon garlic powder
One 28-ounce can diced tomatoes
One 15-ounce can black beans, drained
   and rinsed
One 15-ounce can kidney beans, drained
   and rinsed
One 15-ounce can pinto beans, drained
   and rinsed
2 cups Vegetable Broth (page 270)

OPTIONAL TOPPINGS

Vegan shredded cheese
Vegan sour cream
Chopped chives
Chopped walnuts

TO BAKE THE POTATOES Preheat the oven to 425°F. On a large baking sheet, rub the outside of the sweet potatoes with the olive oil and sprinkle with salt. Prick each potato with a fork and arrange them on the baking sheet. Transfer the baking sheet to the oven and bake until the potatoes are fork-tender, 40 to 45 minutes.

TO MAKE THE CHILI Heat the olive oil in a large pot over medium-high heat. Add the onion and bell pepper and sauté for about 6 minutes, until they turn soft. Stir in the chili powder, cacao powder, cumin, 1½ teaspoons salt, oregano, and garlic powder and cook, stirring occasionally, for 2 minutes. Add the tomatoes, the black, kidney, and pinto beans, and the vegetable broth and simmer, stirring occasionally, until the chili has thickened, about 20 minutes.

TO ASSEMBLE THE DISH To serve, make a lengthwise cut in the top of each potato and pinch the ends, pushing toward the middle to open the potatoes. Ladle the chili onto the potatoes to cover them (you will have chili left over). Serve with the toppings of your choice.

Store the chili in an airtight container in the fridge for up to a week or freeze for up to a month.

Lentil Mushroom Sweet Potato Shepherd's Pie

MAKES 6 SERVINGS | CHEF LESLIE

The world is quickly discovering the healing magic of mushrooms, so I was excited to see Chef Leslie combine mushrooms with sweet potatoes for the perfect hormone healing recipe. I like to use a biodynamic natural wine in this recipe to minimize any added toxins.

TOPPING

1 pound sweet potatoes

¼ to 1 cup cashew milk or another unsweetened nondairy milk

Kosher salt and freshly ground black pepper

FILLING

3 tablespoons extra-virgin olive oil

6 ounces portobello mushrooms, diced

2 carrots, peeled and diced

1 medium yellow onion, diced

4 garlic cloves, chopped

Kosher salt and freshly ground black pepper

2 tablespoons all-purpose gluten-free flour

2 cups Vegetable Broth (page 270)

1 cup full-bodied red wine, such as an organic Cabernet Sauvignon

3 tablespoons tamari

2 tablespoons tomato paste

1 tablespoon fresh oregano

2 cups chopped fresh kale

2 cups black or green cooked or canned lentils

1 cup fresh or frozen peas

TO MAKE THE TOPPING Preheat the oven to 400°F.

Prick the sweet potatoes and bake until they become fork-tender, 40 to 45 minutes.

Once cool enough to handle, peel and transfer them to a bowl. Using a potato masher, mash them with as much cashew milk as needed to achieve your desired consistency. Season with salt and pepper.

TO MAKE THE FILLING Heat the olive oil in a large pot over medium heat. Sauté the mushrooms, carrots, onion, garlic, and a pinch of salt until the vegetables become soft on the edges, 7 to 10 minutes.

Add the gluten-free flour and stir until the veggies are fully coated. Add the vegetable broth, red wine, tamari, tomato paste, and oregano and stir well. Simmer until the carrots become fork-tender, about 10 minutes.

Add the kale, lentils, and peas and stir well. Taste and season with pepper and salt as desired. Set aside.

TO ASSEMBLE THE DISH Preheat the oven to 400°F.

Transfer the filling to a 2-quart ceramic baking dish and distribute it evenly across the bottom of the dish. Using a spatula, spread the mashed sweet potatoes over the top of the filling. Bake until the shepherd's pie is heated through and bubbling at the edges, about 30 minutes. Serve immediately.

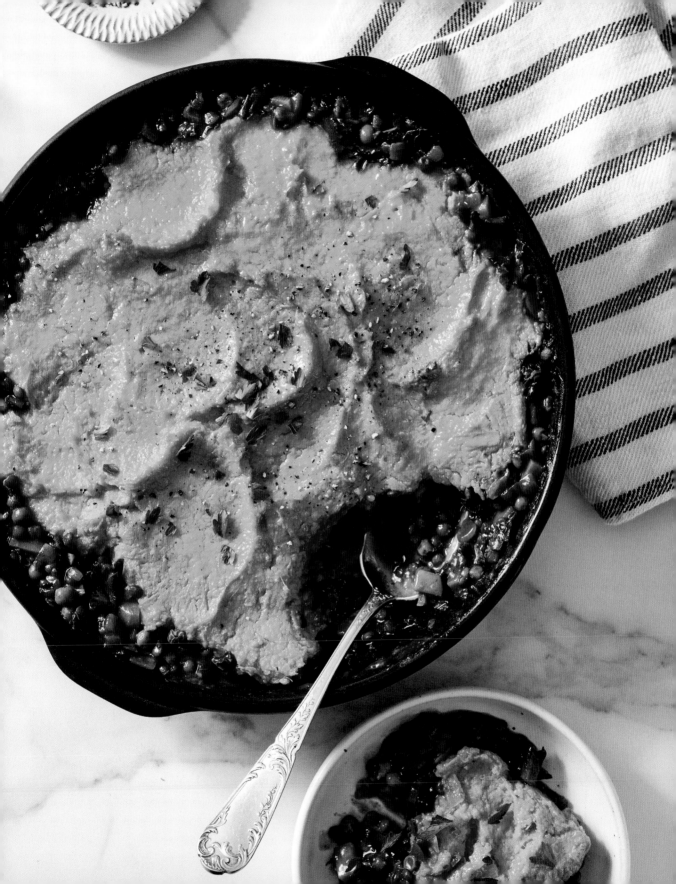

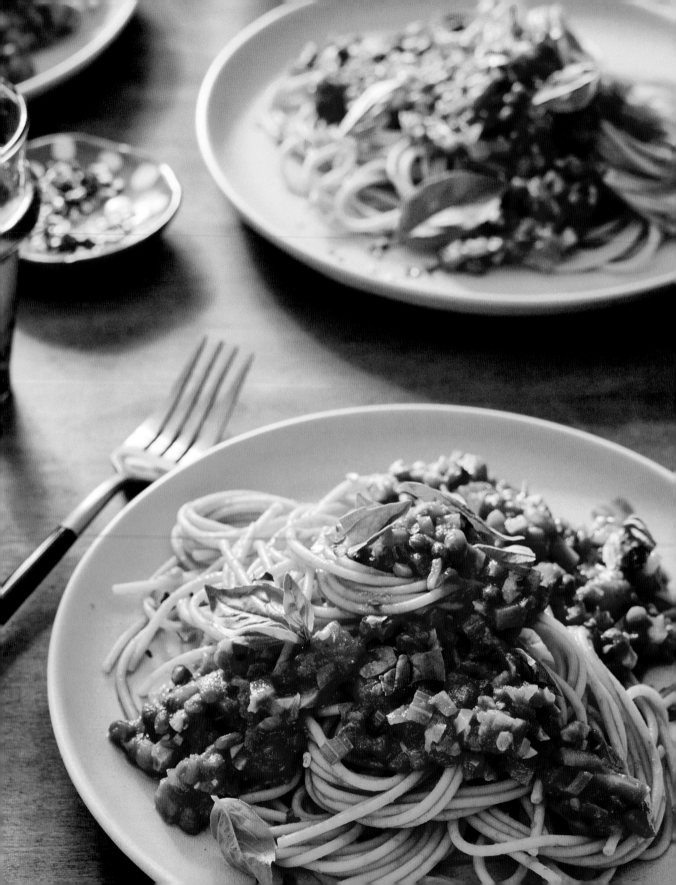

Spaghetti Lentil Bolognese

MAKES 4 SERVINGS | | CHEF LESLIE

This delicious recipe adds the healing benefit of walnuts. Walnuts are food for fueling your brain, while lentils support a healthy microbiome, improve cholesterol levels, and act as an anti-inflammatory. A half cup of organic red wine boosts the flavor of the sauce, but it is optional if you are avoiding alcohol or don't have it on hand.

3 tablespoons extra-virgin olive oil
1 cup diced onion
1 carrot, julienned
1 large celery stalk, julienned
4 to 8 garlic cloves, minced
1 teaspoon dried oregano
1 teaspoon kosher salt
1 pinch red pepper flakes (optional)
One 14½-ounce can crushed tomatoes
½ cup chopped walnuts
½ cup organic red wine (optional)
1 cup cooked lentils
1 pound lentil or chickpea spaghetti
½ cup chopped fresh basil leaves

Heat the olive oil in a large pot over medium heat. Sauté the onion, carrot, celery, and garlic until they turn soft, 6 to 10 minutes. Stir in the oregano, salt, and red pepper flakes (if using).

Add the tomatoes, walnuts, and wine (if using). Decrease the heat to low, cover, and bring to a simmer. Simmer for 10 minutes, then stir in the cooked lentils and let cook for another 5 minutes.

Bring a large pot of water over medium-high heat to a boil and cook the spaghetti according to the package instructions. When the spaghetti is al dente, drain it in a colander and arrange it on serving plates.

Stir the basil leaves into the sauce, then serve immediately over the spaghetti.

Sweet Potato and Tempeh Tacos

MAKES 8 TACOS | | CHEF LESLIE

I love sweet potatoes, and their combination with tempeh makes this a powerful recipe. It is perfect for the middle of your manifestation phase because of tempeh's phytoestrogens and sweet potatoes promoting progesterone production. It's also good at the end of your nurture phase, when your body needs a splash of estrogen. These tacos are delicious with the tomatillo salsa or on their own.

SALSA
¾ pound tomatillos, husks removed, rinsed
1 medium jalapeño, halved, seeds and ribs removed if desired
1 small bunch cilantro
½ teaspoon kosher salt

TACOS
4 tablespoons extra-virgin olive oil
2 sweet potatoes, peeled and cut into ½-inch cubes
One 8-ounce package tempeh, crumbled
½ cup chopped yellow onion
2 garlic cloves, minced
1 tablespoon smoked paprika
1 teaspoon ground cumin
½ teaspoon ground cinnamon
½ teaspoon dried oregano
Kosher salt and freshly ground black pepper
Juice of 1 lime
¼ cup hemp seeds
1 medium avocado, pitted, peeled, and cut into 8 pieces
Eight 6-inch corn tortillas
1 cup coarsely chopped fresh cilantro leaves

TO MAKE THE SALSA In a metal pan, broil the tomatillos and jalapeño halves on the top oven rack until black spots appear, about 6 minutes. Turn the tomatillos over and broil until black spots appear on the other side, about 5 minutes. Cool slightly and pulse in a blender with the cilantro and salt until the cilantro is chopped.

TO MAKE THE TACOS Heat the olive oil in a large skillet over medium heat. Add the sweet potatoes and sauté for 6 minutes, until browned and fork tender. Add the tempeh, onion, garlic, paprika, cumin, cinnamon, and oregano. Season with salt and pepper. Continue to cook and, when the sweet potato becomes fork-tender, add the lime juice and mix well. Set aside.

Pour the hemp seeds into a wide, shallow dish. Press the avocado slices into the hemp seeds so they stick to the avocado.

Heat the tortillas on a hot pan for about 30 seconds on each side until they become pliable and begin to bubble. Wrap in foil.

To serve, fill the tortillas with the sweet potato mixture and top each with an avocado slice, fresh cilantro, and salsa.

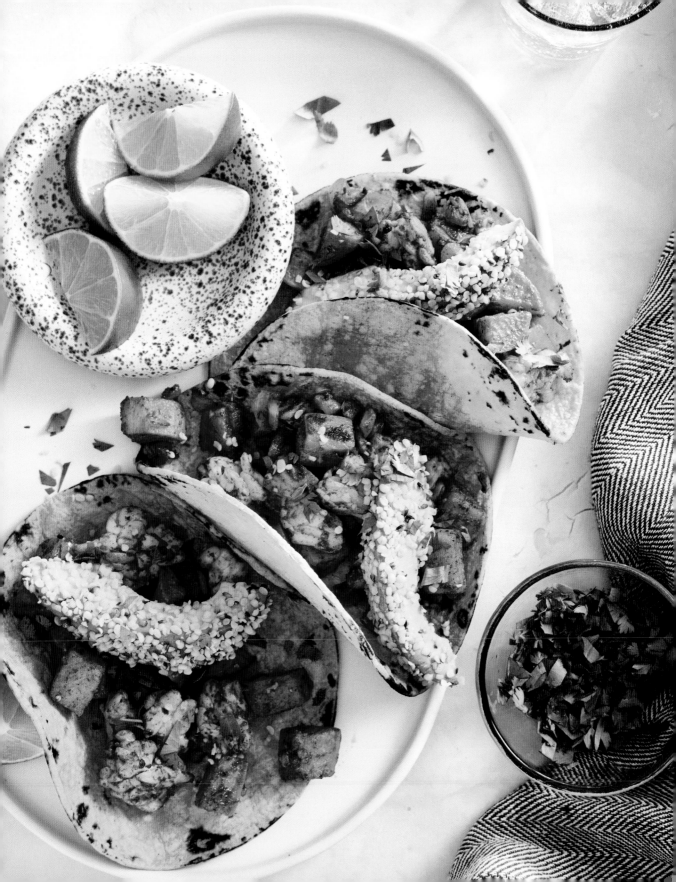

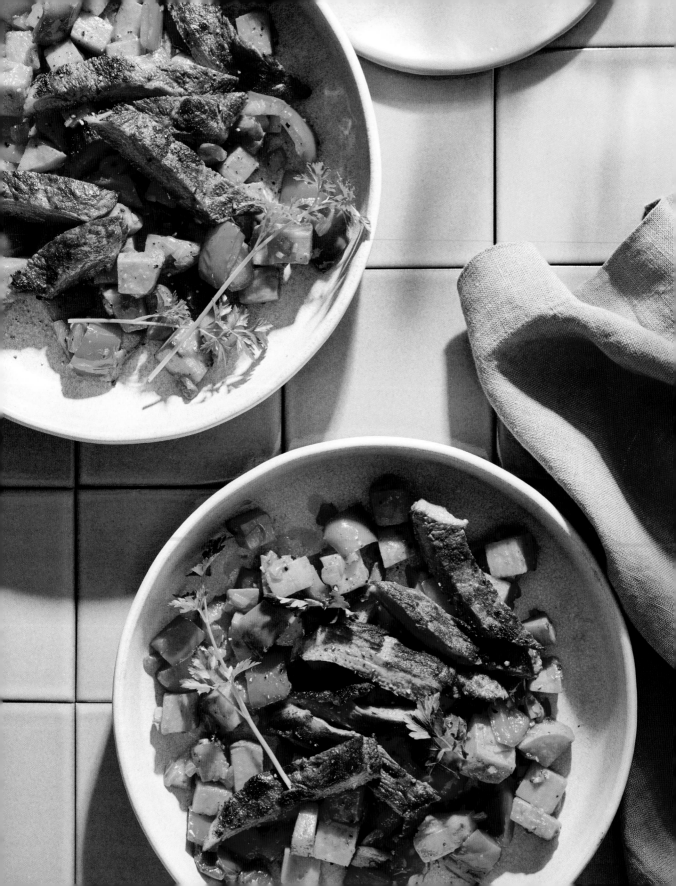

Southwest Steak and Sweet Potato Hash

MAKES 4 SERVINGS | CHEF JEFF

Nothing gives you more of an amino acid punch than steak. I highly encourage you to choose grass-fed steak as it has a better fatty acid profile. You may be surprised to see mesquite sugar here, but it's a lovely addition by Chef Jeff for a smokier sweet taste, plus it is surprisingly easy to find. I also love mesquite sugar's low glycemic index. It spikes your blood sugar very similar to coconut sugar, making it a great sweetening alternative to regular organic sugar.

STEAK RUB

1 teaspoon mesquite or coconut sugar

1 teaspoon kosher salt

1 teaspoon ground cumin

1 teaspoon instant espresso granules

½ teaspoon smoked paprika, preferably Spanish

1¼ to 1½ pounds New York strip steak, about 1 to 1½ inches thick, trimmed of fat

SWEET POTATO HASH

3 tablespoons extra-virgin olive oil, divided

1 small white, yellow, or red onion, chopped

Kosher salt and freshly ground black pepper

1 pound sweet potatoes, peeled and cut into ½-inch cubes

1 small green bell pepper, seeded and chopped

1 small red bell pepper, seeded and chopped

3 large garlic cloves, minced

1 tablespoon tomato paste

½ cup Beef Bone Broth (page 266) or water

Your favorite hot sauce

TO MAKE THE STEAK RUB Set out a large plate. Combine the mesquite sugar, salt, cumin, espresso granules, and paprika in a small, shallow bowl. Rub the steak all over with the spice mixture and place it on the plate. At this point, you can cook the steak immediately, or cover and refrigerate it for up to 24 hours.

TO MAKE THE HASH If the steak has been refrigerated, when you're ready to cook, remove it from the fridge 1 hour ahead of time to allow the meat to come to room temperature. Get a platter ready for holding the cooked meat.

CONTINUED ▶

Southwest Steak and Sweet Potato Hash
CONTINUED

Heat 2 tablespoons of the olive oil in a large sauté pan or skillet over medium-high heat. When the oil is very hot, gently add the steak to the pan. The goal is to sear the outside of the meat and get it evenly caramelized all around. Cook until the first side is nicely browned, about 3 minutes. Turn the steak over and sear the other side until it is cooked to your liking, about 2 minutes for medium. Transfer the steak to a plate and allow it to rest for a few minutes, then slice it.

While the steak rests, add the remaining 1 tablespoon of olive oil to the pan. Decrease the heat to medium and add the onion and a large pinch of salt. Cook, scraping up any browned bits from the bottom of the pan, until the onions become soft, translucent, and lightly browned, 3 to 5 minutes.

Add the sweet potatoes, green and red bell peppers, garlic, and tomato paste and season with salt and pepper. Stir to combine. Increase the heat to medium-high, add the bone broth, and bring the mixture to a boil.

Decrease the heat to medium or medium-low, and simmer, stirring occasionally, until the broth evaporates and the sweet potatoes are tender and lightly browned, 16 to 19 minutes. Add 1 tablespoon of hot sauce and the steak, along with any juices on the plate, to the pan and stir until the steak is heated through.

Taste and season with more salt, black pepper, and hot sauce. Transfer the hash to the platter and serve immediately.

Japanese Savory Pancake (Okonomiyaki)

MAKES 4 SERVINGS | | CHEF JEFF

When I look at this recipe, I see your gut microbes squealing with glee! For those of you who are looking for more protein but need a break from red meat, this combination of seafood and eggs gives you a powerful protein punch.

2 ounces calamari, cut into ½-inch-thick rings and tentacles

2 ounces medium (41/50) shrimp, peeled, deveined, tails removed, and cut into bite-size pieces

4 large eggs, beaten

1 cup (about 2½ ounces) shredded green cabbage

¾ cup store-bought fish bone broth, Dashi (page 271), or water

⅓ cup thinly sliced green onions, white and green parts

¼ cup thinly sliced zucchini or summer squash, quartered lengthwise and thinly sliced

¼ cup thinly sliced cremini or button mushrooms, halved if large

¼ cup almond flour

¼ cup coconut flour

1 packed tablespoon drained and finely chopped Keto Pickled Ginger (page 276)

1 teaspoon xanthan gum (optional)

1 teaspoon baking powder

1 teaspoon kosher salt

½ teaspoon ground white pepper

3 tablespoons unsalted butter, divided

1 cup kimchi

Miso Ginger Dressing (page 288)

Sriracha sauce (optional)

Combine the calamari, shrimp, eggs, cabbage, bone broth, green onions, zucchini, mushrooms, almond flour, coconut flour, pickled ginger, xanthan gum (if using), baking powder, salt, and pepper in a large bowl. Mix well; the batter should be thick. At this point, the batter can be refrigerated for up to 4 hours.

If the okonomiyaki batter is refrigerated, allow it to come to room temperature before cooking.

Heat a 10-inch nonstick skillet over medium heat. Get a round plate that is the same diameter as the top of the skillet.

Melt 1½ tablespoons of the butter in the skillet until it foams. Add the okonomiyaki batter and begin shaking the skillet, alternating between shaking and using a heatproof spatula to loosen the mixture around the edges; the goal is to get the batter to cook without anything sticking to the bottom or sides of the skillet. Decrease the heat to medium-low if the okonomiyaki starts cooking too quickly before its edges have set.

CONTINUED ▶

173

Japanese Savory Pancake (Okonomiyaki)
CONTINUED

Once the okonomiyaki looks mostly set and is browned around the edges (about 7 minutes), remove the skillet from the heat. Using oven mitts, invert the round plate over the top of the skillet. With one hand on the plate and the other holding the skillet, flip the okonomiyaki in one motion onto the plate.

Return the skillet to medium heat and add the remaining 1½ tablespoons of butter. When the butter has melted, slide the okonomiyaki back into the skillet to cook the other side until it is set in the middle and the bottom is nicely browned, about 7 minutes. Decrease the heat to medium-low if it's browning too quickly.

Garnish with kimchi and serve drizzled with Miso Ginger Dressing and sriracha (if using).

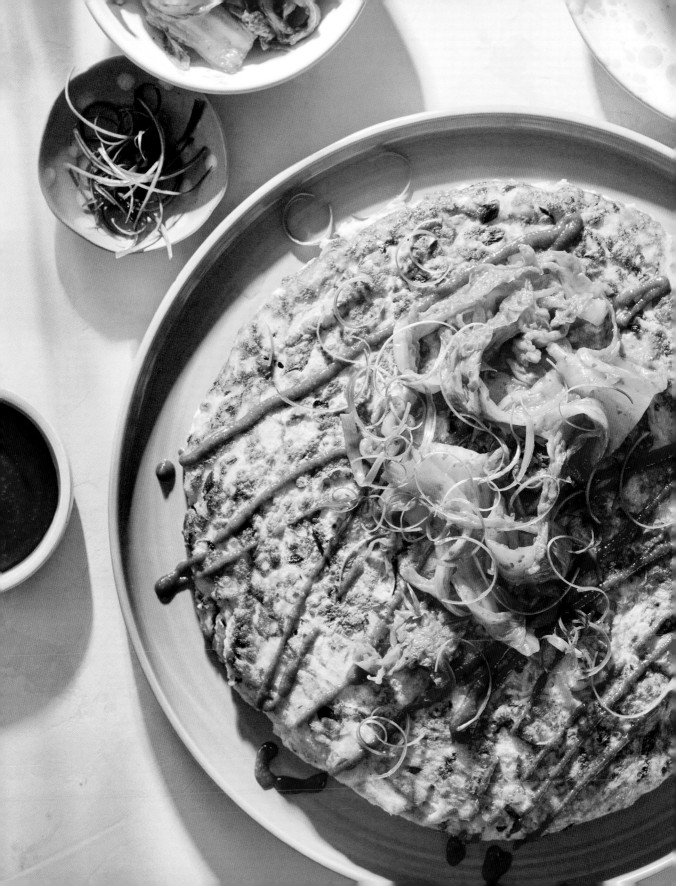

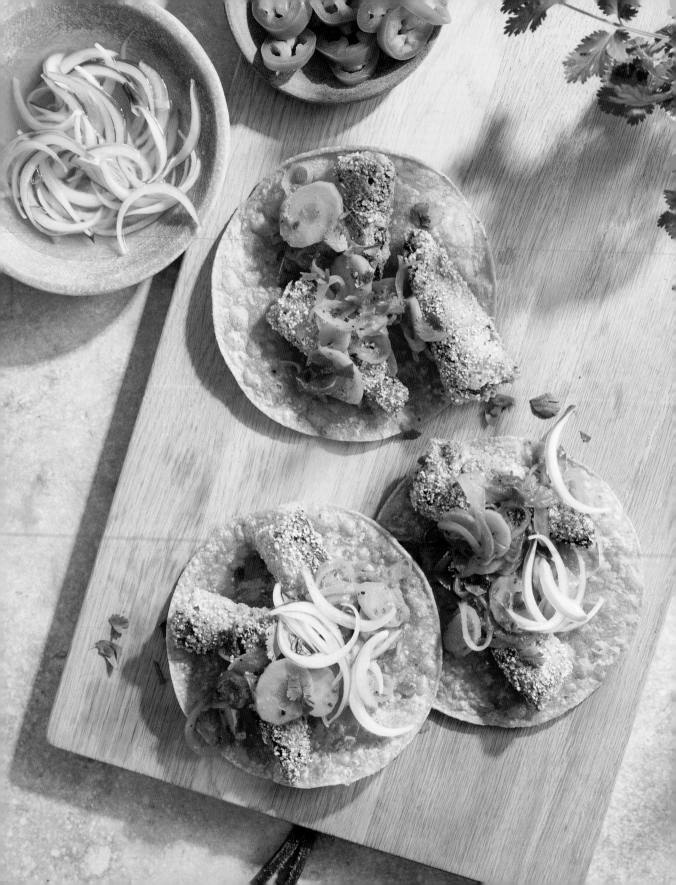

Sardine Tostadas

MAKES 3 SERVINGS (6 MEDIUM TOSTADAS) | CHEF JEFF

This is one of Chef Jeff's recipes that I'm most excited about. Sardines are one of the few foods that give us a good dose of vitamin D, a key nutrient for hormonal health. I don't always gravitate to fattier fishes, but this dish might just turn me into a sardine lover! While you can make this with other types of sardines, Chef Jeff recommends you seek out Spanish ones; they are the gold standard and of the best quality.

ESCABECHE

½ cup fine yellow cornmeal

Kosher salt

Two 4-ounce tins Spanish sardines in olive oil

1 large egg white, beaten with 1 teaspoon water

3 tablespoons extra-virgin olive oil

½ medium white, yellow, or red onion, cut into thin julienne

2 medium carrots, peeled and cut into thin coins

3 large garlic cloves, cut into paper-thin rounds

1½ teaspoons black peppercorns or coarsely ground pepper

1½ teaspoons dried oregano

1 dried bay leaf

3 tablespoons dry white wine

3 tablespoons white wine vinegar

3 tablespoons hot sauce, preferably a vinegary one such as Valentina

TOSTADAS

6 medium (each about 4½ inches) corn tostadas, warmed and then crisped in the oven before serving

½ bunch cilantro, leaves and stems coarsely chopped (about ⅓ cup)

Flake sea salt, such as Maldon

Mexican-Style Pickled Jalapeños and Carrots (page 279) or store-bought jalapeños, minced (optional)

Pickled Red Onions (page 277; optional)

2 limes, cut into quarters

1 medium avocado, halved and sliced thinly

TO MAKE THE ESCABECHE Stir together the cornmeal and ¼ teaspoon salt in a medium bowl. Dip each sardine fillet in the egg white, letting the excess drip off, then dredge in the cornmeal to lightly coat. Set aside on a plate.

Heat the olive oil in a large sauté pan or skillet over medium heat. Set up a large plate lined with paper towels for the fried sardines.

Gently add the sardines to the pan, season them with a little salt, and pan-fry, turning once, until they're browned and crispy on both sides, 2 to 3 minutes. Transfer the sardines to the prepared plate.

CONTINUED ▶

Sardine Tostadas
CONTINUED

In the same pan over medium heat, add the onion, carrots, garlic, peppercorns, oregano, and bay leaf. Add 1 teaspoon salt, stir to combine, and cook until the veggies soften and wilt, 5 to 6 minutes.

Add the wine, white wine vinegar, and hot sauce. Mix well and bring the mixture to a simmer. Turn off the heat.

TO ASSEMBLE THE TOSTADAS Arrange three sardines on top of each tostada, then top them with some of the vegetables and sauce. Garnish with the cilantro and season with sea salt.

Serve with the pickled jalapeños, pickled onions, limes, and avocado slices.

Chicken Cacciatore

MAKES 2 TO 4 SERVINGS | CHEF JEFF

This is an amino acid party! If you want to build muscle, this is your go-to recipe. It's got bone broth to repair your gut, olives to provide a healthy dose of polyphenols, and a vast array of meats to give you all the amino acids you need to make hormones.

MARINADE
Kosher salt and freshly ground black pepper
1½ teaspoons Italian seasoning
1½ teaspoons dried oregano
1 teaspoon red pepper flakes
2 tablespoons extra-virgin olive oil
4 large bone-in, skin-on chicken thighs
  (about 1¾ pounds)

CHICKEN CACCIATORE
¼ cup extra-virgin olive oil
4 ounces pancetta or prosciutto, cut into
  medium dice
1 medium white, yellow, or red onion, peeled
  and cut into medium chunks (avoid
  sweeter Vidalia or Maui onions because of
  their supercharged sugar content)
1 red bell pepper, seeded and cut into
  medium chunks
3 large garlic cloves, chopped
½ pound small cremini or button mushrooms, rinsed and halved
¼ cup pitted olives, such as Spanish queen,
  Gaeta, or kalamata
2 tablespoons capers, drained and rinsed
1 tablespoon coconut sugar
½ cup sherry (any inexpensive bottle from
  the liquor aisle is fine)
One 28-ounce can whole peeled tomatoes
½ cup Chicken Bone Broth (page 268)
  or water

Kosher salt and freshly ground black pepper
½ bunch Italian parsley, coarsely chopped
  (½ cup)
½ lemon, cut in half

TO MAKE THE MARINADE Combine 2 tea-spoons of salt, 1½ teaspoons of black pepper, the Italian seasoning, oregano, and red pepper flakes in a small bowl. Add the olive oil and whisk until the mixture forms a paste. Taste the marinade and season as desired. Spread the marinade all over the chicken thighs. Transfer the chicken to a plate, cover, and refrigerate for at least 2 hours or up to 48 hours.

TO MAKE THE CHICKEN CACCIATORE Preheat the oven to 350°F. Prepare a plate for the cooked chicken.

Heat a large Dutch oven over medium-high heat. When it is hot, add the olive oil to the pot and place the chicken thighs skin side down. Cook until a crust forms on one side, 3 to 5 minutes. Turn over the chicken thighs and repeat on the other side, cooking for about 3 more minutes. Transfer the chicken to the plate.

CONTINUED ▶

Chicken Cacciatore

CONTINUED

Pour out all but 2 tablespoons of the oil. Decrease the heat to medium. Add the pancetta, onion, bell pepper, garlic, and ½ teaspoon of salt. Cook, stirring, until the onions start to become translucent and the vegetables release some liquid, about 7 minutes. Add the mushrooms, olives, and capers, and continue cooking until the mushrooms begin to soften, about 10 to 15 minutes.

Add the coconut sugar and stir to combine. Cook until the vegetables wilt and the onions brown a little, about 2 minutes. Add the sherry and continue cooking until it reduces by half, about 2 minutes. Cut the canned tomatoes into large pieces with a pair of scissors, or crush them into the pot with your hands. Add the tomatoes and bone broth to the vegetables and stir to combine. Bring to a simmer.

Taste and season with salt and pepper as desired, keeping in mind that the sauce will reduce a little more and concentrate the flavors.

Nestle the chicken thighs into the sauce and cover the pot with a lid or aluminum foil. Bake in the oven until an instant-read thermometer inserted into a thigh registers 160°F, about 30 minutes. (The chicken will reach the recommended 165°F with residual heat.)

To serve, transfer the vegetables and sauce to a shallow bowl and top with the chicken. Spoon extra sauce over the chicken, and then sprinkle with the parsley and squeeze some lemon over the top.

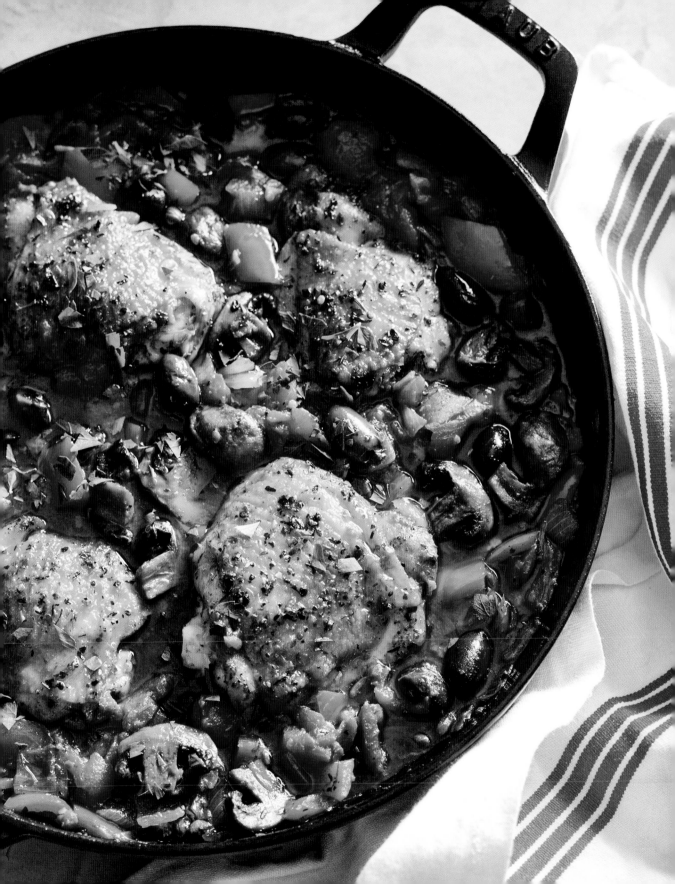

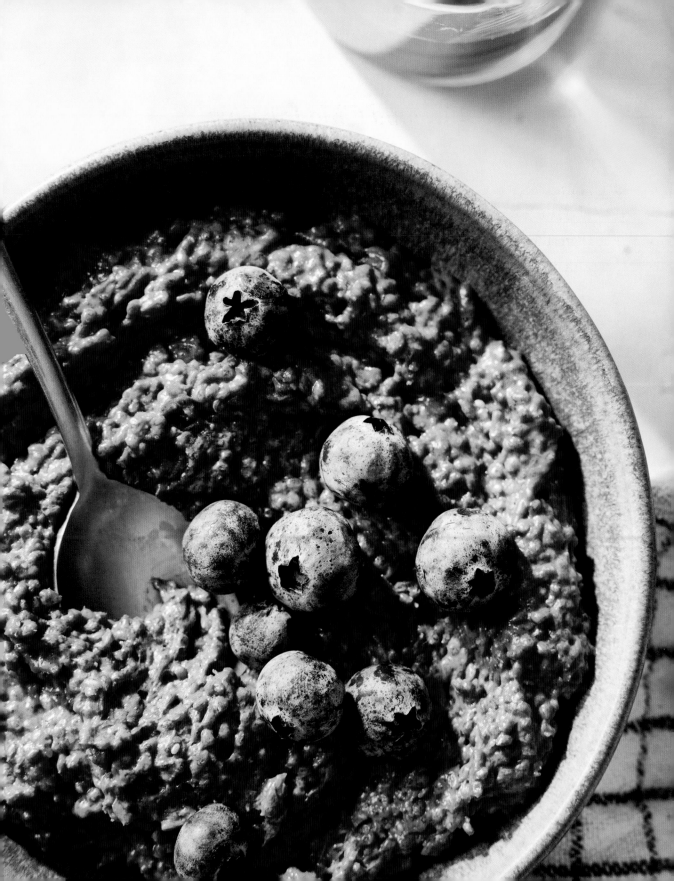

Chocolate Almond Chia Pudding

MAKES 1 TO 2 SERVINGS | CHEF LESLIE

This recipe can be used during many phases. Chia pudding is a fun dish to break your fast with, and the combination of almond milk and maple syrup makes it great for your nurture phase. Chia seeds are nature's detox gift to us. Please note that any milk you use should always be organic.

1 cup unsweetened almond or soy milk
3 tablespoons almond butter or cashew butter
2 tablespoons cacao powder
2 tablespoons maple syrup
5 tablespoons chia seeds
¼ cup raspberries, ½ cup strawberries, or ½ cup blueberries (optional)

Whisk together the almond milk, almond butter, cacao powder, and maple syrup in a medium bowl. Stir in the chia seeds, let sit for 20 minutes, and then stir again.

Refrigerate overnight and garnish with berries, if using.

Maple Peanut Butter Fudge

MAKES 20 FUDGE PIECES | CHEF JEFF

Here's a recipe for those of you with a sweet tooth. Chef Jeff did a phenomenal job of combining the sweeteners with protein and fat so that you'll be satisfied by the sweetness but won't get a huge blood-sugar spike.

½ cup unsalted butter, divided
1 cup natural unsweetened peanut butter
½ cup brown sugar substitute (such as Swerve)
2 tablespoons white miso
2 tablespoons maple syrup
¼ teaspoon kosher salt
1 tablespoon vanilla paste or vanilla extract
2 teaspoons maple extract
2 teaspoons xanthan gum
2 tablespoons heavy cream
¼ cup coarsely chopped roasted peanuts
1 large pinch flake sea salt, such as Celtic or Maldon

Line an 8- or 9-inch square baking pan with parchment paper and set aside.

Heat ¼ cup of the butter in a medium saucepan over medium heat. Cook until the butter begins to darken in color and smells nutty, 4 to 6 minutes. Remove the pan from the heat and let the butter sit in the pan for 1 minute. Add the peanut butter, brown sugar substitute, miso, maple syrup, and salt. Stir to combine and return the pan to the burner over medium heat. Cook, stirring constantly, until the mixture darkens in color, 3 to 4 minutes (be careful it doesn't burn).

Remove from the heat and add the vanilla paste and maple extract to the pan. Stir to combine.

Slice the remaining ¼ cup of butter into cubes. Pour the peanut butter mixture into a blender, add the remaining butter, and blend on low speed, tamping down the mixture to blend. While the blender is running, sprinkle in the xanthan gum; this will help keep the fudge from breaking (when the oil separates from the water) while it cools. Continue to tamp down the mixture to blend.

Increase the blender speed to medium and add the cream while the blender is running. Blend for about 1 minute, tamping as needed to mix the cream into the fudge, until the fudge lightens in color and cools down a little.

Transfer the warm fudge to the prepared baking pan and spread it out evenly with a rubber spatula. Sprinkle with the peanuts and flake salt and allow the fudge to cool completely, 2 to 4 hours.

Slice the fudge into 1½-inch squares and store in an airtight container in the refrigerator. It will last for up to 1 week in the fridge or 2 months in the freezer.

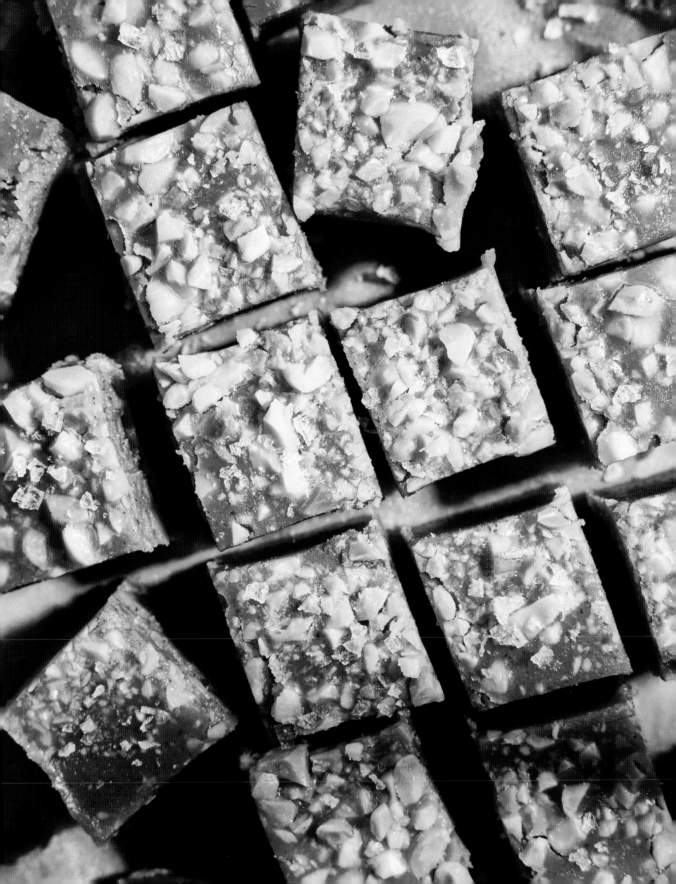

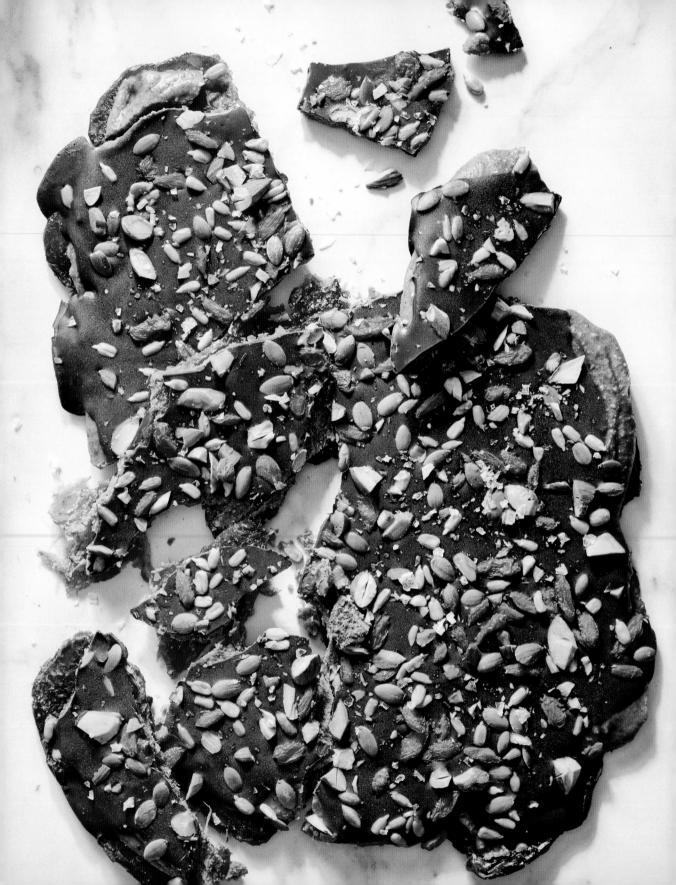

Date Bark

MAKES 12 TO 18 SERVINGS | | CHEF LESLIE

Many consider dates to be a superfood. They are high in antioxidants, minerals, and vitamins, and they are incredibly helpful for brain function. They are a phenomenal sweetener with a higher fiber content than most, which triggers a lower blood-sugar spike.

12 to 14 dates, such as Medjool
½ cup almond butter
1 tablespoon maple syrup (optional)
½ teaspoon ground cinnamon
½ teaspoon vanilla extract
½ cup nondairy dark chocolate chips
1 tablespoon coconut oil or oat milk

TOPPING IDEAS

Sunflower seeds
Pumpkin seeds
Goji berries
Chopped almonds
Flake sea salt, like Maldon

Line a baking sheet with parchment paper. Halve the dates, remove the pits, and splay the dates cup side up and flattened on the baking sheet. Arrange the dates side by side so that they merge together when flattened. Place a sheet of parchment paper on top of the dates. Place another baking sheet on top of the parchment paper and press the top baking sheet to flatten the dates into a single layer about ¼ inch thick. Remove the top sheet of parchment paper and set the dates aside.

Whisk together the almond butter, maple syrup (if using), cinnamon, and vanilla in a small bowl. Using a rubber spatula, spread the mixture evenly over the dates to create a thick layer.

Combine the chocolate chips and coconut oil in a glass bowl and microwave them in 15-second increments, stirring each time, until the chips have dissolved completely and the mixture is smooth.

Pour the chocolate mixture over the almond butter layer and spread it out evenly. Sprinkle with the desired toppings.

Place the baking sheet in the freezer for at least 1 hour. Then cut the date bark into pieces and enjoy! Store in the refrigerator for up to 1 month.

Orange Chia Seed Muffins

MAKES 24 MUFFINS | CHEF LESLIE

This should be your go-to recipe on the days you're craving carbs. The addition of apple cider vinegar ensures a smaller blood-sugar spike while still giving you a sweet treat. I highly recommend you use an all-purpose gluten-free flour to preserve a healthy gut. If you do dairy, spread these muffins with grass-fed butter, or, if you prefer a plant-based alternative, use a nut butter; this creates an even lower blood-sugar spike.

2 cups all-purpose gluten-free flour
½ cup coconut sugar
1 tablespoon baking powder
½ teaspoon sea salt
½ teaspoon ground cinnamon
1 cup orange juice
½ cup melted refined coconut oil
2 tablespoons apple cider vinegar
1 teaspoon vanilla extract
Zest of ½ orange
2 tablespoons chia seeds

Preheat the oven to 375°F. Line two 12-well muffin tins with paper liners.

Whisk together the flour, coconut sugar, baking powder, sea salt, and cinnamon in a large bowl.

Combine the orange juice, coconut oil, apple cider vinegar, and vanilla extract in a separate bowl and whisk together.

Add the wet ingredients to the dry ingredients and whisk to combine. Fold in the orange zest and chia seeds.

Spoon the batter into the prepared muffin cups, filling them three-quarters full. Bake for 25 minutes, or until the muffins are golden brown.

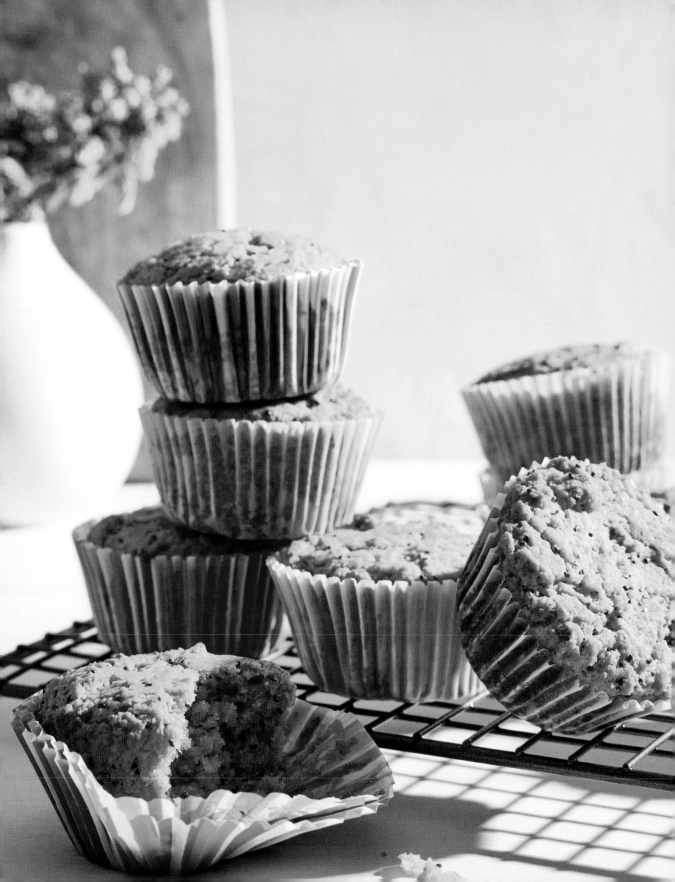

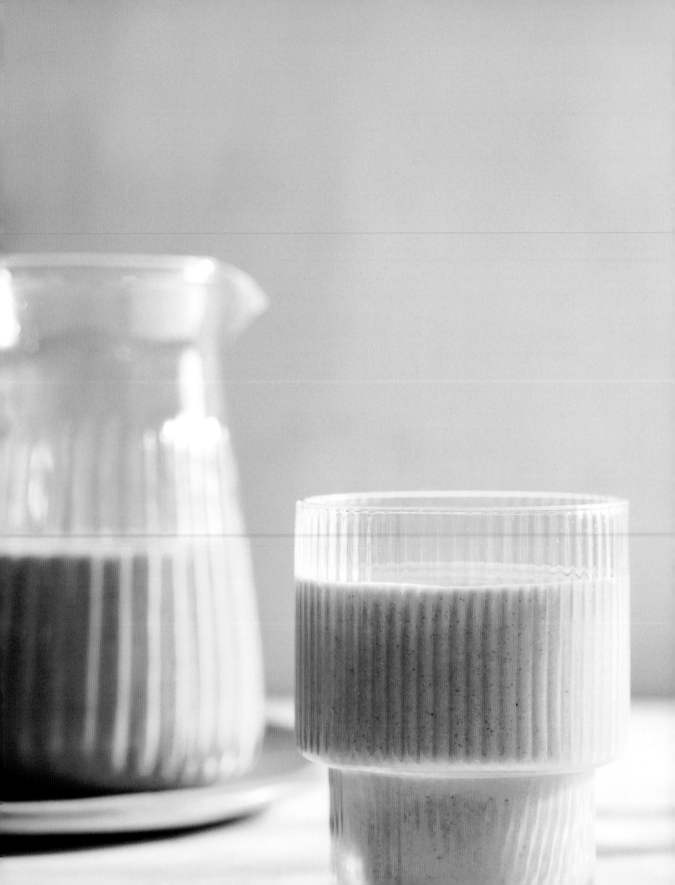

Choco Maca Smoothie

MAKES 1 SERVING | | CHEF LESLIE

Maca is an incredible plant for hormonal health. It is known to improve libido, increase fertility, give you more energy, and improve your moods, making this recipe terrific for your manifestation window. You can find maca powder at any natural food grocery store. An interesting note: Using a green banana instead of a fully ripe one is more beneficial for your microbiome.

2 frozen bananas, chopped
1 cup unsweetened almond milk
2 tablespoons almond butter
1 tablespoon cocoa powder
1 tablespoon maca powder

Combine the bananas, almond milk, almond butter, cocoa powder, and maca powder in a blender and blend on high speed until smooth.

Wild Blueberry Smoothie

MAKES 1 SERVING | | CHEF LESLIE

You have many options with this recipe when it comes to milks and protein powders. If you're on a plant-based diet, I highly encourage you to stick to an organic soy milk, or feel free to add an organic nut milk. Vegan protein powders can be found everywhere. I love the addition of creatine in this recipe because it's excellent fuel for your workouts. This smoothie would make a great pre- or post-workout drink. Use a less-ripe banana to avoid a blood-sugar spike.

1 banana
1½ cups soy milk
1 cup frozen wild blueberries
½ cup vegan protein powder
1 teaspoon maca powder
½ teaspoon creatine

Combine the banana, soy milk, blueberries, protein powder, maca powder, and creatine in a blender and blend on high speed until smooth.

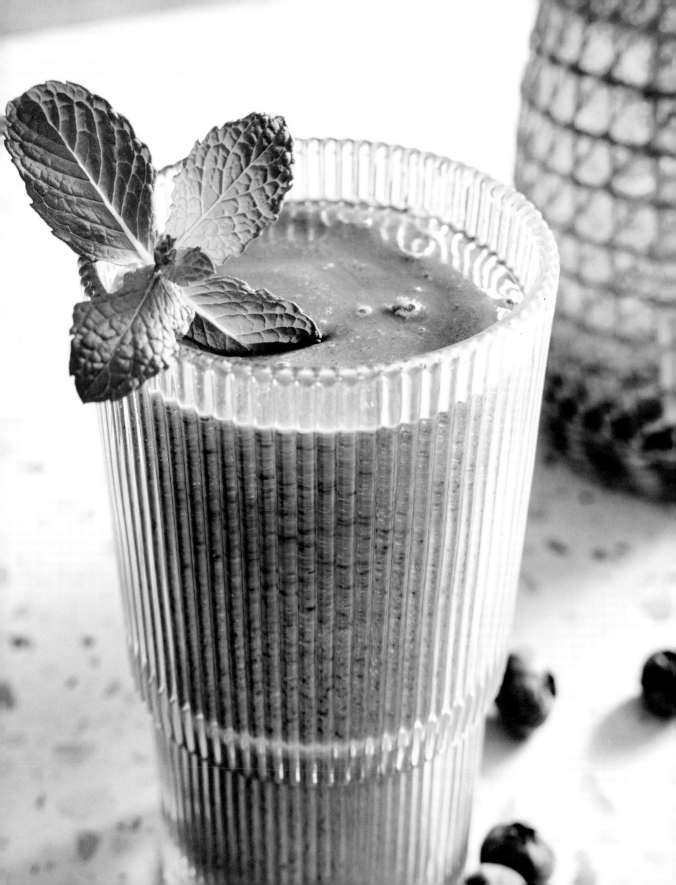

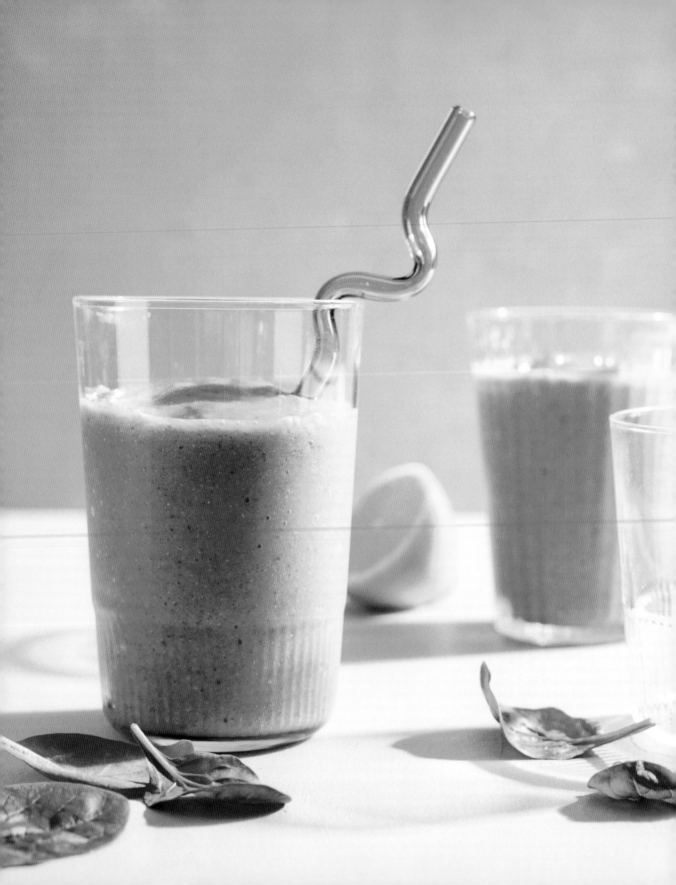

Heal Your Body Smoothie

MAKES 4 TO 5 SERVINGS | | CHEF LESLIE

This recipe is appropriately named! Coconut water is one of the more hydrating liquids you can drink, supplying you with a powerful dose of electrolytes. The ashwagandha and mushroom powders are phenomenal for helping you recover from stressful days. Ashwagandha is a shrub that grows in Asia and Africa. It can support calming the brain, reducing swelling, lowering blood pressure (which helps with fatigue and improves recovery after exercise), and bolstering the immune system. Cordyceps mushrooms support your immune system and may boost your exercise performance, increase antioxidants, and help fight inflammation. The addition of an avocado lessens the blood-sugar spike, while ginger supports healthy digestion, maca helps your body make progesterone, and turmeric is anti-inflammatory.

1 medium apple, Gala or Fuji, peeled and chopped
1 banana
½ avocado
3 cups fresh spinach
2½ cups coconut water
2 cups frozen chopped pineapple
1 cup frozen chopped mango
One 2-inch piece fresh ginger, peeled and chopped
One 2-inch piece fresh turmeric, peeled and chopped
2 tablespoons chia seeds
2 tablespoons maca powder
2 tablespoons ashwagandha powder
2 tablespoons cordyceps mushroom powder
Juice of ½ lemon
1 pinch sea salt
1 pinch cayenne pepper

Combine the apple, banana, avocado, spinach, coconut water, pineapple, mango, ginger, turmeric, chia seeds, maca powder, ashwagandha powder, cordyceps mushroom powder, lemon juice, salt, and cayenne pepper in a blender and blend on high speed until smooth.

Your Best Workout Smoothie

MAKES 1 SERVING | |

This is your go-to smoothie for the week before your period. The mixture of foods in this recipe creates a pretty dramatic blood-sugar spike, which can be necessary days before your period starts. Lean into this recipe when your sweet tooth keeps talking to you or when you start spotting days before your period comes. Chef Leslie loves this smoothie for a pre- or post-workout snack. Beets increase your levels of nitric oxide, which increases blood flow, biogenesis and efficiency, and muscle contraction strengthening.

1 banana
1 cup frozen mixed berries
¾ cup orange juice or water
½ cup chopped raw or cooked beets

Combine the banana, berries, orange juice, and beets in a blender and blend on high speed until smooth.

Cherry-Mint Mocktail

MAKES 1 SERVING | CHEF LESLIE

This simple but mighty drink should be your go-to beverage on days when stress is high. Magnesium lowers cortisol while cherry juice can improve sleep. Pour this delicious mocktail into one of your favorite cocktail glasses for a celebratory drink at the end of a long day. It's perfect for your nurture phase, as progesterone loves a good dose of magnesium.

1 sprig mint
1 cup tart cherry juice (no added sugar)
1 tablespoon magnesium glycinate powder

Muddle the mint at the bottom of a tall glass with a wooden spoon. Add the cherry juice, magnesium glycinate powder, and ½ to ¼ cup of water and stir to combine.

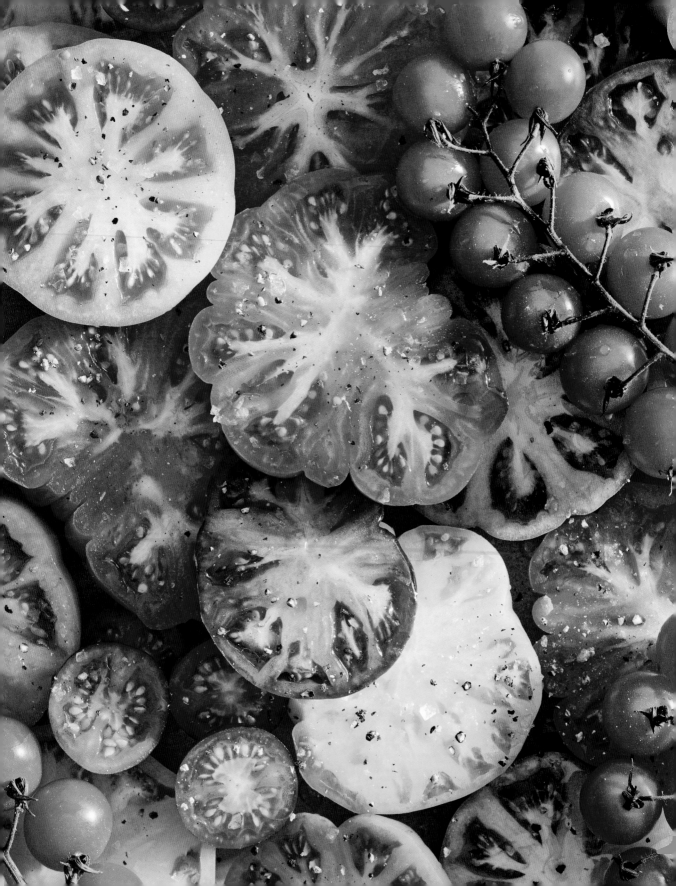

14

Ketobiotic

I AM OVER-THE-MOON THRILLED to introduce you to the ketobiotic recipes in this book. When people lean into a lower-carbohydrate diet, they often assume they have to give up the pleasure that their carb-rich diet has provided them. Nothing could be further from the truth! My ketobiotic approach to food means that not only do we add in what supports a healthy microbiome, but we also have the perfect combination of ingredients to ensure a minimal blood-sugar response. With the ketobiotic eating style, your carbohydrate sources are largely fiber-filled, lowering the blood-sugar spike that accompanies more carb-dense foods.

There are several reasons to make these recipes. First, they taste amazing, and your mind will be blown! Second, if you're still menstruating, these fit superbly into your power phases. And third, if you're in your menopausal years, these recipes are perfect for helping you lose weight and improve mental clarity, and they have the power to lessen those lingering hot flashes.

Not only is a ketobiotic approach to food healing to your metabolic system, but your taste buds will thank you too. I promise, keto never tasted so good!

Keep in mind that the difference between ketobiotic and hormone feasting foods is the carbohydrate count. Ketobiotic is low carb and hormone feasting is higher carb. This means on your hormone feasting days, you could include any ketobiotic recipes—but it doesn't work the other way around.

Guacamole with Vegetable Chips

MAKES 2 SERVINGS | | CHEF LESLIE

I love cumin both for its flavor and its benefits. Cumin is a great source of iron, promotes a healthy digestive system, and helps with weight loss. Consider this recipe to break your fast as it is full of healthy fats, plus the chips offer a variety of vitamins and minerals.

VEGETABLE CHIPS

3 cups thinly sliced veggies of your choice, such as sweet potato, parsnip, celery root, kohlrabi, beets, or yucca (use a mandoline to slice the veggies)

Flake sea salt, like Maldon

1 to 2 tablespoons avocado or extra-virgin olive oil

GUACAMOLE

1 avocado, mashed

¼ cup chopped fresh cilantro leaves

2 tablespoons chopped yellow onion

Juice of ½ lime

¼ teaspoon ground cumin

¼ teaspoon kosher salt

¼ teaspoon garlic powder

TO MAKE THE CHIPS Preheat the oven to 300°F. Line one or two baking sheets with parchment paper.

Lay the vegetable slices in a single layer on paper towels, sprinkle with sea salt, and let sit for 20 minutes. Blot the veggies with more paper towels to absorb most of the moisture.

Lightly toss the veggie slices in a large bowl with the avocado oil. Transfer the slices to the prepared baking sheets in a single layer. Bake for 30 to 40 minutes, until crispy, checking regularly to make sure the chips don't burn. If desired, sprinkle with Maldon salt before serving.

Let cool and serve.

TO MAKE THE GUACAMOLE Mix the avocado, cilantro, onion, lime juice, cumin, salt, and garlic powder in a medium bowl and mash until the guacamole reaches your desired consistency. Transfer to a bowl and serve with the vegetable chips.

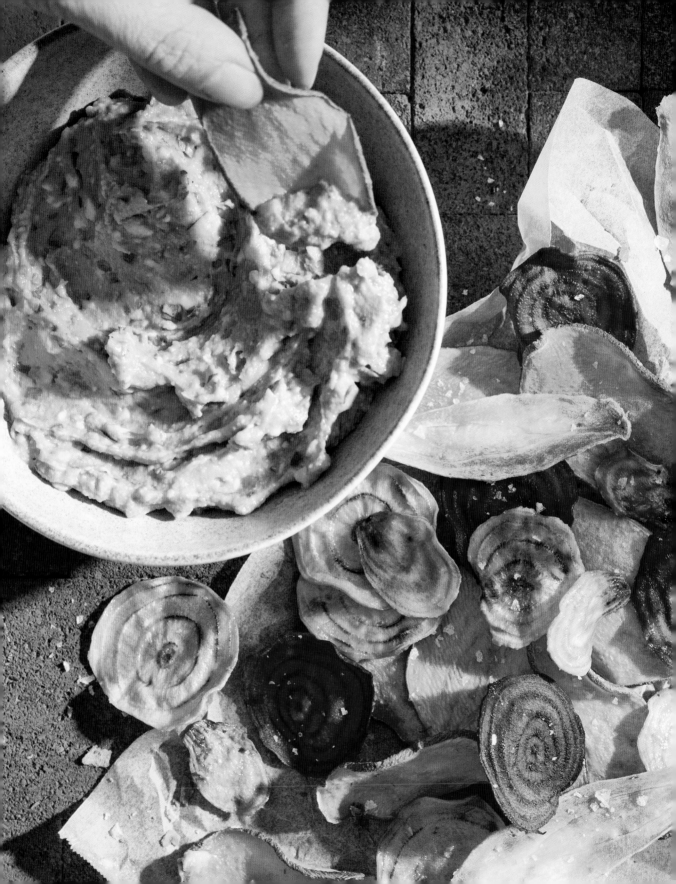

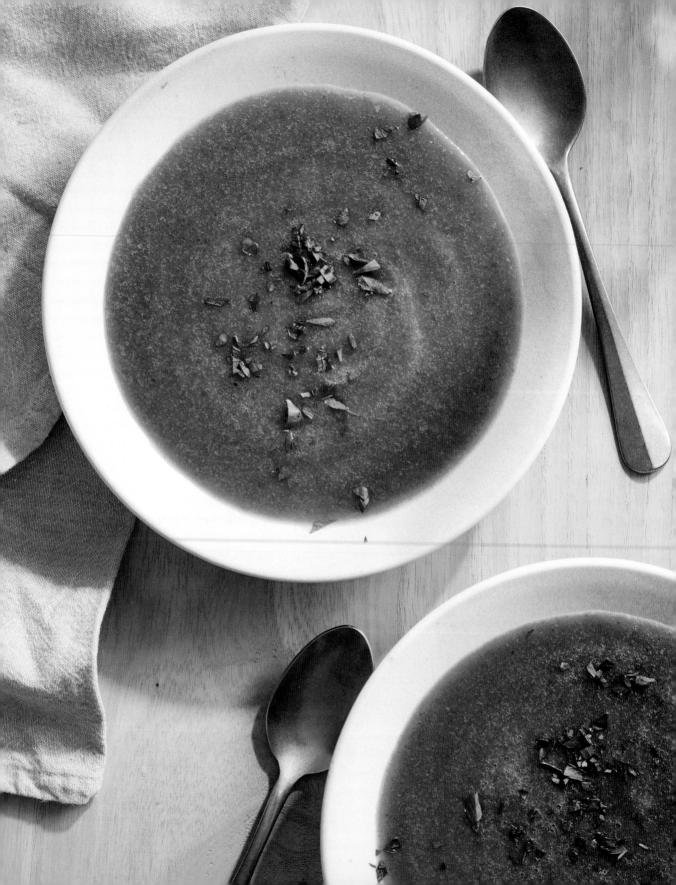

Zucchini String Bean Soup

MAKES 4 TO 6 SERVINGS | CHEF LESLIE

When I was sick as a child, my mom would make a detox soup called Bieler's broth. It was a healing soup that tasted horrible but was so effective at helping my body move through a cold. I asked Chef Leslie if she could devise a tastier version of this broth so you all could get the healing benefit without enduring the harsh flavor of the original Bieler's broth. I was so pleased when I tasted this soup for the first time—it's both healthful and yummy! You can make this ahead of time and freeze it in individual portion sizes so you only have to heat it up to receive its healing benefits.

1 pound green beans, trimmed and cut into 1-inch pieces
3 medium zucchini, quartered and cut into chunks
4 celery stalks, chopped
½ medium yellow onion, diced
1 garlic clove, minced
1 tablespoon kosher salt
1 cup chopped fresh parsley
1 cup chopped fresh spinach

Combine the green beans, zucchini, celery, onion, garlic, salt, and 4 cups of water in a large pot over high heat and bring to a boil. Decrease the heat, stir, cover, and simmer until the vegetables are fork-tender, about 10 minutes.

Remove from the heat, stir in the parsley and spinach, and stir until wilted. Carefully transfer the soup to a high-powered blender and blend on high speed until smooth (you will need to do this in batches). Return the blended soup to the pot, mix well, and serve.

Keep in airtight container in the fridge for up to 5 days or freeze for up to 1 month.

Pumpkin Soup

MAKES 3 TO 4 SERVINGS | | **CHEF LESLIE**

Pumpkin is another hormone hero food. Although it supports all three of your sex hormones, this recipe was designed to keep your blood sugar more stable. It's another dish you may use to break your fast on your power phase days. Add more or less vegetable broth depending on how thick you prefer your soup.

3 tablespoons extra-virgin olive oil
1 medium yellow onion, chopped
6 garlic cloves, minced
6 cups peeled and diced pumpkin
3 cups Vegetable Broth (page 270)
1 large carrot, peeled and coarsely chopped
2 tablespoons curry powder
1 teaspoon ground ginger
1 teaspoon kosher salt
1 pinch freshly ground black pepper
1 pinch cayenne pepper
1 pinch ground cinnamon
1 cup raw unsalted cashews
OPTIONAL GARNISHES
Chopped parsley
Toasted pumpkin seeds (store-bought)

Combine the oil, onion, and garlic in a large stockpot over medium heat and sauté until the onions are soft, about 5 minutes. Add the pumpkin, vegetable broth, carrot, curry powder, ginger, salt, black pepper, cayenne pepper, and cinnamon. Mix well and bring to a boil.

Cover, decrease the heat, and simmer until the vegetables become tender, 20 to 30 minutes.

Transfer the soup to a blender, add the cashews, and blend on high speed until smooth. You may need to blend the soup in batches.

To serve, pour the soup into bowls and garnish with parsley and pumpkin seeds, if desired.

Store in an airtight container in the fridge for up to 5 days or freeze for up to 1 month.

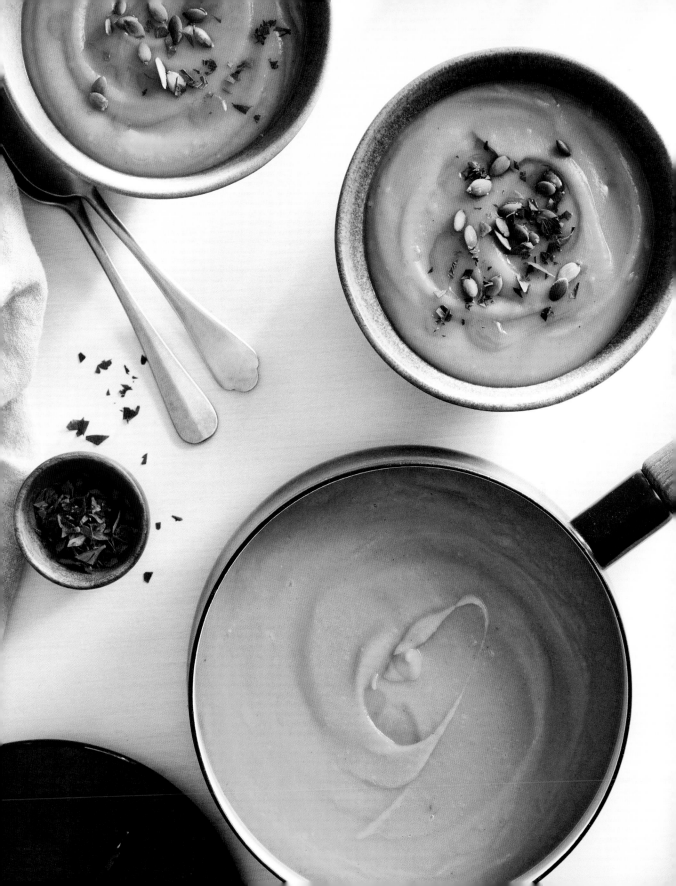

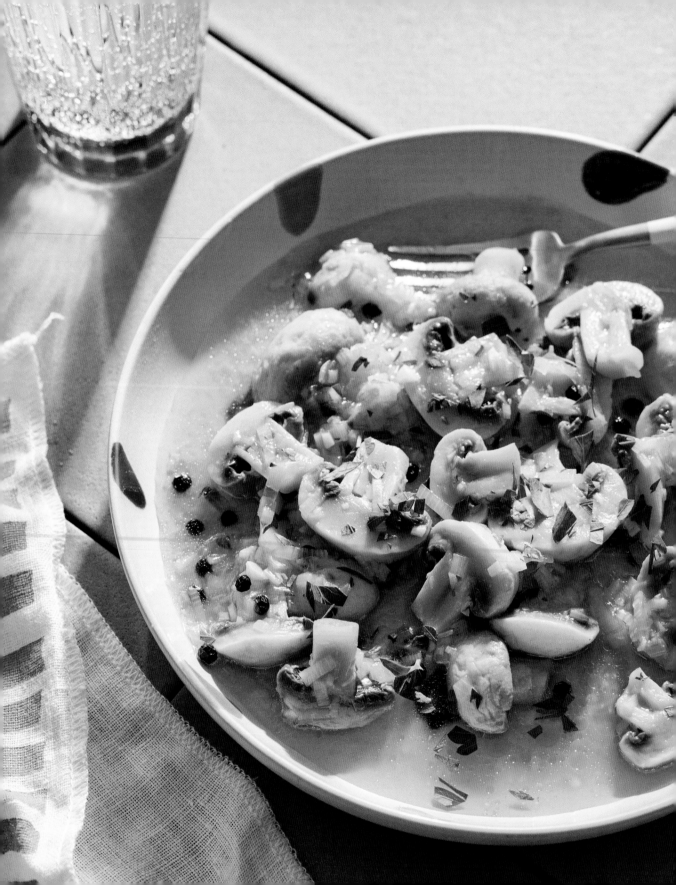

Marinated Mushroom Salad

MAKES 4 SERVINGS | | CHEF JEFF

White button mushrooms are surprisingly powerful for health. They are not only rich in fiber, but also high in protein and have been known to help lessen the risk of conditions like Alzheimer's, heart disease, and diabetes. They are also a great source of selenium for your thyroid. And Chef Jeff's addition of garlic makes it a microbiome-enhancing meal.

MARINADE

1 cup dry white wine

1 cup white wine vinegar

Juice of 1 large lemon

1 medium shallot, coarsely chopped

6 large garlic cloves, coarsely chopped

1 small leek, white and pale green parts halved lengthwise and thinly sliced

5 sprigs Italian parsley

5 sprigs thyme

1 sprig rosemary

Black peppercorns

Kosher salt

MUSHROOMS

1 pound small white button mushrooms, trimmed and halved

1 tablespoon extra-virgin olive oil

¼ cup chopped fresh Italian parsley

Coarse sea salt

TO MAKE THE MARINADE Combine 1 cup of water, the white wine, white wine vinegar, lemon juice, shallot, garlic, leek, parsley, thyme, rosemary, 1 tablespoon of peppercorns, and 1 tablespoon of salt in a medium pot and bring to a boil over medium-high heat. Decrease the heat to low, partially cover, and simmer for 10 minutes.

Taste to see if the flavors have mellowed and season with more salt and pepper if needed. Strain the marinade through a fine-mesh sieve and pour it back into the pot.

TO COOK THE MUSHROOMS Add the mushrooms to the pot with the marinade. Bring to a boil over medium-high heat, then decrease the heat to medium-low and continue to simmer, stirring occasionally, until the mushrooms have shrunk and softened considerably, 10 to 12 minutes. Using a slotted spoon, transfer the mushrooms to a serving bowl.

Increase the heat to medium-high and gently boil until the marinade is reduced to ½ cup, about 10 minutes. Remove the pot from the heat.

Pour 1 to 2 tablespoons of the marinade over the mushrooms, then drizzle with the olive oil and sprinkle with the parsley and coarse salt. Toss to combine.

Taste and season as desired with more marinade or salt.

Spanish Tomato and Tuna Salad

MAKES 4 SERVINGS | | CHEF JEFF

This fabulous tuna recipe calls for bonito del norte white albacore tuna, which is especially flavorful. However, if you want to avoid the high mercury content often found in larger tunas, you might want to use skipjack tuna, which contains lower mercury levels. You may be surprised that this type of tuna is easy to find.

1 medium white, yellow, or red onion, cut into medium julienne

¼ cup Spain's Favorite Sherry Vinaigrette (page 287), divided

Kosher salt

Coconut sugar

4 medium heirloom or beefsteak tomatoes

1 pint heirloom cherry, grape, Sungold, or similar tomatoes

2 tablespoons flake salt, such as Maldon

One 5-ounce can tuna packed in olive oil, preferably bonito del norte (albacore)

2 tablespoons Catalan Plancha Sauce (page 283; optional)

Combine the onion, 2 tablespoons of the sherry vinaigrette, 2 tablespoons of salt, and 2 tablespoons of coconut sugar in a large bowl and mix well. Let sit for 5 minutes to pickle the onion a little.

In the meantime, cut the larger tomatoes into wedges and the smaller tomatoes in half. Add the tomatoes to the onion mixture, drizzle with the rest of the vinaigrette, and toss to combine. Taste and season the salad with more salt and coconut sugar as desired.

To serve, arrange the tomato salad on a large serving plate and sprinkle with the flake salt. Add the tuna to the plate and drizzle everything with the plancha sauce, if using.

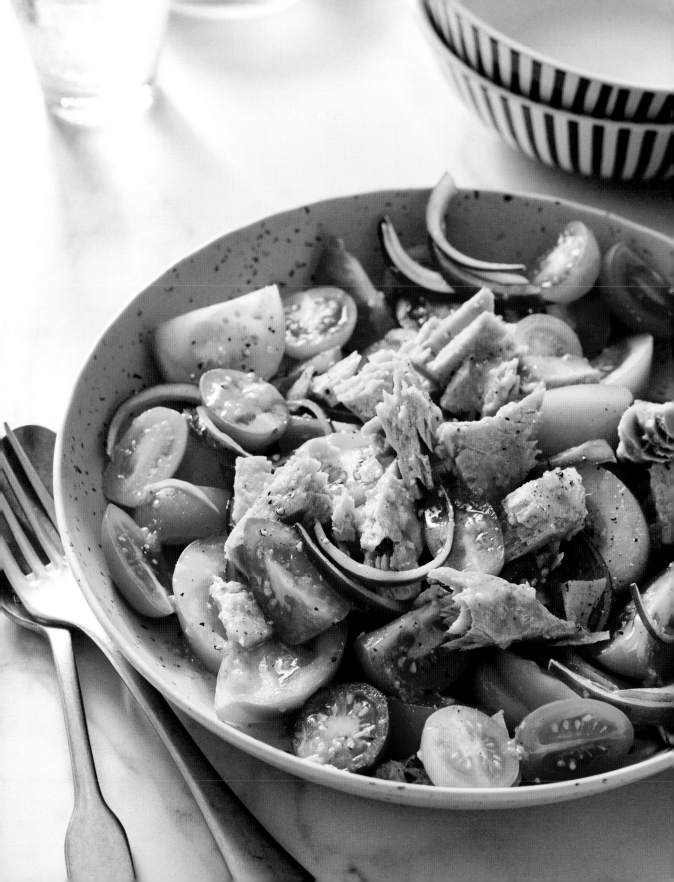

Arugula Salad

MAKES **4** SERVINGS | | CHEF JEFF

Arugula is my absolute favorite salad green and here's why: It's very nourishing to the liver, it's easy to add to any meal, and it showcases salad dressing nicely. Because arugula wilts relatively quickly, dress the leaves right before serving.

4 ounces (about 4 cups) arugula, rinsed and dried

½ cup sliced Parmigiano-Reggiano (slice into paper-thin strips with a veggie peeler)

½ cup Lemon Dressing (page 290)

1½ teaspoons kosher salt

1 tablespoon freshly ground black pepper

Combine the arugula in a large bowl with the Parmigiano-Reggiano cheese. Toss the dressing with the greens and cheese, allowing the cheese to break up into irregular pieces. Season the salad with the salt and pepper.

Tahini Kale Salad

MAKES 4 SERVINGS | CHEF JEFF

I love that Chef Jeff has used three different types of seeds in this salad. Seeds are a phenomenal food for supporting all your hormones. This salad makes a great addition to any of the meat recipes provided in this book for a satisfying meal during your power phases.

SALAD

1 bunch Lacinato kale (about 10 ounces, or 4 tightly packed cups), leaves stripped and coarsely chopped

Juice of ½ lemon

1 pinch kosher salt

¼ to ½ cup Tahini Dressing (page 289)

DUKKAH

2 tablespoons toasted pumpkin seeds

2 tablespoons toasted sunflower seeds

2 tablespoons toasted white sesame seeds

1 teaspoon ground sumac

1 teaspoon za'atar

½ teaspoon freshly ground black pepper

½ teaspoon kosher salt

TO MAKE THE SALAD Combine the kale, lemon juice, and salt in a large bowl. Add ¼ cup of the tahini dressing and toss until well combined. Add additional dressing if you like.

TO MAKE THE DUKKAH Combine the pumpkin seeds, sunflower seeds, sesame seeds, sumac, za'atar, pepper, and salt in a small bowl and toss until well mixed.

To serve, divide the salad between four plates and top each with some of the dukkah.

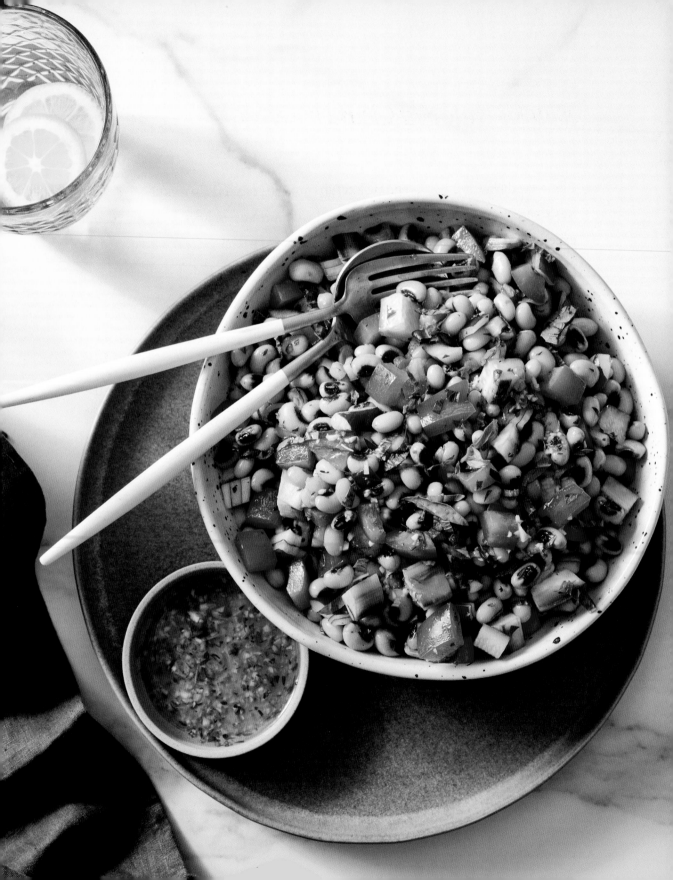

Black-Eyed Pea Crunch Salad

MAKES 4 TO 6 SERVINGS | | CHEF LESLIE

Black-eyed peas are a fun legume known to support weight loss, improve heart health and a healthy microbiome, and provide an incredible protein punch and excellent fiber. They also taste good and look pretty too!

BLACK-EYED PEAS

1½ cups dry black-eyed peas, picked through for stones

DRESSING

½ cup extra-virgin olive oil

Zest and juice of 1 lemon

1 teaspoon dried oregano

1 teaspoon maple syrup

½ teaspoon kosher salt

1 garlic clove, minced

SALAD

1 cup peeled, seeded, and chopped cucumber

⅔ cup chopped red onion

½ cup chopped red bell pepper

2 tablespoons chopped fresh basil

2 tablespoons chopped fresh Italian parsley

2 tablespoons chopped fresh mint

Kosher salt and freshly ground black pepper

TO MAKE THE BLACK-EYED PEAS Combine the black-eyed peas and 5 cups of water in a large bowl and soak overnight.

The next day, drain and rinse the black-eyed peas and transfer them to a large pot. Cover them with water and bring to a boil over high heat. Boil for 5 minutes, then decrease the heat and simmer until the black-eyed peas are tender, 20 to 30 minutes.

Drain and rinse the black-eyed peas in cool water. Set aside.

TO MAKE THE DRESSING Whisk together the olive oil, lemon zest and juice, oregano, maple syrup, salt, and garlic in a small bowl and set aside.

TO MAKE THE SALAD Combine the black-eyed peas, cucumber, onion, bell pepper, basil, parsley, and mint in a large bowl.

Add the dressing and toss until well mixed. Taste and season with salt and pepper.

This salad is terrific served at room temperature or chilled. Will keep in the fridge for up to 4 days.

Avocado and Brazil Nut Salad

MAKES 1 SERVING | | CHEF LESLIE

Brazil nuts are incredible for thyroid health—only six Brazil nuts a day are needed to support a healthy thyroid. The added seeds in this salad support hormone production, making this meal an endocrine-system dream.

DRESSING

1 tablespoon extra-virgin olive oil

1 teaspoon freshly squeezed lemon juice

1 pinch kosher salt

1 pinch freshly ground black pepper

SALAD

1 cup baby kale or baby spinach

½ medium avocado, sliced lengthwise

4 to 6 almonds, chopped

1 to 3 Brazil nuts, chopped

1 teaspoon pepitas

1 teaspoon chopped fresh parsley

1 teaspoon chopped fresh dill

½ teaspoon sunflower seeds

TO MAKE THE DRESSING Whisk together the olive oil, lemon juice, salt, and pepper in a small bowl and set aside.

TO MAKE THE SALAD Arrange the kale on a small plate or in a bowl. Top with the sliced avocado, almonds, Brazil nuts, pepitas, parsley, dill, and sunflower seeds.

Drizzle with the dressing and serve.

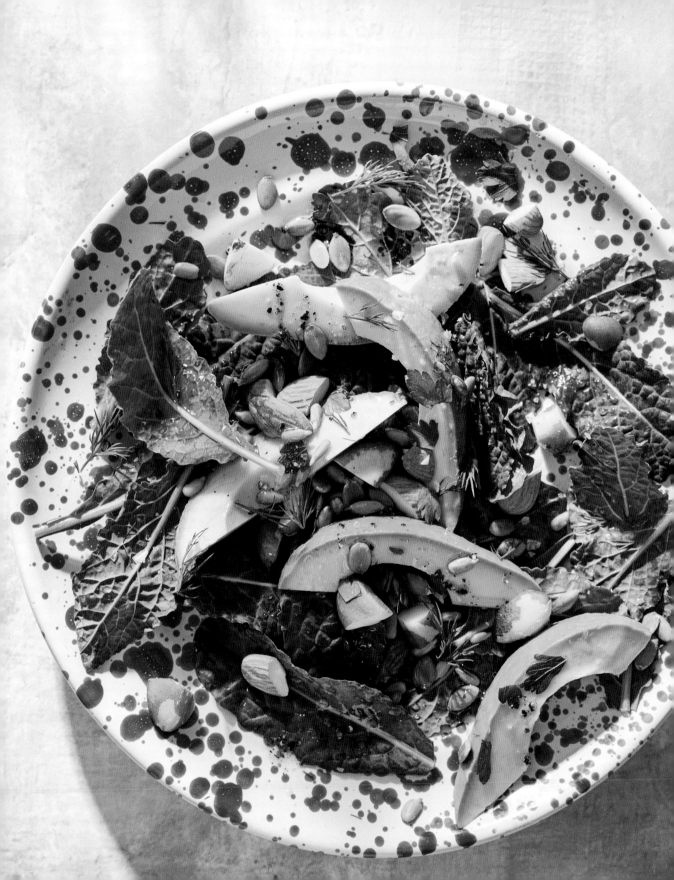

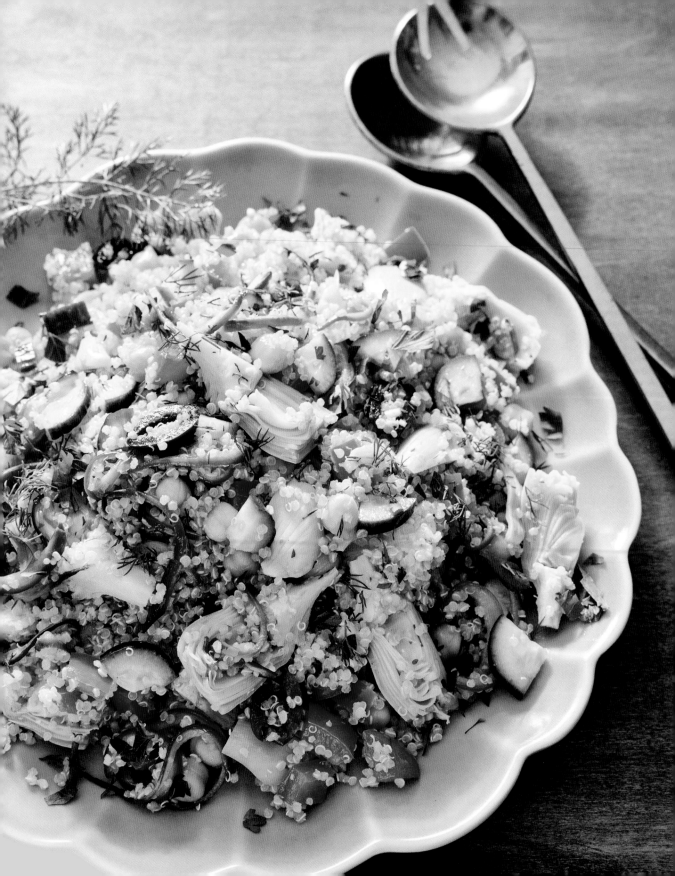

Mediterranean Quinoa Salad

MAKES 6 SERVINGS | | CHEF LESLIE

I use quinoa all the time to replace rice. It triggers a lower glucose response and is packed with protein. Artichoke hearts are a great prebiotic, whereas kalamata olives are an incredible polyphenol food. Make sure your artichoke hearts and olives are packed in water or olive oil, not canola oil.

SALAD

1 cup dry quinoa, rinsed
1 red bell pepper, seeded and diced
½ cup sliced red onion, cut into medium julienne
Extra-virgin olive oil
Kosher salt
One 15-ounce can chickpeas, drained
One 15-ounce can artichoke hearts, packed in water, drained
½ cup diced cucumber
½ cup halved and pitted kalamata olives
¼ cup minced fresh dill
¼ cup minced fresh parsley

VINAIGRETTE

¼ cup extra-virgin olive oil
2 tablespoons lemon juice
2 tablespoons red wine vinegar
1 teaspoon dried oregano
1 garlic clove, finely minced

TO MAKE THE SALAD Preheat the oven to 400°F. Line a baking sheet with parchment paper.

Bring 2 cups of water to a boil in a medium pot over high heat. Add the quinoa, cover, and decrease the heat to medium-low. Let it simmer for 15 minutes, or until the quinoa has absorbed all the water. Remove from the heat and let sit for 5 minutes with the lid on. Fluff with a fork and set aside.

Arrange the bell pepper and onion on the prepared baking sheet. Drizzle the veggies with olive oil and sprinkle with salt.

Roast for 15 minutes, or until the veggies are soft. Set aside.

TO MAKE THE VINAIGRETTE Whisk together the olive oil, lemon juice, red wine vinegar, oregano, and garlic in a small bowl until thoroughly combined.

TO ASSEMBLE THE SALAD Combine the quinoa, roasted veggies, chickpeas, artichoke hearts, cucumber, olives, dill, and parsley in a large bowl. Add as much vinaigrette as you like and toss until well mixed.

Kimchi Edamame Bowl

MAKES 1 SERVING | CHEF LESLIE

This is a great recipe on the days you need a little more estrogen, as the edamame gives you a dose of nature's estrogen. It's perfect for my menopausal friends who are experiencing signs of low estrogen, like hot flashes, brain fog, joint pain, or migraines.

DRESSING
2 tablespoons coconut aminos
2 tablespoons extra-virgin olive oil
1 tablespoon grated fresh ginger
1 teaspoon freshly squeezed lime juice

BOWL
1 cup dry quinoa, rinsed
1 cup edamame, thawed if frozen
1 cup diced cucumber
½ cup diced store-bought baked tofu
½ cup thinly sliced purple cabbage
½ medium avocado, sliced
½ cup vegan kimchi
1 sheet nori, cut into strips

TO MAKE THE DRESSING Whisk together the coconut aminos, olive oil, ginger, and lime juice in a small bowl.

TO MAKE THE BOWL Bring 2 cups of water to a boil in a medium pot over high heat. Add the quinoa, cover, and decrease the heat to medium-low. Let it simmer for 15 minutes, or until the quinoa has absorbed all the water. Remove from the heat, let it sit 5 minutes with the lid on, fluff with a fork, and set aside.

To serve, scoop 1 to 2 cups of quinoa into a bowl. Arrange the edamame, cucumber, baked tofu, cabbage, avocado, kimchi, and nori in wedges around the bowl and drizzle with the dressing.

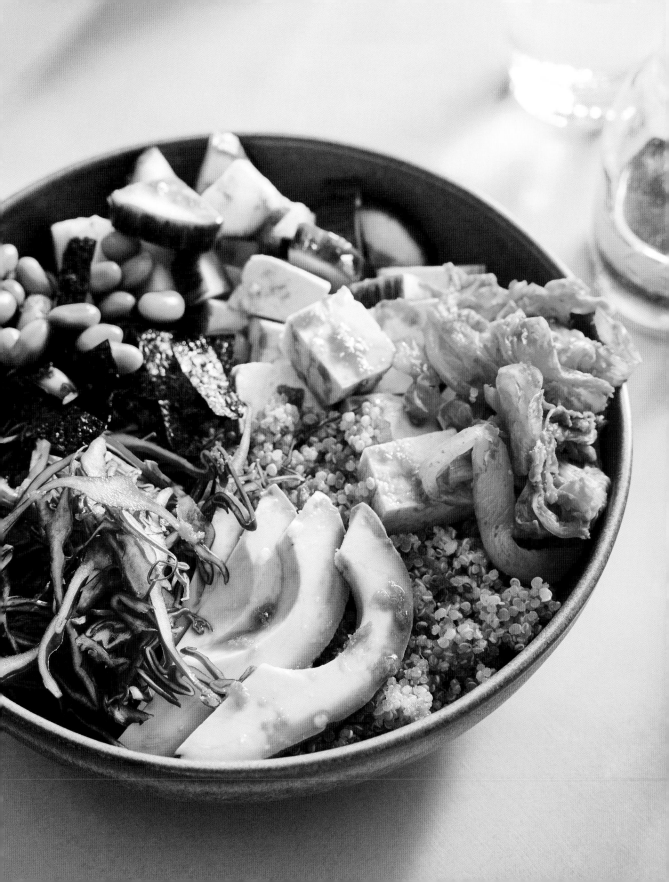

Cauliflower Rice Bowl

MAKES 2 SERVINGS | CHEF LESLIE

Cauliflower rice is a fun twist on regular rice that many lean into when they want a lower glucose response. If you love rice and are looking for a good alternative, give cauliflower rice a try.

TAHINI DRESSING
2 tablespoons tahini
2 tablespoons freshly squeezed lemon juice
½ teaspoon kosher salt
¼ teaspoon garlic powder
¼ teaspoon freshly ground black pepper

BOWL
3 tablespoons tamari
1 tablespoon nutritional yeast
½ teaspoon kosher salt
¼ teaspoon garlic powder
7 ounces firm tofu, cubed
2 tablespoons extra-virgin olive oil, divided
3 cups torn Swiss chard leaves (3-inch pieces)
1 garlic clove, thinly sliced
4 ounces cremini mushrooms, sliced
2 cups hot cooked cauliflower rice, prepared according to the package directions
1 avocado, diced
1 tablespoon hemp seeds
8 cherry tomatoes, halved

TO MAKE THE DRESSING Whisk together 1 teaspoon of water, the tahini, lemon juice, salt, garlic powder, and pepper. Add a bit more water if you need to thin it out. Set aside.

TO ASSEMBLE THE BOWL Preheat the oven to 400°F. Line a baking sheet with parchment paper.

Whisk together the tamari, nutritional yeast, salt, and garlic powder in a medium bowl until thoroughly combined. Add 1 teaspoon of water, if needed, to thin the dressing. Add the tofu and toss until it is well coated with the dressing.

Spray the parchment paper with avocado oil nonstick cooking spray and arrange the tofu on the prepared baking sheet. Bake for 15 minutes, or until the tofu turns golden brown. Set aside.

Heat 1 tablespoon of the olive oil in a medium skillet over medium heat. Add the Swiss chard and garlic and cook until the chard is wilted, about 1 minute. Transfer to a bowl.

Add the remaining 1 tablespoon of olive oil to the same skillet over medium heat. Add the mushrooms and sauté until they become soft, about 5 minutes.

TO SERVE Spoon the cooked cauliflower rice into a bowl. Top with the Swiss chard, mushrooms, baked tofu, and avocado in individual sections. Sprinkle with the hemp seeds, add the cherry tomatoes, and drizzle with tahini dressing.

Quinoa Tabbouleh and Grilled Tofu

MAKES 4 SERVINGS | CHEF LESLIE

I've recently brought tofu back into my life, and what I love about it is that it not only provides a phytoestrogen burst, but also absorbs all the flavors you put it with. This recipe is spectacular for your power phases because of the added edamame and the protein boost from the quinoa.

TABBOULEH

1 cup dry quinoa, rinsed

3 cups chopped fresh curly parsley

½ cup pre-cooked edamame, thawed if frozen

¼ cup hemp seeds

2 Roma tomatoes, diced

3 green onions, green and white parts chopped

4 tablespoons extra-virgin olive oil

3 tablespoons chopped fresh mint

Juice of 1 lemon

Kosher salt and freshly ground black pepper

TOFU

2 14-ounce packages extra-firm tofu

2 tablespoons tamari

1 pinch kosher salt

4 tablespoons avocado oil

TO MAKE THE TABBOULEH Bring 2 cups of water to a boil in a medium pot over high heat. Add the quinoa, cover, and decrease the heat to medium-low. Let it simmer for 15 minutes, or until the quinoa has absorbed all the water. Remove from the heat and let sit for 5 minutes with the lid on. Fluff with a fork.

Combine the parsley, quinoa, edamame, hemp seeds, tomatoes, green onions, olive oil, mint, and lemon juice in a large bowl and mix well. Season with salt and pepper, cover, and refrigerate.

TO MAKE THE TOFU Wrap the tofu in paper towels or a kitchen towel, add a weight on top, and let sit for 30 minutes. Drain. Preheat a grill or a grill pan to medium-high heat.

Cut each block of tofu lengthwise into quarters. Sprinkle both sides with tamari and salt.

Brush the grill or grill pan with the avocado oil and place the tofu directly on the hot oiled surface. Grill for 3 minutes. Using tongs, flip the tofu. If it sticks to the grill, let it cook a little longer. Once it releases easily, flip the tofu and grill until the second side releases easily, about 3 minutes. Both sides should have grill marks.

Spoon tabbouleh into bowls and top with the tofu.

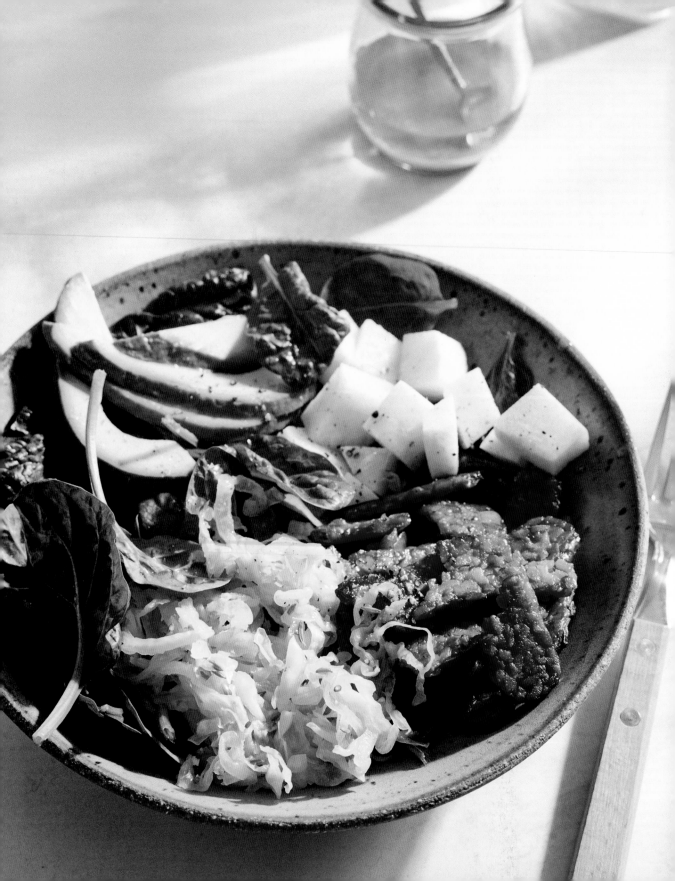

Probiotic Bowl

MAKES 1 SERVING | CHEF LESLIE

This recipe is a massive gift to your gut microbiome. I recommend having this dish at the end of Power Phase 1, right before you enter your manifestation stage, when your gut microbiome is important for breaking down hormones. If you're going through perimenopause and are experimenting with bioidentical hormones, this meal is a good partner in helping you get those hormones to your cells.

SAUERKRAUT DRESSING

1 tablespoon extra-virgin olive oil

1 tablespoon sauerkraut liquid

½ teaspoon Dijon mustard

¼ teaspoon monk fruit sweetener

TEMPEH

3 tablespoons coconut oil

4 ounces smoky tempeh, cut into bite-size cubes

BOWL

2 cups baby spinach

½ cup Turmeric Sauerkraut (page 282) or store-bought sauerkraut with 1 pinch grated turmeric added

½ medium avocado, diced

¼ cup diced fresh jicama

TO MAKE THE SAUERKRAUT DRESSING Whisk together the olive oil, sauerkraut liquid, mustard, and monk fruit sweetener in a small bowl. If the mixture is too thick, add 1 teaspoon of water and whisk well.

TO MAKE THE TEMPEH Heat the coconut oil in a frying pan over medium-high heat. When the oil is hot, add the tempeh. Sear the tempeh until it turns golden, 3 to 5 minutes on each side.

TO ASSEMBLE THE BOWL Put the spinach in a bowl and arrange the tempeh, turmeric sauerkraut, avocado, and jicama in separate sections on top. Drizzle with the sauerkraut dressing.

Spinach, Kale, and Goat Cheese Frittata

MAKES 2 TO 4 SERVINGS | CHEF JEFF

Goat cheese is often thought of as adding a unique taste to any dish, but I like that it's an easily digested form of dairy. You may even consider using goat's whole milk and heavy cream in this dish. Frittatas are very versatile, so feel free to swap out the veggies or cheeses listed here and add your own favorites. Serve this creamy frittata with leaves of radicchio or our Arugula Salad on page 210.

2 tablespoons whole milk

2 teaspoons white miso

6 large eggs

2 tablespoons heavy cream

2 tablespoons grated Parmigiano-Reggiano cheese

Kosher salt

1 teaspoon ground white pepper

Zest of ½ lemon

½ cup crumbled goat cheese

2 tablespoons extra-virgin olive oil

¼ medium white, yellow, or red onion, cut into thin julienne

1 medium leek, white and pale green parts only, thinly sliced (save the dark green parts for another use)

1 cup finely chopped curly green kale, leaves stripped from stems

1 cup coarsely chopped baby spinach

Preheat the oven to 400°F.

Whisk together the milk and miso in a medium bowl until smooth. Add the eggs, cream, Parmigiano-Reggiano cheese, 1 teaspoon of salt, pepper, and lemon zest and whisk until combined. Add the goat cheese, mix well, and set aside.

Heat the olive oil in a well-seasoned 8-inch oven-safe skillet over medium heat. Add the onion and leek; season them lightly with salt and cook, stirring often, until the onion softens and becomes translucent, about 8 minutes. (Decrease the heat to medium-low if the onion-leek mixture starts to brown too quickly.)

Add the kale and cook, stirring often, just until it starts to wilt and soften, about 2 minutes.

Add the spinach and stir to combine, then add the egg mixture. Stir the greens and eggs, gently shaking the skillet. Once the eggs are about halfway set, transfer the skillet to the oven and cook to your desired level of firmness, 6 to 8 minutes. (If you like, you can turn on the broiler and pop the frittata under the broiler to brown it a little.)

Let the frittata cool slightly before cutting it into wedges and serving it from the pan.

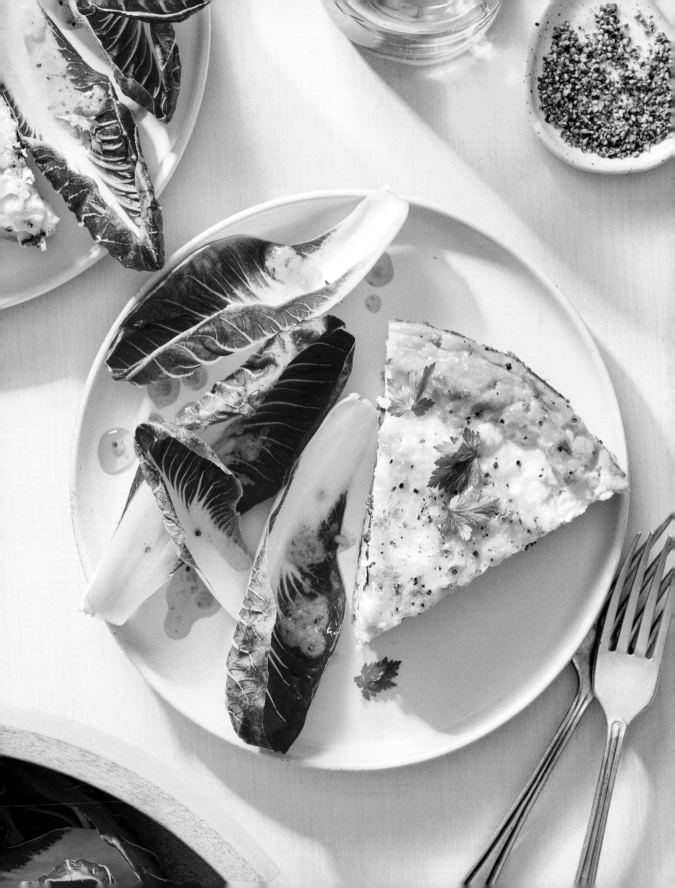

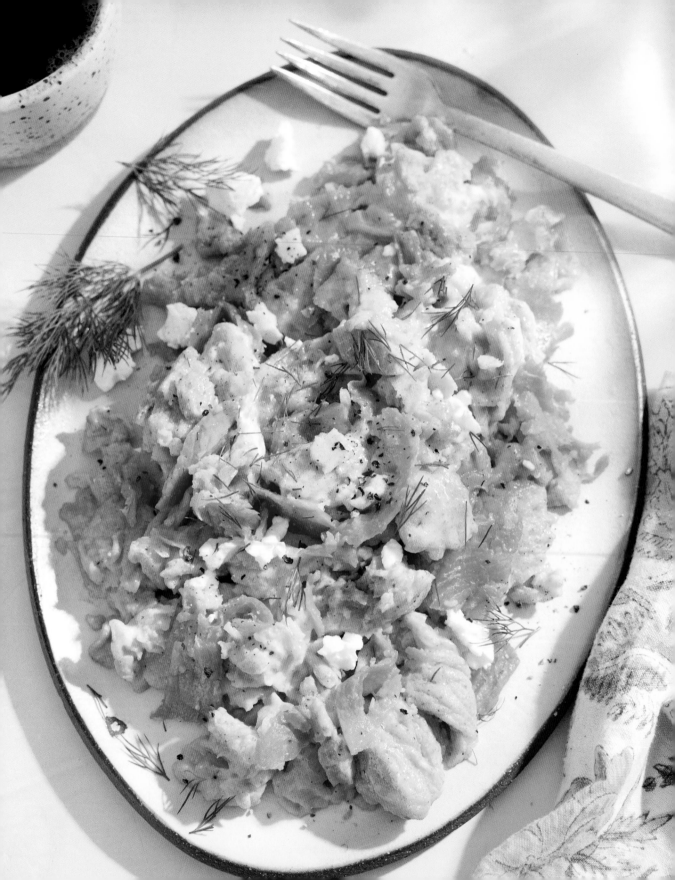

Turmeric Eggs with Smoked Salmon and Goat Cheese

MAKES 2 TO 4 SERVINGS | | CHEF JEFF

If you prefer to break your fast in the morning, I highly recommend using this as your first meal to open up your eating window during your ketobiotic days. The turmeric is great as an anti-inflammatory, and the salmon provides a good dose of omega-3s.

8 large eggs
1 teaspoon ground turmeric
1 teaspoon kosher salt
1 teaspoon freshly ground black pepper
2 tablespoons unsalted butter, cut into cubes
3 ounces smoked salmon, cut into strips
6 tablespoons crumbled goat cheese
3 sprigs dill (including tender stems), coarsely chopped

Combine the eggs, turmeric, salt, and pepper in a medium bowl and whisk until well combined. Set aside.

Add the butter to a medium sauté pan over medium heat. As the butter melts, add the eggs. As the eggs start to cook, begin whisking the mixture; the goal is to break up the egg curds without browning or anything sticking to the bottom or sides of the pan.

When the eggs are about halfway set, switch to a rubber or silicone spatula and continue stirring until the eggs reach the consistency you prefer. Remove the pan from the heat, add the smoked salmon and goat cheese, and stir until combined.

Transfer the eggs to a platter, garnish with dill, and serve.

Turkish Eggs with Yogurt and Chili Brown Butter

MAKES 2 TO 4 SERVINGS | | CHEF JEFF

This pretty breakfast dish is a great twist on a fried egg! The chili brown butter is to die for, and the addition of Greek yogurt makes this a power protein meal, perfect for your muscle-building days.

YOGURT

1 cup plain full-fat Greek yogurt
2 garlic cloves, minced
1 tablespoon finely chopped fresh dill
1 tablespoon finely chopped fresh mint
½ teaspoon kosher salt
½ teaspoon freshly ground white pepper

CHILI BROWN BUTTER

2 tablespoons unsalted butter, cut into cubes
1½ teaspoons extra-virgin olive oil
1 teaspoon chili powder, such as Urfa biber, Aleppo, or ancho
¼ teaspoon cayenne pepper
Juice of ¼ lemon
Kosher salt

EGGS

4 eggs
8 tablespoons extra virgin olive oil
4 tablespoons unsalted butter
Sea salt, such as Maldon

TO MAKE THE YOGURT Combine the yogurt, garlic, dill, mint, salt, and white pepper in a small saucepan and set aside.

TO MAKE THE CHILI BROWN BUTTER Melt the butter in a small saucepan over medium-high heat. Cook until it starts to smell nutty and just begins to turn a light brown color, about 4 minutes.

Remove the pan from the heat and add the olive oil, chili powder, and cayenne pepper. The butter will bubble a little and then subside. Add the lemon juice and 1 pinch of salt and stir to combine. Set aside.

TO MAKE THE EGGS Heat a medium skillet over medium-high heat, and set up a plate with a paper towel for the cooked eggs. Crack each egg into a small ramekin, ensuring the yolk doesn't break. Once the skillet is heated, pour in 2 tablespoons of the olive oil, and tip the pan forward so the oil pools away from you. Slip the cracked egg into the oil, and allow it to fry for 10 seconds before laying the pan flat on the burner. Season the egg with salt and pepper.

Add 1 tablespoon butter to the pan, and allow it to foam and melt. If you would like, spoon some of the hot buttery oil over the egg, cooking it to your desired doneness.

Remove the egg to the prepared dish, and repeat for the remaining eggs.

To serve, gently warm the yogurt over low heat until it loses its chill. Spoon some of the yogurt onto each serving plate, then top it with some of the warm chili butter. Top each plate with an egg and a pinch of sea salt.

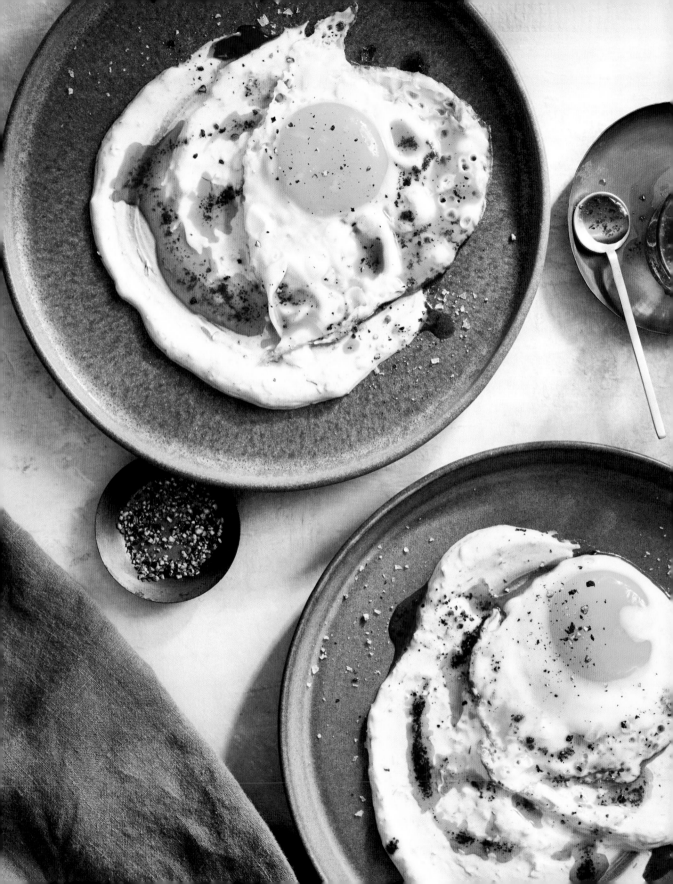

Soft Scrambled Eggs with Za'atar and Feta

MAKES 2 TO 4 SERVINGS | | CHEF JEFF

One thing I love about eggs is how dense they are in nutrients needed for healthy cartilage, organs, skin, muscles, and hair. Sheep's cheese is easier to digest than other dairy, making this an excellent break-fast meal on your ketobiotic days. Depending on how creamy you like your eggs, you can use milk or not.

8 large eggs
2 tablespoons whole milk
1 teaspoon kosher salt
2 tablespoons unsalted butter, cut into cubes
3 tablespoons crumbled sheep's milk feta
   (I like Valbreso)
1 tablespoon za'atar
1 tablespoon sumac
1 tablespoon extra-virgin olive oil

Beat the eggs with the milk and salt in a medium bowl. Pour the egg mixture into an unheated medium nonstick skillet, then turn on the heat to medium and add the butter. As the eggs start to cook, begin whisking the mixture; the goal is to break up the egg curds without browning or anything sticking to the bottom or sides of the skillet.

Once the eggs are about halfway set, switch to a rubber or silicone spatula and continue stirring until the eggs reach the consistency you like. Remove the skillet from the heat and keep stirring until the eggs are fully cooked.

Transfer the eggs to a platter and top with the feta, za'atar, and sumac. Drizzle with the olive oil and serve.

Tempeh and Broccoli with Forbidden Rice

MAKES 4 TO 6 SERVINGS | CHEF LESLIE

Tempeh is an incredible plant-based source of protein. It's high in phytoestrogens, so it's excellent for those of you going through the menopausal experience. This recipe is also good for your power phases because its combination of ingredients keeps your blood sugar very stable. The forbidden rice is higher in fiber than other types of rice, which is critical for helping you break down hormones.

¼ cup Functional Mushroom Broth (page 272)

2 tablespoons arrowroot powder

4 tablespoons avocado oil, divided

1 pound tempeh, cut into 1-inch cubes

6 cups broccoli, cut into ½-inch florets and stems

½ cup low-sodium tamari

4 garlic cloves, minced

One 2-inch piece fresh ginger, peeled and minced

Kosher salt and freshly ground black pepper

4 cups cooked forbidden rice, cooked according to package instructions

2 green onions, green and white parts thinly cut on the diagonal

Whisk together the mushroom broth and arrowroot powder in a small bowl to create a slurry. Set aside.

Heat 2 tablespoons of the avocado oil in a large skillet or wok over medium-high heat. Add the tempeh cubes and cook, stirring often, until they are golden and crisp, about 4 to 5 minutes for each side. Transfer the tempeh to a plate.

Add the remaining 2 tablespoons of avocado oil, the broccoli, and ¼ cup of water to the same skillet and cook until the liquid has evaporated and the broccoli is almost tender, 3 to 5 minutes.

Add the tempeh, tamari, garlic, ginger, and 1 pinch each of the salt and pepper to the skillet and stir to combine. Add the mushroom slurry, stir, and cook until the sauce is thickened and the broccoli is tender, about 3 minutes.

Serve in bowls over the forbidden rice and garnish with green onions.

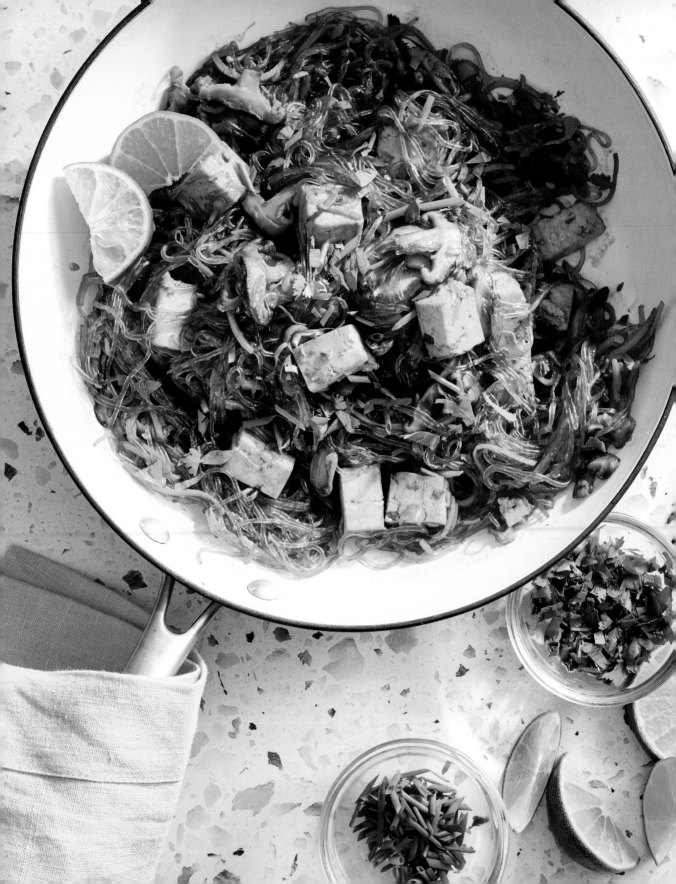

Kelp Noodle Pad Thai

MAKES 2 SERVINGS | | CHEF LESLIE

This fun twist on pad Thai swaps in kelp noodles, which are fantastic for your power phases. If you want to lessen your blood-sugar spike, you may dial back on the palm or brown sugar.

2 tablespoons Thai tamarind paste
2 tablespoons palm sugar or brown sugar
2 tablespoons tamari
1 pinch red pepper flakes (optional)
One 12-ounce package kelp noodles
¼ cup lemon juice
2 teaspoons baking soda
3 tablespoons coconut oil
1 cup sliced shiitake mushrooms
½ cup shredded carrots
1 shallot, chopped
3 garlic cloves, chopped
One 14- to 16-ounce package firm tofu,
    drained and cut into ½-inch cubes
1 cup fresh bean sprouts
1 cup fresh cilantro leaves
½ cup chopped fresh chives

Whisk together the tamarind paste, palm sugar, tamari, and red pepper flakes (if using) in a small bowl. Set aside.

Combine the kelp noodles, lemon juice, and baking soda in a bowl and massage the noodles with your hands. Rinse the noodles in water and set aside.

Heat the coconut oil in a wok or large frying pan over high heat. Add the mushrooms, carrots, shallot, garlic, and tofu. Cook until the garlic becomes golden, 3 to 5 minutes. Add the kelp noodles and tamarind sauce and toss until the sauce evenly coats everything.

To serve, top with the bean sprouts, cilantro, and chives.

Socca Pizza

MAKES ONE 10-INCH PIZZA | CHEF LESLIE

A pizza that is low carb?! Thank you, Chef Leslie! There are so many reasons I love this recipe, but perhaps the greatest is that it fits in perfectly with your power phases, when you are trying to minimize your blood-sugar spikes.

TOMATO SAUCE
1 tablespoon extra-virgin olive oil
3 garlic cloves, minced
One 14½-ounce can crushed tomatoes
6 to 8 fresh basil leaves

VEGAN BÉCHAMEL SAUCE
½ cup raw unsalted cashews
2 tablespoons nutritional yeast
2 teaspoons tapioca starch
½ teaspoon white miso paste
¼ teaspoon garlic powder
¼ teaspoon kosher salt

CRUST
1 cup chickpea flour
1 cup sparkling water
3 tablespoons extra-virgin olive oil, divided
1 pinch kosher salt

OPTIONAL TOPPINGS
Sliced onion
Sliced mushrooms
Baby spinach
Sliced garlic

TO MAKE THE TOMATO SAUCE Heat the olive oil in a medium pot over medium heat. Add the garlic and cook until it starts sizzling. Add the crushed tomatoes, decrease the heat to low, and simmer for 15 minutes. Right before using, stir in the fresh basil leaves.

TO MAKE THE BÉCHAMEL SAUCE Combine 1 cup water, the cashews, nutritional yeast, tapioca starch, miso paste, garlic powder, and salt in a blender and blend on high speed until smooth and pureed.

Pour the sauce into a small saucepan over medium heat and bring to a boil. Whisk constantly until the sauce thickens. Remove from the heat and set aside.

TO MAKE THE CRUST Place a 10-inch cast-iron skillet in the oven and preheat to 450°F.

Whisk together the chickpea flour, sparkling water, 2 tablespoons of the olive oil, and salt in a medium bowl until smooth. Place a tea towel over the bowl and let it rest for 20 to 30 minutes.

Carefully remove the cast-iron skillet from the oven and add the remaining olive oil to the skillet. Pour the batter into the skillet and bake until the crust is golden brown and crisp on the edges, 15 to 20 minutes.

Using a spatula, loosen the crust from the skillet and spread the top of it with tomato sauce. Dollop with spoonfuls of the béchamel sauce and top with your favorite veggies. Return the skillet to the oven and cook until the béchamel has lightly browned.

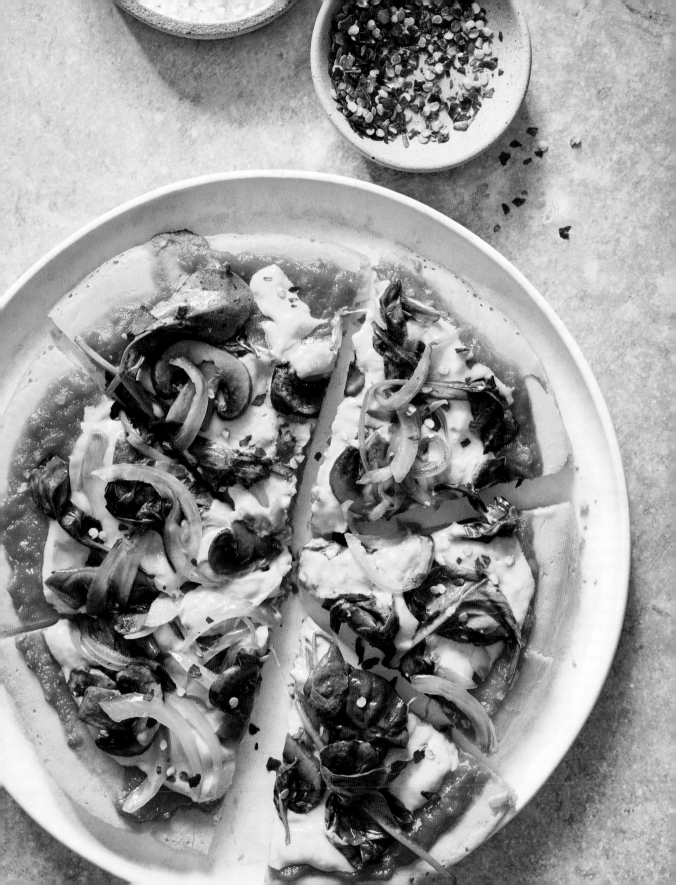

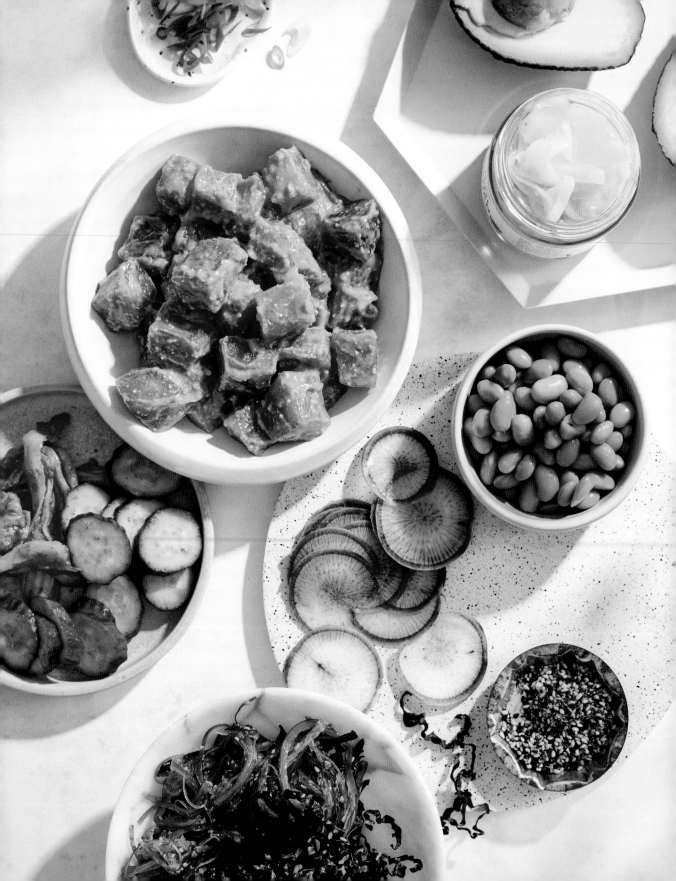

Miso and Ginger Poke Bowl

MAKES 4 SERVINGS | | CHEF JEFF

Who doesn't love a good poke? This refreshing meal provides tons of protein if you're trying to build muscle. Always look for fish that are wild, as they typically have more fatty acids and can be lower in toxins. Choose your favorite store-bought or homemade toppings to make this bowl your own.

MARINADE

¼ cup white or yellow miso

One 1-inch piece fresh ginger, peeled and chopped

1 large garlic clove

2 tablespoons toasted sesame oil

1 tablespoon tamari

1 tablespoon rice wine vinegar or white vinegar

1 tablespoon raw honey

1 tablespoon Sriracha sauce or Keto Chili Sauce (page 284)

Kosher salt

POKE

1 pound sushi-grade ahi tuna, salmon, or your favorite fish, cut into ½-inch cubes (see Note)

2 tablespoons Nori Komi furikake or sesame seeds

OPTIONAL TOPPINGS

2 cups chopped kale leaves

1 cup Keto Pickled Ginger (page 276) or store-bought

1 cup Korean-Style Pickled Cucumbers (page 275)

1 cup Pickled Daikon and Carrot Slaw (page 280)

1 cup kimchi

1 cup store-bought prepared seaweed salad

1 cup edamame

½ cup thinly sliced green onions, green and white parts

1 avocado, pitted, peeled, cut into quarters, and thinly sliced

Sriracha sauce, Miso Ginger Dressing (page 288), or Keto Chili Sauce (page 284)

TO MAKE THE MARINADE Combine the miso, ginger, garlic, sesame oil, tamari, rice wine vinegar, honey, Sriracha sauce, and salt to taste in a blender and blend on high speed until the marinade is a chunky paste. Taste and season with more salt as desired.

TO MAKE THE POKE Combine the marinade, furikake, and the fish in a large bowl and toss until the poke is well coated. Add your preferred toppings. Enjoy immediately.

NOTE Fish that is served raw is almost always frozen for a specific period of time and at a specific temperature to kill parasites and other baddies that might cause you problems. This is a law from the FDA Food Code that many sushi bars and most poke joints must follow, even if it's not talked about. If you buy fish labeled "sushi grade," it has likely undergone this process and is safe to eat raw. If you buy fresh fish or catch your own, take a look at the recommended flash-freezing guides to decide how you would like to proceed.

Salmon with Furikake

MAKES 4 SERVINGS | CHEF JEFF

Salmon is an interesting protein source because, if you choose the right type, you can get a very nutrient-dense experience. Always look for wild salmon as it contains far more healthy fatty acids than farmed fish. Chef Jeff loves to serve this dish alongside Korean pickled cucumbers.

Kosher salt

2 teaspoons coconut sugar

4 wild salmon fillets, 4 to 6 ounces each, skin and pin bones removed

2 tablespoons raw honey

2 tablespoons Dijon mustard

2 tablespoons extra-virgin olive oil, divided

1 tablespoon furikake (preferably Nori Komi) or toasted sesame seeds

Korean-Style Pickled Cucumbers (page 275; optional)

Combine 2 teaspoons of salt and the coconut sugar in a small bowl.

Place the salmon fillets on a plate and sprinkle them generously with the salt-sugar mixture. Refrigerate the salmon for at least 1 hour and up to 4 hours.

Remove the salmon from the refrigerator before cooking to allow the fish to come to room temperature. Rinse off the salmon, pat dry, and set aside for 30 minutes.

Mix the honey and mustard together in a small bowl and set aside.

Preheat the oven to the highest broil setting and place the rack on the top shelf. Meanwhile, brush a large sheet pan with 1 tablespoon of olive oil.

Place the salmon on the prepared sheet pan, skinned side down, and rub it with the remaining 1 tablespoon of olive oil.

Broil until the salmon turns pink and is mostly cooked through, 5 to 6 minutes, depending on the thickness of the fillets.

Remove the sheet pan from the oven and, using a spoon, smear the honey-mustard mixture all over the top of the fillets, dividing it evenly. Broil until this glaze has baked on and is slightly toasted, 1 to 2 minutes.

Remove the salmon from the oven and immediately sprinkle liberally with the furikake.

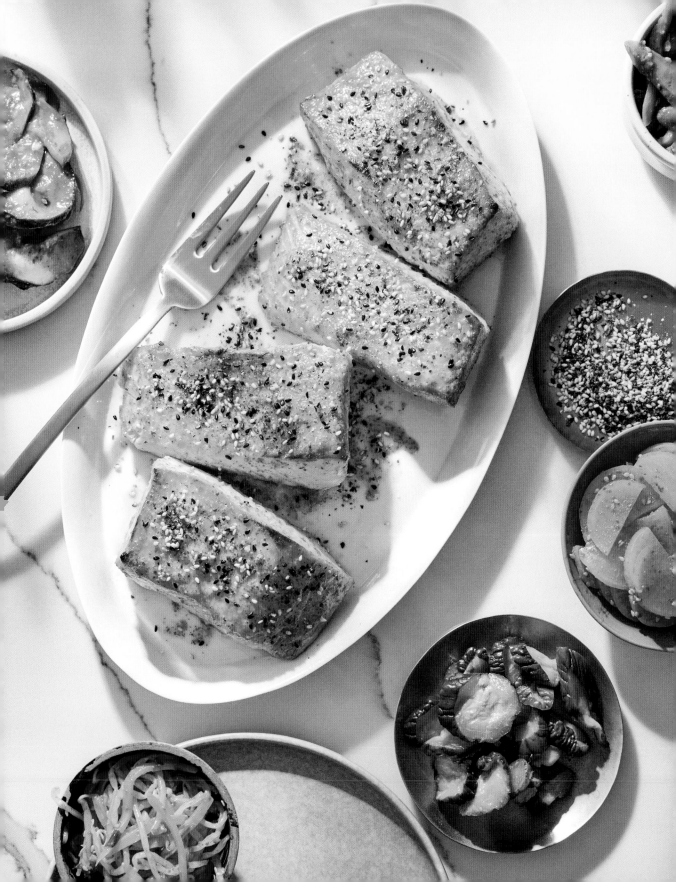

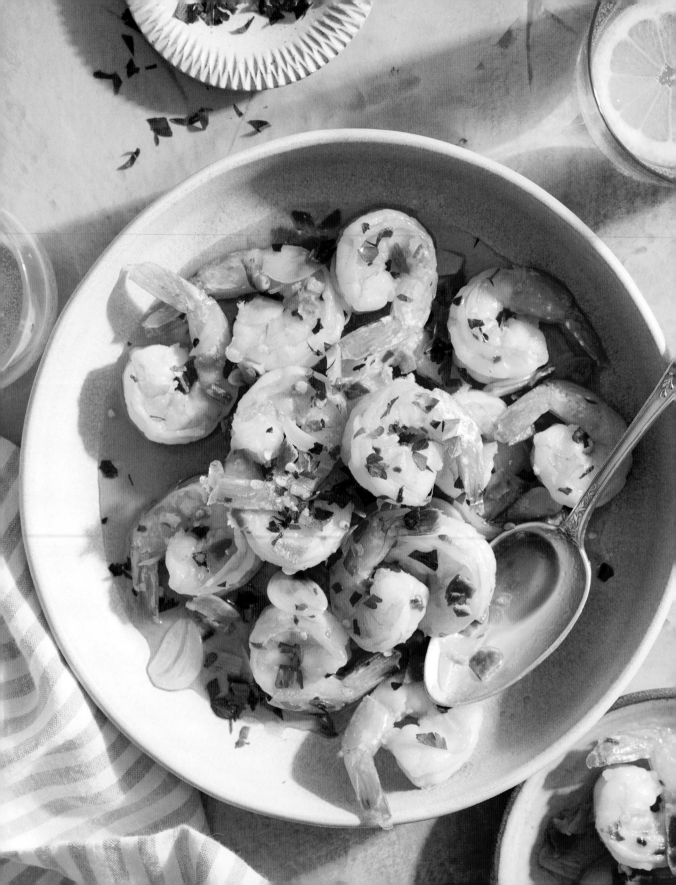

Spanish Garlic Shrimp

MAKES 4 SERVINGS | | CHEF JEFF

This is a great power protein recipe—perfect if you are trying to build more muscle or just looking for more foods with a high amino acid profile. I love all the garlic Chef Jeff put in this recipe, both because it's delicious and because it supports your immune system and provides your gut microbes with a healthy treat. Chef Jeff recommends having your ingredients ready to go before you start cooking because this dish moves quickly.

½ cup extra-virgin olive oil

Kosher salt

15 garlic cloves, thinly sliced into paper-thin rounds

1 chile de árbol, seeded and minced, or 1 teaspoon red pepper flakes

¼ cup cured ham, such as jamón ibérico, minced (optional)

1 pound extra-large (26/30) shrimp, peeled and deveined

Juice of 1 lemon

1 tablespoon unsalted butter

¼ cup coarsely chopped Italian parsley

Sea salt, such as Maldon

Heat the olive oil and 1 teaspoon of salt in a medium skillet over medium heat until the oil just begins to smoke. Carefully add the garlic; it will immediately begin to sizzle. Immediately add the chile and cured ham (if using) and stir until combined. Add the shrimp and stir them around in the hot oil until they turn a light pink, 2 to 3 minutes. Remove the skillet from the heat.

Add the lemon juice and stir to combine. Add the butter and gently shake and swirl the skillet to emulsify the butter into the sauce. Taste and season the shrimp with more kosher salt as desired.

To serve, spoon the shrimp and sauce into shallow bowls; top with the parsley and a sprinkling of sea salt.

Lemongrass Chicken

MAKES 4 SERVINGS | | CHEF JEFF

I love the taste of lemongrass mixed with ginger in this protein-dense meal. This recipe is ideal for your power phases and makes great use of avocado oil, one of the healthiest anti-inflammatory fats.

MARINADE

½ small yellow onion, chopped

2 lemongrass stalks, white base only, thinly sliced

3 large garlic cloves

3 tablespoons coconut sugar

3 tablespoons avocado oil

2 tablespoons peeled, chopped fresh ginger

1½ tablespoons fish sauce

1½ tablespoons tamari

Juice of 3 limes

2 teaspoons freshly ground black pepper

Kosher salt

CHICKEN

4 large boneless, skinless chicken thighs (about 1½ pounds total), or 4 small boneless, skinless chicken breasts (about 1½ pounds total)

Kosher salt and freshly ground black pepper

1 lime, cut in half

DIPPING SAUCE

2 tablespoons coconut sugar

2 tablespoons fish sauce

Zest and juice of 2 limes

1 garlic clove, minced

1 small chili pepper (ideally a Thai bird's eye, Fresno, or jalapeño pepper), seeded and minced (optional)

TO MAKE THE MARINADE Combine the onion, lemongrass, garlic, coconut sugar, avocado oil, ginger, fish sauce, tamari, lime juice, black pepper, and 1½ teaspoons of salt in a food processor and process on high speed until the marinade becomes a chunky puree. Taste the marinade and season with more salt as desired.

TO MAKE THE CHICKEN Place the chicken in a large nonreactive bowl with a lid or a large ziploc plastic bag and pour the marinade over the chicken. Turn the chicken in the bowl or seal the bag and turn over a few times to coat the chicken in the marinade. Cover the bowl or seal the bag and refrigerate for 2 hours or up to overnight.

Take the chicken out of the refrigerator 1 hour ahead of cooking to allow it to come to room temperature. Remove the chicken from the marinade, season it with salt and pepper, and set aside.

CONTINUED ▶

Lemongrass Chicken
CONTINUED

TO MAKE THE DIPPING SAUCE Combine ¼ cup of water, the coconut sugar, fish sauce, lime zest and juice, garlic, and the pepper (if using) in a small bowl and mix well. Taste the sauce and season with more lime as desired. Set aside.

TO GRILL Preheat a grill to high heat, ideally with a hotter side to sear the chicken and a cooler side to finish cooking. Set a platter alongside the grill to hold the cooked chicken.

Place the chicken on the hotter side of the grill. If your grill has a cover, close it and allow the chicken to get a good sear on the first side, about 4 minutes. Flip the chicken, sear for another 2 minutes, then move it to the lower heat side. Continue cooking until an instant-read thermometer inserted in the thickest part registers an internal temperature of 160°F, 4 to 6 minutes longer. Transfer the chicken to the platter. As the chicken sits, it will reach the recommended 165°F.

Squeeze the lime over the chicken. Cut the chicken into slices and drizzle with some of the dipping sauce.

TO OVEN-ROAST Preheat the oven to 425°F.

Place the chicken onto a sheet pan without crowding the pieces and bake for 30 to 40 minutes, depending on the size of the chicken, or until an instant-read thermometer inserted in the thickest part registers an internal temperature of 160°F. Transfer the chicken to the platter. As the chicken sits, it will reach the recommended 165°F.

Squeeze the lime over the chicken. Cut the chicken into slices and drizzle with some of the dipping sauce.

Miso-Marinated Grilled Pork

MAKES 4 SERVINGS | | CHEF JEFF

Pork is a beneficial meat because it contains a powerful combination of iron, selenium, vitamin B12, zinc, and magnesium—key nutrients you need to make hormones. It's also very dense in protein; one steak provides 43 grams. Chef Jeff specifically recommends ibérico pork because of its high monounsaturated fat content, but if you can't find it, boneless pork loin chops will work in a pinch.

MARINADE

½ medium white, yellow, or red onion, coarsely chopped

1 medium carrot, peeled and coarsely chopped

5 large garlic cloves, coarsely chopped

One 1½-inch piece fresh ginger, peeled and chopped

½ cup white or yellow miso

Freshly ground black pepper

PORK

4 ibérico pork steaks (look for secreto, loin chops, blade steaks, or another grilling cut)

Kosher salt and freshly ground black pepper

1 lemon, cut in half

Sea salt, such as Maldon

Extra-virgin olive oil (if pan-searing)

TO MAKE THE MARINADE Combine the onion, carrot, garlic, ginger, miso, and 1 teaspoon of pepper in a mini food processor and process on high speed, scraping down the mixture from the sides of the processor once or twice, until the marinade becomes a thick, chunky paste. Taste the marinade and season with more pepper as desired.

TO MAKE THE PORK Place the pork in a shallow baking dish and, using a spatula, spread the marinade all over the meat. Cover and refrigerate for at least 4 hours or up to overnight.

Take the pork out of the refrigerator 1 hour ahead of cooking to allow the meat to come to room temperature. Remove the pork from the marinade and scrape off the excess. Season the pork with salt and pepper and set aside.

TO GRILL Preheat a grill to medium-high heat (about 400°F), ideally with a hotter side to sear the pork and a cooler side to finish cooking. Set a platter alongside the grill to hold the cooked pork.

CONTINUED ▶

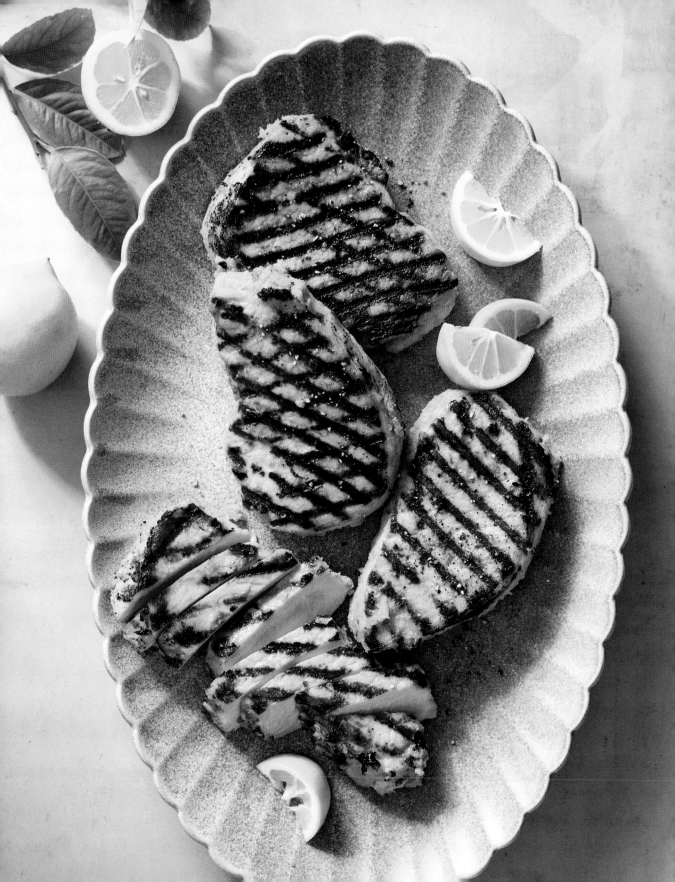

Miso-Marinated Grilled Pork

CONTINUED

Place the pork on the hotter side of the grill and cook, turning once, until it is seared and grill-marked on both sides, about 10 minutes. Move the pork to the cooler side of the grill and continue cooking until an instant-read thermometer inserted in the thickest part registers an internal temperature of 140°F, 3 to 5 minutes longer. Transfer the pork to the platter. As the pork sits, it will reach the recommended 145°F.

Squeeze the lemon over the pork. Cut the pork into slices against the grain and season with sea salt and a few grinds of pepper before serving.

TO PAN-SEAR Place a sheet pan in the oven and preheat to 425°F. Get a platter ready for the cooked pork.

Heat a large sauté pan over medium-high heat. When the pan is hot, add 2 to 3 tablespoons of olive oil and 1 or 2 pieces of pork, or whatever will fit without crowding. Cook the pork until a crust forms on one side, 5 to 8 minutes. Flip over the pork and repeat on the other side, cooking for about 5 more minutes. Transfer the pork to the sheet pan in the oven and brush the meat with olive oil. If you're searing the pork in batches, pour off the oil in the sauté pan, wipe the pan with a paper towel, and repeat the process for the remaining pork, placing the cooked pork onto the sheet pan.

Bake for 5 to 7 minutes, or until the pork is cooked through and an instant-read thermometer inserted in the thickest part registers an internal temperature of 140°F. Transfer the pork to the platter. As the pork sits, it will reach the recommended 145°F.

Squeeze the lemon over the pork and season with sea salt and a few grinds of pepper before serving.

NOTE This recipe works great with almost any of the marinades or dressings in this book (see Pantry, page 265).

The recommended temperature to cook pork has been lowered in recent years, so we no longer need to overcook pork at 160°F. This is especially true with Ibérico pork, which is typically treated more like a steak and is best served medium-rare—just like a steak.

Greek Lamb T-Bones with Whipped Feta

MAKES 4 SERVINGS | | CHEF JEFF

In my family, we like to diversify our red meat sources, and lamb is one of our favorite go-tos. I encourage you to get grass-fed lamb. There are 26 grams of protein in just one lamb chop. Red meats generally give you the densest amino acid profile.

WHIPPED FETA

8 ounces sheep's milk feta in brine, brine reserved
Zest of 1 lemon
2 tablespoons extra-virgin olive oil
Freshly ground black pepper

MARINADE

¼ cup extra-virgin olive oil
¼ cup lemon juice
¼ cup feta brine, reserved from the whipped feta
2 teaspoons dried oregano
2 teaspoons red pepper flakes

LAMB

8 lamb loin (T-bone) chops, each about 1 inch thick (about 2 pounds total weight; about 2 meaty chops per person)
Kosher salt and freshly ground black pepper
Juice of 1 lemon
Extra-virgin olive oil
Chopped fresh parsley

TO MAKE THE WHIPPED FETA Combine the feta, lemon zest, olive oil, and black pepper in a mini food processor, along with a splash of the reserved feta brine, and process until it reaches a creamy, smooth consistency. You may need to scrape down the sides of the processor a few times to get all the feta incorporated into the mixture. Taste and season the whipped feta with more black pepper as desired. Set aside.

TO MAKE THE MARINADE Combine the olive oil, lemon juice, feta brine, oregano, and red pepper flakes in a small bowl. Set aside.

TO MAKE THE LAMB Place the lamb T-bones in a large nonreactive bowl with a lid or a large ziplock plastic bag and pour the marinade over the meat. Turn the lamb in the bowl or seal the bag and turn over a few times to coat the lamb in the marinade. Refrigerate for at least 4 hours or up to 48 hours.

CONTINUED ▶

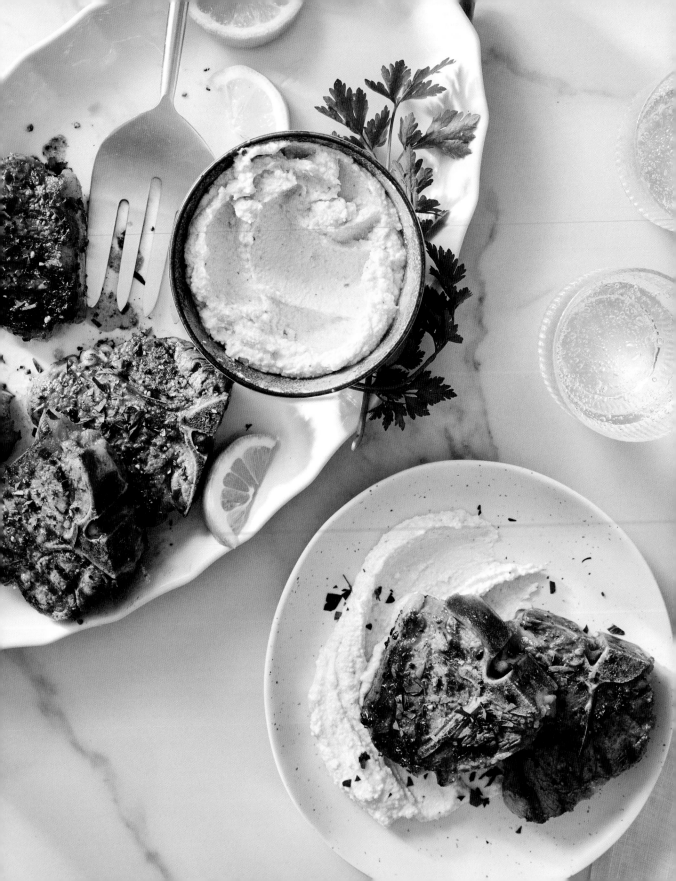

Greek Lamb T-Bones with Whipped Feta
CONTINUED

Take the lamb out of the refrigerator 1 hour ahead of cooking to allow the meat to come to room temperature. Remove the lamb from the marinade and discard the marinade. Season the lamb with salt and pepper and set aside.

TO GRILL Preheat a grill to high heat (about 300°F), ideally with a hotter side to sear the lamb and a cooler side to finish cooking. Set a platter alongside the grill to hold the cooked lamb.

Place the lamb on the hotter side of the grill. If your grill has a cover, close it and allow the lamb to get a good sear on the first side, about 5 minutes. (If you want to get fancy, at about the 4-minute mark, give the lamb a 45-degree turn to create crosshatch marks.) Once it is ready, flip the lamb and move it to the lower heat side. Continue cooking until an instant-read thermometer inserted in the thickest part registers an internal tempera-ture of 130°F for medium-rare or 135°F for medium, 4 to 5 minutes longer. Transfer the lamb to the platter.

To serve, drizzle the lamb with lemon juice and a little olive oil, sprinkle with parsley, and serve with the whipped feta.

TO PAN-SEAR Preheat the oven to 425°F. Get a sheet pan ready for holding the seared lamb, as well as a platter for the finished cooked lamb.

Heat a large sauté pan over high heat. When the pan is hot, add ¼ cup of olive oil to the pan. Add as much lamb as will fit without crowding. Cook the lamb until a crust forms on one side, 4 to 6 minutes. Flip over the lamb and repeat on the other side, cooking for about 4 to 6 more minutes. Transfer the lamb to the sheet pan. If you're searing the lamb in batches, pour off the oil in the sauté pan, wipe the pan with a paper towel, and repeat the process for the remaining lamb, placing the cooked lamb onto the sheet pan.

Bake for 6 to 10 minutes, or until an instant-read thermometer inserted in the thickest part registers an internal temperature of 130°F for medium-rare or 135°F for medium. Transfer the lamb to the platter.

For bonus points, discard the oil in the pan, place the pan back over the heat, and carefully add ¼ cup of water or broth. Scrape up any crusty brown bits, stir, and reduce the liquid by half. While the lamb is resting, drizzle it with these juices.

To serve, drizzle the lamb with lemon juice and a little olive oil, sprinkle with parsley, and serve with the whipped feta.

Pomegranate Grilled Asparagus with Cashew "Ricotta" and Roasted Garlic Dressing

MAKES 2 TO 4 SERVINGS   CHEF LESLIE

Pomegranates are packed with nutrients and antioxidants, have several anti-cancer properties, and are a terrifically anti-inflammatory food. Their many antimicrobial properties support a healthy gut microbiome. I love their texture and crunch, and their brightness makes this dish look so beautiful on a plate. Cashews have a richer, more complex taste than many other nuts, and they are a great source of magnesium, zinc, and iron—all incredibly beneficial to the female body.

ROASTED GARLIC DRESSING

1 whole garlic bulb

Extra-virgin olive oil

Freshly squeezed lemon juice

1 teaspoon Dijon mustard

Kosher salt and freshly ground black pepper

CASHEW RICOTTA

7 ounces firm tofu, drained

¼ cup raw cashews

2 tablespoons nutritional yeast

2 tablespoons extra-virgin olive oil

1 teaspoon white miso paste

¼ teaspoon onion powder

¼ teaspoon garlic powder

Lemon juice

Kosher salt

ASPARAGUS

1 bunch medium-thick asparagus, tough ends snapped and discarded (12 ounces after snapping; 1¼ pounds presnapped)

Extra-virgin olive oil

Kosher salt and freshly ground black pepper

¼ cup pomegranate seeds

2 tablespoons coarsely chopped Marcona almonds

2 tablespoons pepitas, toasted

TO MAKE THE ROASTED GARLIC DRESSING
Preheat the oven to 350°F.

Slice the garlic bulb in half crosswise, drizzle with a little olive oil, and then wrap the garlic bulb halves in aluminum foil. Bake until very tender, about 45 minutes.

Unwrap the garlic and let it cool completely.

Squeeze the roasted garlic out of each clove into the jar of an immersion blender. Add 3 tablespoons of olive oil, 1 tablespoon of lemon juice, and the mustard. Season with salt and pepper and blend until the dressing becomes smooth. Set aside.

TO MAKE THE CASHEW RICOTTA Place the tofu in a large bowl and mash it with a fork or a potato masher.

CONTINUED ▶

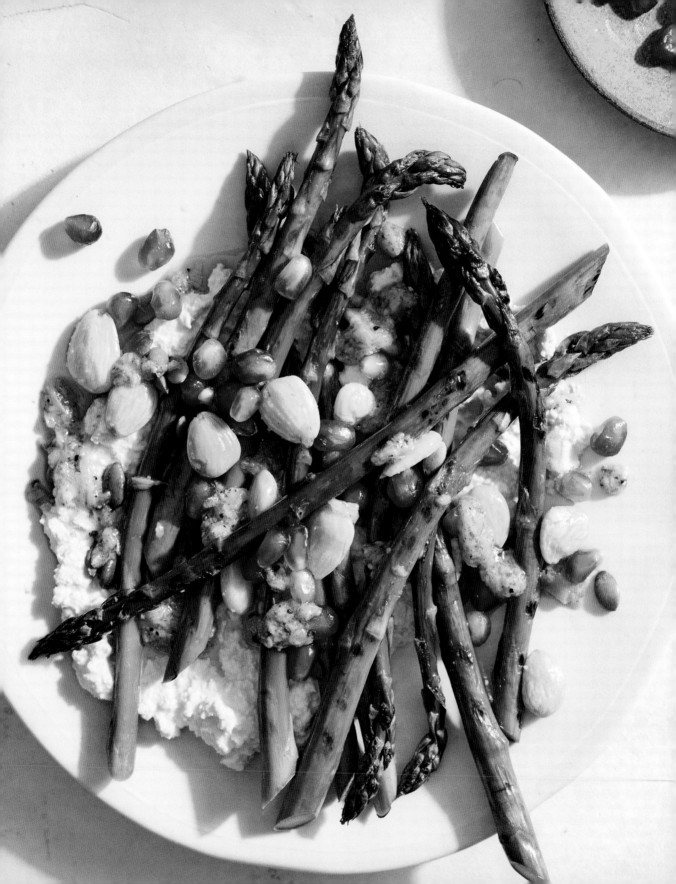

Pomegranate Grilled Asparagus with Cashew "Ricotta" and Roasted Garlic Dressing
CONTINUED

Transfer 2 tablespoons of the mashed tofu to the jar of an immersion blender. Add the cashews, 2 tablespoons of water, the nutritional yeast, olive oil, miso paste, onion powder, garlic powder, 1 teaspoon of lemon juice, and salt to taste, and blend until smooth. Pour the cashew mixture over the tofu and mix well. Taste and season with more salt and lemon juice, if you like. Set aside.

TO COOK THE ASPARAGUS Prepare a grill for direct cooking over medium heat (400°F). Drizzle the asparagus with olive oil and season with salt and pepper. Lay the asparagus on the grill, perpendicular to the grate. Grill, turning occasionally with tongs, until nicely grill-marked and crisp-tender, about 4 minutes. Transfer to a baking sheet.

TO FINISH THE DISH Divide the cashew ricotta between two to four plates. Top each plate with asparagus and sprinkle with the pomegranate seeds, almonds, and pepitas. Drizzle with the roasted garlic dressing and serve.

Walnut Pâté

MAKES 4 SERVINGS (2 CUPS) | CHEF LESLIE

Walnuts are excellent brain food. For those of you who eat a plant-based diet, this is a good recipe to combine with our Fasting Crackers (page 107) for a low-glycemic snack. It's also terrific to munch on when your brain needs some extra fuel on long days.

PÂTÉ

1 cup walnut pieces
2 tablespoons extra-virgin olive oil
8 ounces cremini mushrooms, sliced
½ cup chopped shallots
4 garlic cloves, minced
Kosher salt and freshly ground black pepper
2 sun-dried tomatoes, not packed in oil
1 tablespoon tamari
½ teaspoon thyme
½ cup chopped fresh parsley

OPTIONAL GARNISHES

Sun-dried tomatoes, chopped
Chopped toasted walnuts

Toast the walnuts in a large dry skillet over medium heat until they turn slightly brown and fragrant, about 2 minutes. Transfer the walnuts to a plate.

Heat the olive oil in the same pan over medium heat. Add the mushrooms, shallots, garlic, and 1 pinch of salt and cook, stirring often, for 5 minutes. Add the sun-dried tomatoes, tamari, and thyme and cook until the veggies become soft, about 5 minutes. Turn off the heat, add the parsley, and stir until it wilts.

Transfer the mixture to a food processor and pulse until it is almost but not quite completely smooth (a pâté texture). Add the walnuts and pulse until all the large pieces are broken up, but the pâté is not totally smooth. Pause to scrape down the sides of the processor occasionally. Taste and add more salt and pepper if desired.

Press the pâté into a 2-cup serving dish, cover, and refrigerate for at least 3 hours or up to overnight.

Serve with Fasting Crackers (page 107) and garnish with sun-dried tomatoes or toasted chopped walnuts.

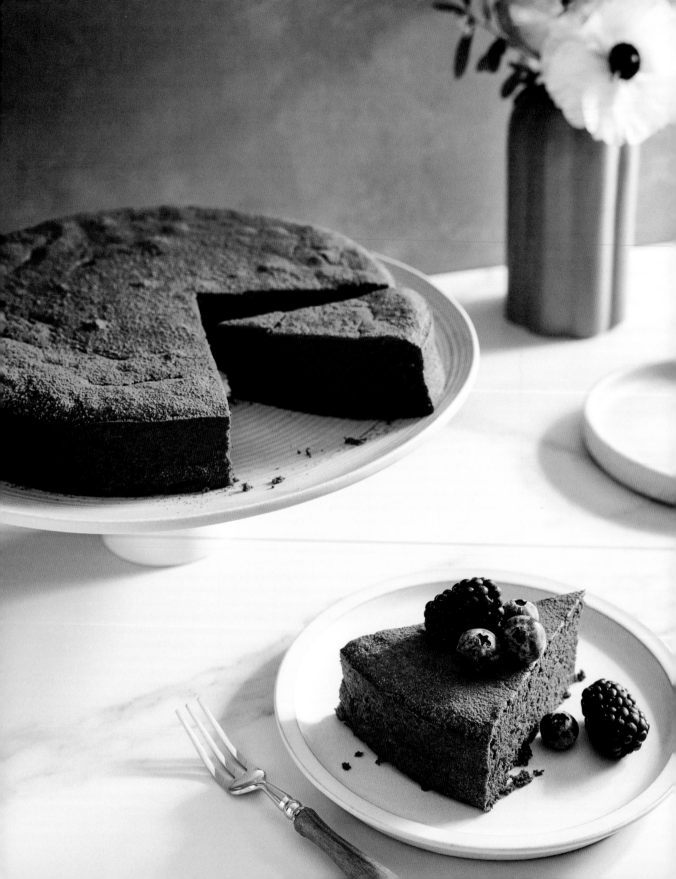

Flourless Chocolate Almond Torte

MAKES 8 SERVINGS | CHEF JEFF

Bring this delicious torte the next time you're invited to a friend's house for dinner. Oftentimes when you're trying to stay low carb and you're eating out at a social occasion, you learn to just skip the dessert. But Chef Jeff made this recipe very blood-sugar friendly, making it a great keto dessert that everyone will devour.

1 cup keto chocolate chips, such as Guittard Santé 72% Cacao Chocolate
1 cup unsalted butter, cut into chunks
¼ cup almond butter
2 tablespoons white miso
6 large eggs, separated
1 cup coconut sugar, divided
1 cup almond flour
2 tablespoons Dutch-processed cocoa powder, such as Guittard or Valrhona
2 tablespoons instant espresso granules
2 tablespoons brandy or vodka
1 tablespoon vanilla bean paste or vanilla extract
¼ teaspoon kosher salt

Preheat the oven to 350°F. Spray a 9-inch springform cake pan with avocado oil non-stick cooking spray.

Fill a medium pot halfway with water and place it over medium-high heat.

Combine the keto chocolate chips, butter, almond butter, and miso in a metal or glass bowl. Place the bowl over the pot of hot water, creating a double boiler. (Make sure the bottom of the bowl doesn't touch the water, or it will be too hot.) Heat, stirring often, until the chocolate and butters have melted. Turn off the heat and let the bowl sit, keeping the chocolate mixture warm with the residual heat.

Beat the egg whites in a large bowl with a whisk or electric mixer for about 2 minutes, or until fluffy peaks form. Add 2 tablespoons of the coconut sugar and continue beating for about 4 minutes until the peaks become stiff. Set aside.

CONTINUED ▶

Flourless Chocolate Almond Torte
CONTINUED

Combine the egg yolks and the remaining ¾ cup plus 2 tablespoons coconut sugar in another large bowl and beat with a whisk or electric mixer until the yolks become pale in color and thick, about 4 to 6 minutes. Add the almond flour, cocoa powder, espresso granules, brandy, vanilla, and salt and stir until well combined. Stir in the chocolate-butter mixture until well combined.

Add one-third of the beaten egg whites to the yolk mixture and stir to combine. Add another one-third of the whites and gently fold them in with a rubber spatula. (Some streaks of egg white in the mixture are fine.)

Add the remaining one-third of the whites and gently fold them in, trying to smooth out as many white streaks as possible without deflating the whites.

Pour the batter into the prepared springform cake pan, smooth out the top with the spatula, and bake for 30 to 35 minutes, or until a toothpick inserted in the center of the cake comes out clean.

Set the cake on a wire rack and allow it to cool completely for about 1 hour before unmolding.

Salted Caramel Sauce

MAKES 6 TO 8 SERVINGS (1 CUP) | CHEF JEFF

When Chef Jeff devised this recipe, he was so excited about how it turned out that he had to text me right away. Finding sweet treats that don't elicit a high blood-sugar response is hard to do, but he created one for us all to enjoy. Try this caramel sauce on our Flourless Chocolate Almond Torte (page 255) or Keto Basque Cheesecake (page 263), or spooned over your favorite treat.

6 tablespoons unsalted butter
6 tablespoons brown sugar substitute
  (such as Swerve) or coconut sugar
6 tablespoons heavy cream
1 tablespoon plus 1 teaspoon white miso
Kosher salt
2 teaspoons instant espresso granules
2 teaspoons vanilla extract

Combine the butter and brown sugar substitute in a small saucepan over medium-high heat. Bring the mixture to a vigorous simmer while whisking, until it is bubbling heavily and combined, about 1 minute. Continue to cook until the sauce turns a shade darker, about 3 minutes. Remove from the heat and carefully add the heavy cream—the sauce will sputter and boil a little, then calm down.

Whisk in the miso, ½ teaspoon of salt, and espresso granules and return the pan to medium heat. Bring to a simmer, stirring often, until the mixture thickens slightly, 1 to 3 more minutes. Remove the pan from the heat, add the vanilla, and mix well. Taste and season with more salt as desired. Let cool.

The sauce can be refrigerated in an airtight container for up to 1 week.

Coconut Oil Fudge

MAKES 28 BITE-SIZE PIECES | | CHEF LESLIE

This fun recipe provides a quick bite-size treat to satisfy your chocolate cravings. Coconut oil offers so many incredible healing properties; it turns off your hunger hormone, helps you get into ketosis more easily, and heals your gut microbiome. If you want to make sure your blood sugar stays really stable with this recipe, be sure to use grade-B maple syrup.

½ cup refined coconut oil
½ cup cacao powder
½ cup almond butter
¼ cup maple syrup
⅛ teaspoon kosher salt

Line an 8 x 8-inch baking pan with parchment paper.

Combine the coconut oil, cacao powder, almond butter, maple syrup, and salt in a small saucepan over medium heat and whisk until smooth.

Pour the mixture into the prepared baking pan and spread it out evenly with a rubber spatula. Allow the fudge to cool completely, 2 to 4 hours, or refrigerate overnight. Cut into 1½-inch squares and store in an airtight container for up to 1 week in the fridge or 2 months in the freezer.

Fat-Bomb Smoothie

MAKES 1 SERVING   CHEF LESLIE

Make this smoothie on those busy days when you want to kill hunger while keeping your blood sugar stable. It's effortless to prepare and super easy to drink. It tastes great and is handy when you need a go-to meal that gives you energy.

One 13.5-ounce can full-fat coconut milk
1 ripe medium avocado
½ cup ice
¼ cup cacao powder
¼ cup almond butter

Combine the coconut milk, avocado, ice, cacao powder, and almond butter in a blender and blend on high speed until smooth.

Strawberry-and-Cream Protein Pops

MAKES 6 TO 9 PROTEIN POPS | | CHEF LESLIE

This is the recipe you eat to show all your friends that you are not deprived on your low-carbohydrate days! These pops look fun and they taste delicious. If you're trying to minimize the blood-sugar impact, I encourage you to cut the banana in half or use a fairly unripe one.

1½ cups unsweetened nondairy milk
⅔ cup vegan protein powder
8 strawberries, halved
1 banana
5 strawberries, chopped

Combine the nondairy milk, protein powder, halved strawberries, and banana in a blender and blend on high speed until smooth.

Stir in the chopped strawberries and pour the mixture into a Popsicle mold.

Freeze overnight. To unmold the protein pops, run the mold under hot water for a few seconds until the pops loosen.

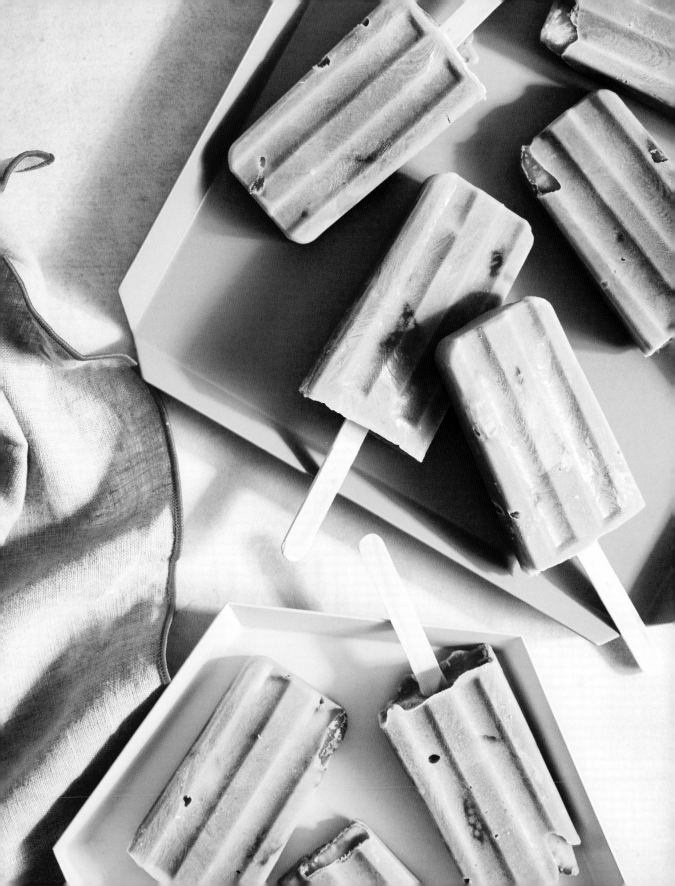

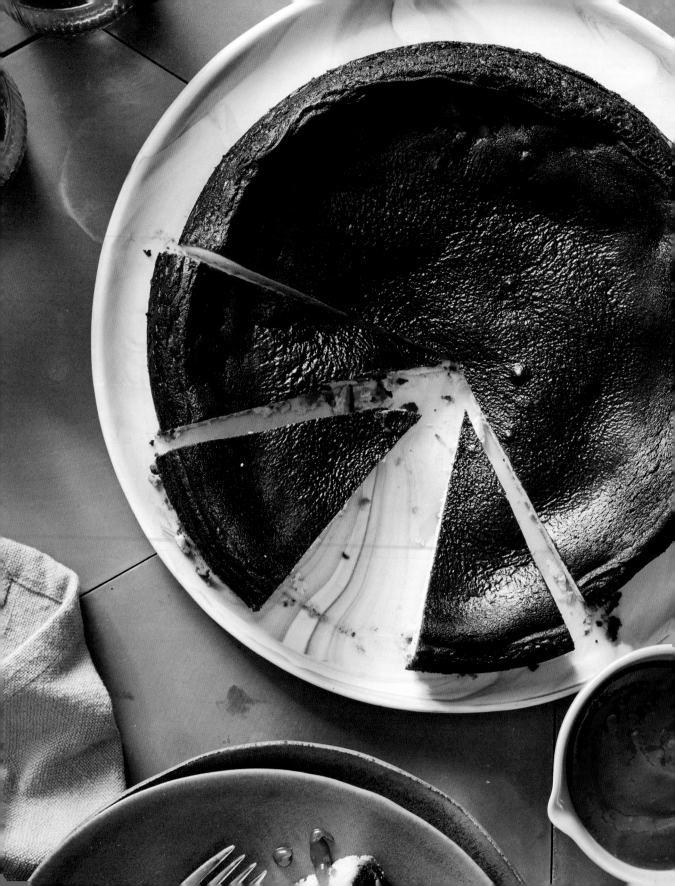

Keto Basque Cheesecake

MAKES 10 TO 12 SERVINGS | CHEF JEFF

All the yummy fat in this dessert is likely to keep your blood sugar stable. I highly encourage you to use raw honey, as it contains more enzymes, which helps prevent a large blood-sugar spike. Swerve is a great sweetener because it offers incredible support to your gut microbiome. It is a delicious combination of fermented sugar along with prebiotic fibers and a burst of citrus for flavor. Serve with Salted Caramel Sauce, page 257.

17 ounces fresh goat cheese
1 pound cream cheese
½ cup powdered sugar substitute, such as Swerve
¼ cup raw honey
2 tablespoons white miso
½ teaspoon kosher salt (optional)
1½ cups heavy cream
5 large eggs
1 tablespoon vanilla bean paste or vanilla extract
½ cup fine almond flour

Preheat the oven to 350°F.

Grease a 9 x 3-inch heavy cheesecake pan or a springform pan with a removable bottom with avocado oil nonstick cooking spray. Line the bottom of the pan with parchment paper and also spray it with cooking spray. Place the cheesecake pan on a sheet pan.

Combine the goat cheese, cream cheese, sugar substitute, honey, miso, and salt (if using) in the bowl of a stand mixer fitted with a paddle attachment. Beat until fluffy and combined, scraping down the sides as needed with a spatula, about 2 minutes.

Whisk together the cream, eggs, and vanilla in a separate bowl until thoroughly combined.

Pour the egg mixture into the cream cheese mixture. Beat on low speed until everything is thoroughly combined, scraping down the sides as needed. Increase the speed to high and whip for 5 minutes to aerate the mixture.

Add the almond flour and beat on low speed one more time until just combined.

Pour the batter into the prepared cheese-cake pan and place it on the center rack of the oven.

Bake for 10 minutes at 350°F, and then increase the heat to 375°F and bake the cheesecake for 20 minutes. Increase the heat to 400°F and bake for 30 more minutes.

When done, the top of the cheesecake should be very brown, and a toothpick inserted into the center should come out clean.

Remove the cheesecake and cool in the sheet pan on a wire rack to room temperature and then chill, covered, overnight before serving.

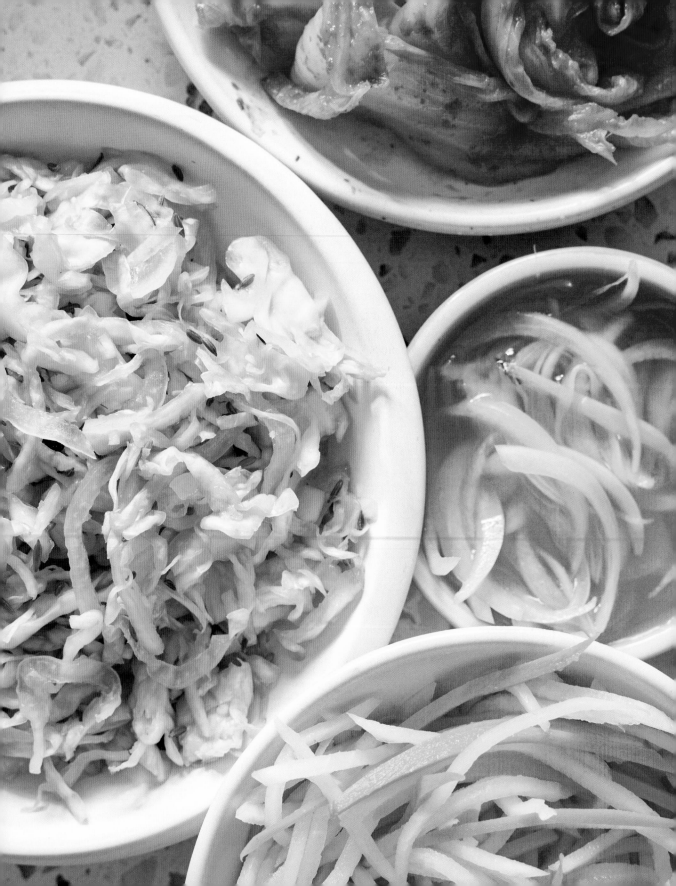

15

Pantry

STORE-BOUGHT DRESSINGS and soups are packed with all kinds of obesogens. It's nearly impossible to find a chemical-free dressing or condiment. That's why I'm so pleased to offer you some healthy homemade pantry items that are easy to make, tasty, and free of toxins.

Make a huge batch of broth and freeze into individual portions to use in recipes or sip on their own. Snack on these delicious and gut-friendly pickles. Drizzle these yummy dressings over a salad or mix into a stir-fry. You'll be amazed at the delicious and toxin-free variations available to you throughout the month and sometimes even while fasting!

Beef Bone Broth

MAKES 2 QUARTS | | CHEF JEFF

Broths are a faster's dream. Some broths you can consume in your fasting window, while others are good for your first meal in your eating window. There are many ways you can use broth to build a fasting lifestyle unique to you. I love the idea of dividing this broth into individual portions to reheat for sipping or cooking. Chef Jeff recommends using a smoked ham bone, which adds great oomph and flavor. For the sherry, you can use any inexpensive bottle. The alcohol will be largely cooked out, but if you're avoiding alcohol, just leave it out.

MEAT AND BONES

2½ pounds meaty beef bones, such as oxtails

2½ pounds beef shank (sometimes called beef soup bones)

2½ pounds beef marrow bones or knuckle-bones

½ ham bone or ham hock (optional)

¼ cup extra-virgin olive oil

¼ cup tomato paste

½ cup sherry

2 tablespoons sherry vinegar or red or white wine vinegar

STOCK

2½ pounds carrots, peeled and cut into large chunks

2 large yellow onions, peeled and cut into large chunks

2 large celery stalks, cut into large chunks

One 28-ounce can crushed tomatoes

1 cup garlic cloves, peeled

1 cup fresh shiitake, white button, or cremini mushrooms

½ cup red miso (optional)

1 tablespoon black peppercorns

1 dried bay leaf

5 to 10 sprigs thyme

1 sprig rosemary

One 5- to 6-inch piece Parmesan rind (optional)

TO ROAST THE MEAT AND BONES Preheat the oven to 425°F.

Place the meat and bones (except the ham bone or ham hock, if using) on several sheet pans. Coat the bones in the olive oil, then roast for 20 minutes. Once the bones turn golden on one side, flip them over and spread the tomato paste on the bones.

Continue roasting for another 20 to 30 minutes until the bones turn very brown.

Place the bones into a very large stockpot, along with the ham bone (if using). Return the empty sheet pans to the oven. Add the sherry to the pans and bake for 10 minutes to warm up the sherry. Carefully remove the sheet pans from the oven. Use a wooden spoon to scrape up any crusty meaty bits (fond) that accumulated on the pans. Pour the sherry liquid and fond into the stockpot. Add the sherry vinegar and stir well.

TO MAKE THE STOCK Pour enough cold water into the stockpot to cover the bones by 1 to 2 inches. Turn the heat to medium-high and bring the mixture to a simmer.

As the stock approaches a boil, fat and impurities will be released. Continuously skim the stock until it comes to a light boil. Decrease the heat to a low boil. Keep skimming the stock until it is relatively clear, approximately 30 minutes.

Fill the pot to the top with hot tap water, and let it simmer for at least 12 hours, skimming occasionally, until no more foam and floaties pop up.

Add the carrots, onions, celery, tomatoes, garlic, mushrooms, miso (if using), peppercorns, and bay leaf, and simmer for another 2 to 3 hours. At this point, the meat and bones should be falling apart, and the veggies will be very soft.

Turn off the heat and add the thyme, rosemary, and Parmesan rind (if using). Let the stock sit for 30 minutes.

Using tongs, discard the larger bones and chunks, then strain the stock through a fine-mesh sieve set over a large food-safe container. If the stock is still cloudy or contains floating particles, strain it a few more times through the sieve or through a cheesecloth or muslin until it runs clearish.

Return the stock to the pot, bring it to a boil over medium-high heat, and cook until it reduces to about 2 quarts.

Pour the stock into a vessel that fits in your fridge and chill it overnight. When cold, it should look like a wobbly mass of meat Jell-O that can be frozen in usable portions. It can be heated, seasoned, and sipped for a delicious and very nutritious snack. Refrigerate for up to 7 days or freeze for up to 3 months.

Chicken Bone Broth

MAKES 3 QUARTS | | CHEF JEFF

From a delicious snack to sip on while breaking your fast to its protein-and-taste punch in a range of recipes, this chicken broth is one I adore. Chicken has more protein than beef, so those of you wanting to build muscle may find this is the perfect broth to sip on during your fasting window. You can use a smoked ham hock for extra flavor. Any inexpensive sherry can be used, or left out if you are avoiding alcohol. It's fine to use cremini or white button mushrooms, but the shiitake provide more flavor.

MEAT AND BONES

2½ pounds chicken wings

2½ pounds chicken backs, necks, or carcasses; whole chickens or stewing hens are fine

2½ pounds turkey thighs or wings

½ ham bone or ham hock

½ cup sherry

2 tablespoons sherry vinegar or red or white wine vinegar

STOCK

1 pound carrots, peeled and cut into large chunks

1 large yellow onion, peeled, cut into large chunks

4 celery stalks, cut into large chunks

½ cup garlic cloves, peeled

½ cup fresh shiitake, white button, or cremini mushrooms

¼ cup white miso (optional)

½ tablespoon black peppercorns

1 dried bay leaf

2 sprigs thyme

1 sprig rosemary

One 3-inch piece Parmesan rind (optional)

TO COOK THE CHICKEN AND BONES Place all the bones into a very large stockpot, along with the ham hock, if using.

Pour enough cold water into the stockpot to cover the bones by 1 to 2 inches. Turn the heat to medium-high and bring the mixture to a simmer. Once the bones come to a simmer, turn off the heat, carefully remove the pot from the stove, and dump out the water. Pour cold water over the bones, and then dump out that water too to clean the bones of any residual particles. Finally, fill the pot with cold water one more time to just above the bones and set it on the stovetop.

Add the sherry and sherry vinegar to the pot.

TO MAKE THE STOCK Heat the pot over medium-high heat to bring it to a simmer.

As the stock approaches a boil, fat and impurities will be released in the form of foam and little floaties. Using a ladle, skim them off constantly until the stock slowly reaches a light boil. Once it boils, lower the heat so the stock gently boils for about 30 minutes, continuing to ladle off any impurities as they come up.

Keep skimming the stock until it is relatively clear or once the impurities aren't appearing as often; decrease the heat to medium-low or low, where just a few bubbles rise up every few seconds.

Add the carrots, onion, celery, garlic, mushrooms, miso (if using), peppercorns, and bay leaf, and simmer for another 2 to 3 hours. At this point, the meat should be falling off the bones, and the veggies will be very soft.

Turn off the heat and add the thyme, rosemary, and Parmesan rind (if using). Let the stock sit for 30 minutes.

Using tongs, discard the larger bones and chunks, then strain the stock through a fine-mesh sieve set over a large food-safe container. If the stock is still cloudy or contains floating particles, strain it a few more times through the sieve or through a cheesecloth or muslin until it runs clearish.

Return the stock to the pot, bring it to a boil over medium-high heat, and cook until it reduces to about 3 quarts, which should take about 20 minutes, or you can take it down further and just add water to the concentrated stock later when you are cooking with it.

Let the stock cool to room temperature, and then pour the stock into a vessel that fits in your fridge and chill it overnight. When cold, it should look like a wobbly mass of chicken Jell-O that can be frozen in usable portions. It can be heated, seasoned, and sipped for a delicious and very nutritious snack. Refrigerate for up to 7 days or freeze for up to 3 months.

Vegetable Broth

MAKES 2 QUARTS | **CHEF LESLIE**

There are so many reasons why you want to incorporate broth into your fasting lifestyle. For some of you, broth works in your fasting windows (always test your blood sugar). Others will find it the perfect go-to when opening up your eating window. No one rocks a plant-based broth like Chef Leslie! This recipe contains so many prebiotic nutrients that your gut microbes will be singing with glee.

2½ medium carrots, sliced
2 medium yellow onions, peeled and quartered
1½ large red bell peppers, seeded and cut into 3- to 4-inch pieces
5 medium celery stalks, sliced, leaves included
1 Roma tomato, halved
¼ pound cremini mushrooms, quartered
½ bunch parsley, leaves and stems
3 garlic cloves
1 dried bay leaf
1½ teaspoons tomato paste
½ teaspoon dried thyme
½ teaspoon kosher salt
¼ teaspoon freshly ground black pepper

Put the carrots, onions, bell peppers, celery, tomato, mushrooms, parsley, garlic, bay leaf, tomato paste, thyme, salt, pepper, and 8 cups of water in a large stockpot over medium-high heat. Bring to a boil, then reduce the heat to low and simmer for 1 hour.

Remove from the heat and let cool completely.

Strain the broth and pour it into airtight containers. Refrigerate for up to 7 days or freeze for up to 1 month.

Dashi

MAKES 2 QUARTS | | CHEF JEFF

This broth is incredibly healing for your thyroid. Kombu is dried seaweed that is packed with iodine, a key nutrient for proper thyroid function. What's wonderful about this dashi is that not only can it be used in other recipes, but also, if you drink a warm cup of this broth a couple times a week, it can fire up your metabolism while nourishing your thyroid.

1 large piece of kombu (2 ounces), broken in half
2 cups loosely packed bonito flakes

Add 8 cups of cold water and the kombu in a large pot over low heat. Slowly bring the water to just below a simmer; this should take 30 minutes and finish with bubbles just barely breaking the surface.

Remove the pot from the heat and remove the kombu; if it's just starting to disintegrate as you pluck it out, you're on the right track. Pour in the bonito flakes and push them down under the liquid without stirring or agitating them too much.

Once the bonito flakes sink, let the dashi steep for about 10 minutes, then strain the stock and chill. Refrigerate for up to 7 days or freeze for up to 3 months.

Functional Mushroom Broth

MAKES 3 QUARTS | | CHEF LESLIE

I have received so many requests from fasters on plant-based diets for a broth that would be incredibly healing in both your fasting window and as a go-to to break your fast. So one of my first requests I had for Chef Leslie was to create a delicious, beneficial broth for those of you who prefer plant-based options. I love breaking fasts (especially longer ones) with broths, but there aren't many good plant-based ones. Functional mushrooms bring so much more than taste to your body. Feel free to experiment with different mushrooms and mushroom powder to fit your own budget.

32 ounces high-nutrient dried mushrooms of any type (shiitake, maitake, cordyceps, turkey tail, reishi, lion's mane, white, portobello, cremini)

1 medium yellow onion, ends trimmed and quartered with skin on

1 large celery stalk, cut into 1-inch pieces

1 large carrot, peeled and cut into 1-inch pieces

9 to 12 bulbs of garlic, cut in half with the paper attached

One 1-inch piece fresh ginger

One 1-inch piece fresh turmeric

3 sprigs thyme

1 tablespoon dried parsley

1 dried leaf of kombu seaweed (optional)

Kosher salt and freshly ground black pepper

Combine the mushrooms, onion, celery, carrot, garlic, ginger, turmeric, thyme, parsley, salt and pepper, and kombu (if using) in a large pot and add 1 gallon of water. Bring to a boil over medium-high heat, stirring occasionally.

Decrease the heat to low, cover, and simmer until your broth is full of flavor, 4 to 6 hours.

Let cool to room temperature. Strain the mixture through a fine-mesh sieve into glass jars with screw-top lids.

The broth can be refrigerated for 1 week or frozen for up to 3 months. If freezing the broth, pour the broth into ice cube trays and freeze. Once frozen, transfer the cubes to an airtight container and store in the freezer.

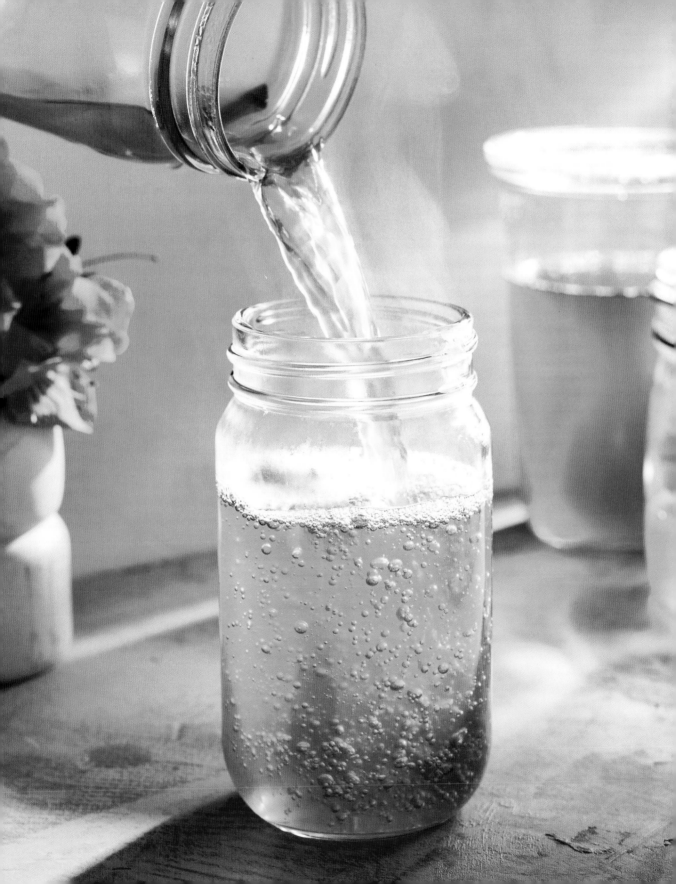

Basic Pickling Liquid

MAKES ABOUT 2 CUPS | | CHEF JEFF

Any food that is pickled is a blessing to your body. Personally, I love the salty crunch a pickled cucumber offers. But pickled vegetables of all kinds can provide the extra electrolytes often needed before a longer fast. Pickled vegetables are also known to ease muscle cramping, slow down blood-sugar spikes, and, when fermented, provide your gut with new healthy microbes for metabolizing hormones. To begin with, here is a great recipe for pickling liquid, and then in the pages that follow, you'll find some excellent ways to pickle vegetables. You may try a couple of these pickles as a fasted snack (always be sure to test it with your blood sugar reader).

Keto sweetener, such as monk fruit, coconut sugar, or keto maple syrup
2 teaspoons raw honey
Kosher salt
1¼ cups rice wine vinegar or your vinegar of choice
½ cup crushed ice

Combine ¾ cup of hot water, 2 tablespoons of keto sweetener, honey, and 2 teaspoons of salt in a large bowl and stir until everything is dissolved. Add the rice wine vinegar and ice and stir to combine. Taste and season with more keto sweetener and salt as desired.

NOTE Raw honey minimizes the blood-sugar spike that normally comes with honey and is also needed for the fermentation process.

This pickling liquid will improve as it sits overnight, so feel free to make it ahead of time and refrigerate for up to 1 month.

Korean-Style Pickled Cucumbers

MAKES 2 CUPS | | CHEF JEFF

Let's talk about spice for a hot moment. Many spicy ingredients are packed with capsaicin, which has been known to help speed up metabolism. Korean chili powder is also rich in three bioactive compounds—carotenoids, capsaicinoids, and flavonoids. These compounds pack a serious antioxidant punch and can help protect you from the cellular damage that environmental toxins bring.

1 tablespoon sesame seeds (if you buy them already toasted, skip the first step)
1 pound kirby or slicing cucumbers, peeled (if desired) and cut into ¼-inch-thick rounds
Coconut sugar
Kosher salt
2 garlic cloves, peeled
1 tablespoon red or white miso
1 tablespoon raw honey
1 tablespoon tamari
1 tablespoon sesame oil
Gochugaru (Korean chili powder) or finely ground red pepper flakes
2 tablespoons Basic Pickling Liquid (page 274), made with rice wine vinegar

Toast the sesame seeds in a small dry skillet over medium-high heat until they are slightly browned and fragrant. Remove from the heat and set aside.

Combine the cucumber, 1 tablespoon coconut sugar, and 1 teaspoon salt in a medium bowl and toss to mix well. Let the cucumbers sit for 10 minutes, then drain off their liquid.

Using a microplane or the small holes of a box grater, grate the garlic and add it to a small bowl. Add the miso, honey, tamari, sesame oil, and 1 teaspoon of gochugaru and stir to mix well. Stir in the pickling liquid until well combined. Pour the mixture over the cucumbers and toss to combine. Taste and season the cucumbers with more salt, coconut sugar, and gochugaru as desired. Stir in the toasted sesame seeds.

Refrigerate for 1 hour before serving. Serve within 1 to 2 days.

NOTE The longer they sit in the pickling liquid, the softer and more pickled these pickles become. Depending on how thickly they are cut, the cucumbers typically lose their crunch and texture after 48 hours.

Keto Pickled Ginger

MAKES ½ CUP | | CHEF JEFF

This recipe should have been called Gut Hero. Ginger is one of the most healing foods for your gut. It has the power to soothe an upset stomach, help nausea, and even fight bacterial and fungal infections. When you pickle it, you amplify all those healing effects. But pickling ginger can also bring extra sugar, so the fact that Chef Jeff created a keto version of pickled ginger is a metabolic miracle!

2 ounces fresh ginger, approximately
   8 inches
½ cup Basic Pickling Liquid (page 274),
   made with rice wine vinegar
Kosher salt

Using a knife, slice off the uneven nubs on the sides of each ginger piece. Using the back of the knife or a spoon, scrape off the skin and discard it.

Using a vegetable peeler, peel the ginger into strips; it should yield about ½ cup.

Transfer the ginger to a jar.

FOR A QUICK PICKLE Warm up the pickling liquid in a small pot over medium-high heat and bring to just under a simmer. Pour the liquid over the ginger and set the jar aside to cool. Cover and refrigerate for at least 1 hour.

FOR A SLOWER PICKLE Pour the pickling liquid over the ginger. Cover the jar and refrigerate for at least 8 hours.

Taste and season with salt as desired.

NOTE These pickles will improve as they sit for a few days, so feel free to make them ahead of time and refrigerate for up to 1 month.

Pickled Red Onions

MAKES ABOUT 3 CUPS | | CHEF JEFF

Pickled red onions offer you many health benefits, providing a powerful dose of both probiotics and prebiotics and a healthy infusion of folate, which is a key nutrient needed for hormone production.

1 large red onion, cut into a thin julienne, onion skins reserved
1½ cups Basic Pickling Liquid (page 274)
1 teaspoon coriander seeds
1 teaspoon cumin seeds
1 teaspoon black peppercorns
1 teaspoon whole cloves
1 small bay leaf
Kosher salt

Place the onions in a heatproof bowl or container fitted with a lid.

FOR A QUICK PICKLE Combine the pickling liquid, coriander, cumin, peppercorns, cloves, and bay leaf in a small pot over medium-high heat and bring to just under a simmer. Pour the mixture over the onions. Place the onion skins on top (so they are easy to remove later) and set the bowl aside to cool. Cover and refrigerate for at least 1 hour. Remove the onion skin after 24 hours.

FOR A SLOWER PICKLE Whisk the pickling liquid, coriander, cumin, peppercorns, cloves, and bay leaf in a medium bowl and pour it over the onions. Toss to combine. Place the onion skins on top (so they are easy to remove later) and cover and refrigerate for at least 24 hours.

Taste and season with salt as desired.

NOTE These pickles will improve as they sit for a few days, so feel free to make them ahead and refrigerate for up to 1 month.

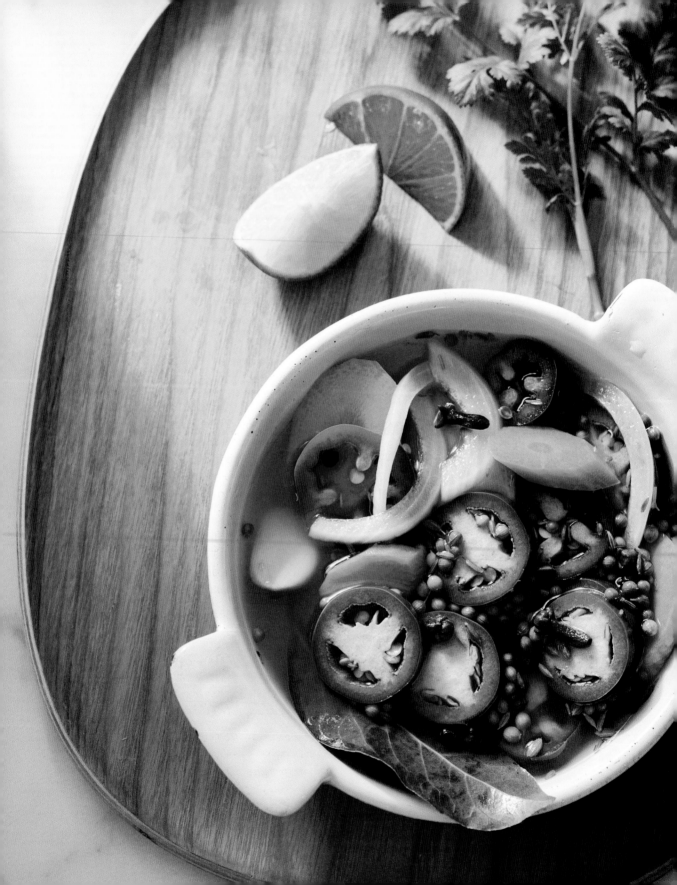

Mexican-Style Pickled Jalapeños and Carrots

MAKES 2 CUPS   CHEF JEFF

One of the most important eat-like-a-girl principles is to diversify your food choices. The same goes for the vegetables you pickle. Pickling different vegetables will yield different probiotics. Pickled carrots are also high in vitamin C, while pickled jalapeños give you a burst of capsaicin that will help you burn fat. It's a beautiful combination for the female body.

1 medium carrot, peeled and cut into
  ¼-inch-thick slices on the diagonal
½ small white onion, cut into thin julienne
3 garlic cloves, peeled
2 large jalapeños, stems trimmed and cut
  into ¼-inch-thick slices
2 teaspoons coriander seeds
2 teaspoons cumin seeds
2 teaspoons black peppercorns
1 teaspoon whole cloves
1 dried bay leaf
2 cups Basic Pickling Liquid (page 274)
Kosher salt

Combine the carrot, onion, garlic, and jalapeños in a nonreactive bowl or container fitted with a lid.

FOR A QUICK PICKLE Combine the coriander, cumin, peppercorns, cloves, bay leaf, and pickling liquid in a small saucepan over medium-high heat and bring to just under a simmer. Pour the mixture over the vegetables. Set aside to cool. Cover and refrigerate for at least 1 hour.

FOR A SLOWER PICKLE Combine the coriander, cumin, peppercorns, cloves, bay leaf, and pickling liquid in a medium bowl and pour the mixture over the vegetables. Cover and refrigerate for at least 24 hours.

Taste and season with salt as desired.

NOTE If you don't want to buy a bunch of whole spices, most stores sell an inexpensive spice blend called "pickling spices." Two tablespoons of this mix make a perfectly fine substitute.

These pickles will improve as they sit for a few days, so feel free to make them ahead of time and refrigerate for up to 1 month.

Pickled Daikon and Carrot Slaw

MAKES 2 CUPS | | CHEF JEFF

Gut dysbiosis is a term often used for an imbalance between good and bad bacteria in the gut. Pickled daikon brings balance back to even the most troubled gut. Years of birth control, multiple rounds of antibiotics, and nonstop chronic stress may have your gut microbiome in a disoriented state. Add pickled daikon to any recipe and you take a major step forward in healing. Enjoy!

1 small daikon radish (about 7 ounces total weight), peeled and cut into medium julienne

2 medium carrots, peeled and cut into medium julienne

1½ cups Basic Pickling Liquid (page 274), ideally made with rice wine vinegar

Kosher salt

Place the daikon and carrots in a bowl or container fitted with a lid.

FOR A QUICK PICKLE Place the pickling liquid in a small pot over medium-high heat and bring to just under a simmer. Pour the liquid over the radish mixture and set aside to cool. Cover and refrigerate for at least 1 hour.

FOR A SLOWER PICKLE Pour the pickling liquid over the radish mixture. Cover and refrigerate for at least 8 hours.

Taste and season with salt as desired.

NOTE These pickles will improve as they sit for a few days, so feel free to make them and refrigerate for up to 1 month.

A strong sulfurous smell is normal when you first open this container of pickles.

Korean-Style Pickled Radishes

MAKES 2 CUPS | | CHEF JEFF

Radishes are packed with potassium and are known to help support a healthy immune system, increase hydration, improve blood flow, detoxify, and lower blood pressure. Pickle them and you amplify all those healing effects!

1 Korean radish (8 ounces) or 1 small daikon radish (8 ounces), peeled, trimmed, and cut into thick julienne, or 14 to 16 (8 to 9 ounces) trimmed standard round radishes, cut into bite-size chunks
1 cup Basic Pickling Liquid (page 274), ideally made with rice wine vinegar
½ teaspoon ground turmeric (optional)
Kosher salt

Place the radishes in a bowl or container fitted with a lid.

FOR A QUICK PICKLE Combine the pickling liquid and turmeric (if using) in a small pot over medium-high heat and heat to just under a simmer. Pour the mixture over the radishes and set aside to cool. Cover and refrigerate for at least 1 hour.

FOR A SLOWER PICKLE Whisk together the pickling liquid and turmeric (if using) in a medium bowl and pour the mixture over the radishes. Cover and refrigerate for at least 8 hours.

Taste and season with salt as desired.

NOTE These pickles will improve as they sit for a few days, so feel free to make them ahead and refrigerate for up to 1 month.

Turmeric Sauerkraut

MAKES 1 QUART | CHEF LESLIE

Oooooo . . . turmeric with fermented cabbage! That is an anti-inflammatory win for your body. I would recommend you make a large batch of this recipe and add to all your favorite meals. Your gut will thank you!

2 pounds green cabbage, 1 leaf reserved, the rest shredded
1 tablespoon kosher salt
4 garlic cloves, minced
¼ white onion, thinly sliced
1 teaspoon black peppercorns
½ teaspoon caraway seeds
One 1-inch piece fresh ginger, peeled and grated
One 1-inch piece fresh turmeric, peeled and grated

Combine the shredded cabbage and salt in a large bowl. Massage the cabbage with your hands and then let sit at room temperature for 15 minutes.

Massage the cabbage again and squeeze it to release its juices. Add the garlic, onion, peppercorns, caraway seeds, ginger, and turmeric and, using tongs, mix well.

Using a spoon, very tightly pack the cabbage mixture into a quart-size jar; you don't want any oxygen in it. Leave 2 inches at the top of the jar, and place the cabbage leaf on top. Make sure it covers the mixture below and press down firmly.

Fill a small ziplock bag with 1 cup of water and seal it. Place it on top of the cabbage leaf and press down to make sure there is zero oxygen in the jar. Place the lid on the jar loosely, and do not seal it!

Store the jar in a dark place for 1 week. The cabbage will look noticeably softer. The color will change from a light green to yellowish green. After that, the cabbage is ready to eat.

NOTE If the water level drops at any point, make a salt mixture with 6½ tablespoons water to just under ½ teaspoon of salt and pour it over the cabbage.

You can continue to ferment your cabbage another week, or you can seal the jar and store the sauerkraut in the fridge for up to 6 months.

Catalan Plancha Sauce

MAKES ABOUT 2 CUPS   CHEF JEFF

Garlic is an amazing prebiotic that fuels the happy microbes in your gut. A great go-to on the days you want to give your gut the fuel it needs to break down hormones, make neurotransmitters, and support a healthy immune system. This sauce is also a great add to many of Chef Jeff's meat dishes.

Zest and juice of 3 lemons
5 large garlic cloves, peeled
1 bunch curly parsley, leaves and stems separated, stems coarsely minced
Kosher salt
Monk fruit sweetener
2 cups extra-virgin olive oil

Combine the lemon zest and juice, garlic, and parsley stems in a blender and blend on medium speed until the garlic is coarsely chopped.

Add the parsley leaves, 2 tablespoons of salt, and 1 tablespoon monk fruit sweetener and pulse on high speed until the parsley leaves are coarsely chopped.

Add the olive oil and blend on low speed until the sauce is a smooth puree. Taste and season with more salt and monk fruit sweetener as desired.

NOTE It's completely natural for the sauce to separate once it settles. Before using, give it a solid stir or shake it in a lidded container.

This sauce will keep up to 24 hours, but after that, it will lose its brightness—so it's best to whip it up right before using.

Keto Ketchup and Chili Sauce

MAKES 2 CUPS | | CHEF JEFF

Dear ketchup—I have tried to find a healthy version of your delicious taste but keep coming up short. Not to mention that you are packed with sugar. So thank you, Chef Jeff, for nailing this recipe. Keto ketchup?! This is a huge win for women everywhere.

KETCHUP

One 14-ounce can tomato puree
2 tablespoons apple cider vinegar
2 tablespoons white vinegar
2 tablespoons raw honey
Brown sugar substitute (such as Swerve) or coconut sugar
Kosher salt

ADD FOR THE CHILI SAUCE

1½ teaspoons chili powder
1 teaspoon onion flakes
1 teaspoon garlic powder

TO MAKE THE KETCHUP Combine the tomato puree, ¼ cup of water, the apple cider vinegar, white vinegar, honey, 2 tablespoons of brown sugar substitute, and 1 tablespoon of salt in a medium saucepan over medium-high heat. Bring the mixture to a boil.

Decrease the heat to low to maintain a simmer until the mixture thickens to a ketchup-like consistency, about 30 minutes.

Taste and season with more salt, sugar substitute, or vinegar as desired.

TO MAKE THE CHILI SAUCE Make the ketchup as directed above, but add the chili powder, onion flakes, and garlic powder when you add all the other ingredients. Proceed with the rest of the ketchup recipe.

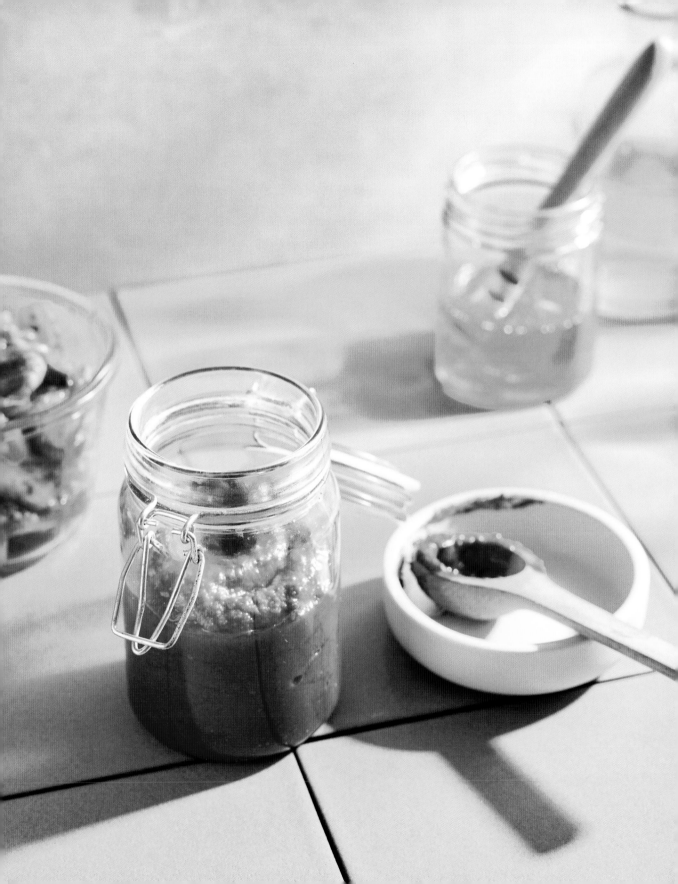

Chimichurri

MAKES 2 CUPS | | CHEF JEFF

Chimichurri is one of my favorite sauces. I love to drip it over steak—talk about a dopamine hit! Although any honey will do, the addition of raw honey provides you with nutrients needed to prevent allergies, suppress a cough, and support healthy brain function. This is a fabulous recipe by Chef Jeff!

2 tablespoons dried oregano
1 teaspoon sweet paprika
1 teaspoon red pepper flakes
1 teaspoon ground cumin
Kosher salt
Raw honey
5 large garlic cloves, peeled
1 cup red wine vinegar, divided
1 bunch Italian parsley, stems minced
1 bunch cilantro, stems minced
1 bunch fresh oregano
½ cup extra-virgin olive oil

Combine the dried oregano, paprika, red pepper flakes, cumin, 2 tablespoons of salt, and 1 tablespoon of honey in a small bowl. Pour in ¼ cup of hot water, stir, and let steep for 10 minutes.

Combine the garlic and ½ cup of the red wine vinegar in a food processor and process on high speed until the garlic is minced. Add the rest of the vinegar and process.

Add the parsley, cilantro, oregano, and the steeped spice mixture to the food processor and process on high speed until the herbs are broken up into smaller pieces.

Add the olive oil and pulse until the chimichurri is thoroughly blended. Taste and season with more salt and honey as desired.

NOTE It's completely natural for the chimichurri to separate once it settles. Before using, give it a solid stir or shake it in a lidded container.

This chimichurri will keep up to 24 hours, but after that, it will lose its brightness, so it's best to whip it up right before using.

Spain's Favorite Sherry Vinaigrette

MAKES ¾ CUP 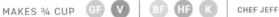 CHEF JEFF

I love all the garlic in this vinaigrette recipe! Garlic is not only a great prebiotic that will feed your gut microbes, but it's also a great go-to when you need immune support.

¼ cup Spanish sherry vinegar
2 large garlic cloves, peeled
2 teaspoons Dijon mustard
½ Roma tomato
1½ teaspoons raw honey
Coconut sugar
Kosher salt
½ cup extra-virgin olive oil

Combine the sherry vinegar, garlic, and mustard in a blender.

Cut the tomato in half and grate the cut side on a grater down to the skin. Add the tomato pulp to the blender, along with the honey, 1½ teaspoons of coconut sugar, and 1 teaspoon of salt. Discard the tomato skins.

Blend on high speed until the garlic is minced.

With the blender running on low speed, add the olive oil in a stream to emulsify the dressing. Taste and season with more coconut sugar and salt as desired.

NOTE It's completely natural for the vinaigrette to separate once it settles. Before using, give it a solid stir or shake it in a lidded container.

This vinaigrette will improve as it sits overnight, so feel free to make it ahead of time and refrigerate for up to 1 week.

Miso Ginger Dressing

MAKES ABOUT 1 CUP | CHEF JEFF

Vinegar is an incredibly healing food. Rice wine vinegar is specifically known to promote blood circulation, dispel a cold, promote a healthy metabolism, and nourish blood and the skin. It is also rich in vitamins B1, B2, niacin, and vitamin E, key nutrients you need to make hormones.

1 small carrot, peeled and chopped
One 1-inch piece fresh ginger, peeled and chopped
2 tablespoons chopped yellow or white onion
2 tablespoons white or yellow miso
2 tablespoons rice wine vinegar
2 tablespoons keto maple syrup or raw honey
1 tablespoon tamari
1 teaspoon Dijon mustard
Kosher salt
Coconut sugar
¼ cup avocado oil
1 tablespoon sesame oil

Combine the carrot, ginger, onion, miso, vinegar, maple syrup, tamari, mustard, ½ teaspoon of salt, and 1 tablespoon of coconut sugar in a blender and blend on high speed until mostly smooth and creamy.

With the blender running on low speed, add the avocado oil and sesame oil in a stream to emulsify the dressing. Taste and season with more salt and coconut sugar as desired.

This dressing will improve as it sits overnight, so feel free to make it ahead of time and refrigerate for up to 1 week.

Tahini Dressing

MAKES ABOUT 1 CUP | CHEF JEFF

Another healing dressing by Chef Jeff! Tahini is made from ground sesame seeds and has many health benefits. It can lower cholesterol, supports healthy liver and kidney function, protects brain health, improves bone mineral density, and helps prevent many hormonal cancers. Not to mention it's packed with magnesium—the mineral hero for hormones!

¼ cup rice wine vinegar
2 tablespoons tahini
1½ teaspoons raw honey
1 teaspoon peeled and grated fresh ginger
1 garlic clove, chopped
Coconut sugar
Kosher salt
½ cup avocado oil

Combine the vinegar, tahini, honey, ginger, garlic, 1½ teaspoons of coconut sugar, and ½ teaspoon of salt in a blender and blend on high speed until mostly smooth.

With the blender running on low speed, add the avocado oil in a stream to emulsify the dressing. If the dressing is too thick, add a little water, 1 teaspoon at a time, to thin to your desired consistency.

Taste and season with more coconut sugar and salt as desired.

NOTE This dressing will improve as it sits overnight, so feel free to make it ahead of time and refrigerate for up to 1 week.

Lemon Dressing

MAKES 1½ CUPS | CHEF JEFF

The lemon is one of the most versatile foods in nature. It has so many healing qualities, including detoxification, hydration, weight-loss promotion, and healthy gut support. Lemon also boosts energy and can help calm an anxious brain. I highly recommend using local honey in this recipe as it can help with allergies.

Zest and juice of 2 lemons
3 large garlic cloves, peeled
1½ teaspoons Dijon mustard
1½ teaspoons raw honey
Kosher salt
Monk fruit sweetener
1 cup extra-virgin olive oil

Combine the lemon zest and juice, garlic cloves, mustard, honey, 1 teaspoon of salt, and 1½ teaspoons of monk fruit sweetener in a blender and blend on medium speed until the dressing is a smooth puree.

With the blender running on low speed, add the olive oil in a stream to emulsify the dressing. Taste and season with more salt and sweetener as desired.

NOTE It's completely natural for the dressing to separate once it settles. Before using, give it a solid stir or shake it in a lidded container.

This dressing will keep up to 24 hours, but after that, it will lose its brightness, so it's best to whip it up right before using.

Italian Stallion Calabrian Chili Dressing

MAKES 1½ CUPS | | CHEF JEFF

I love the name Chef Jeff gave this dressing! If you are not familiar with Calabrian chili peppers, they originally came from the Calabria region in Italy. They have a robust flavor, making this a beautiful dressing to just drizzle over a bowl of mixed greens. These peppers are also rich in antioxidants, have incredible anti-inflammatory properties, will fire up your metabolism, and even have the power to clear your nasal passages when your sinuses act up.

½ cup jarred sweet cherry peppers, stems removed

¼ cup white wine vinegar

¼ cup red onion, coarsely chopped

2 large garlic cloves, peeled

2 teaspoons finely chopped jarred Calabrian chili peppers

2 teaspoons Italian seasoning

1 teaspoon dried oregano

1 teaspoon dried basil

½ teaspoon freshly ground black pepper

Kosher salt

Raw honey

¾ cup extra-virgin olive oil

Combine the sweet cherry peppers, vinegar, onion, garlic, Calabrian chili peppers, Italian seasoning, oregano, basil, black pepper, ½ teaspoon of salt, and 2 teaspoons of honey in a blender and blend on high speed until mostly smooth.

With the blender running on low speed, add the olive oil in a stream to emulsify the dressing.

Taste and season with more salt and honey as desired.

NOTE It's completely natural for the dressing to separate once it settles. Before using, give it a solid stir or shake it in a lidded container.

This dressing will improve as it sits overnight, so feel free to make it ahead of time or keep it in the refrigerator for up to 1 week.

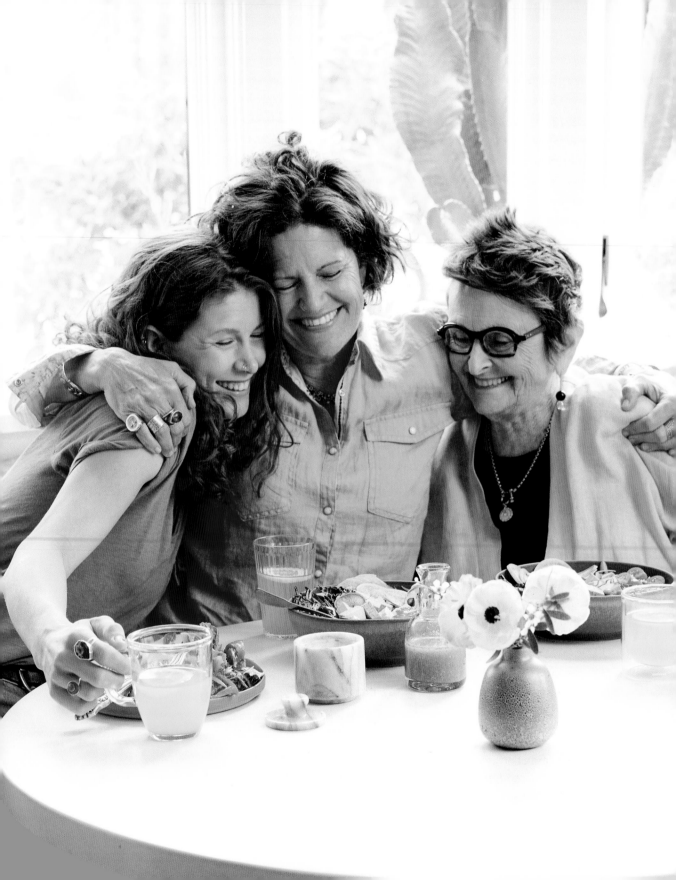

CONCLUSION

WHEN WOMEN HEAL, THE WHOLE WORLD HEALS

BEING A WOMAN IS A GIFT. I hope you see that now. Learning how to honor this miraculous body you are blessed to live in is critical not only for your well-being, but for the well-being of humanity. It has been said "When women heal, the whole world heals." The well-being of women has a massive impact on the health and harmony of the world at large. Women play a crucial role in the social, economic, and environmental aspects of societies. When women are healthy, educated, and empowered, they can make significant contributions to the well-being of their families, communities, and beyond, leading to positive changes on a global scale. The time has come to get women healthy. The world needs us!

As you take this information and play with it, be gentle with yourself. Too many of us have conditioned our brains to adapt to the rigidity of new information. We've learned to sacrifice, push through, and ignore the signals our bodies give us. We have been taught there is a right and wrong way. Today is the day you get to let go of that agenda. It's time to soften and listen to the wisdom your hormones are whispering to you. There is no wrong way, there is only your way.

Be playful with the concepts I've laid out for you. If you find yourself overwhelmed with all the information presented here, pick one or two concepts that resonate with you. Get to know those for a while. Be curious about how your body responds to these new ideas. Once you feel comfortable with them, add a few more concepts into your lifestyle. Before you know it, you will be living congruently with your feminine body.

As you discover new aspects of yourself through the art of eating and fasting like a girl, share them with others. Too many women are suffering. These women need us. When one woman wins, we all win. As you learn how to live in harmony with your hormones, you become a beacon of hope for other women. Reach around you and find those who need a lifeline with their health. We can heal one another and create a new paradigm of health. A version of healthcare that works for all women. A paradigm where women heal women. The nurturing feminine way is one of collaboration, not competition. Let's rally around one another and honor the uniqueness we each bring to the world.

I am so honored to have been your guide on this *Eat Like a Girl* journey. Please know I am cheering you on. You can always reach out and find me on my socials or in my Reset Academy, where I am guiding thousands of women to better health. Keep believing in yourself! The world is ready for you to shine!

Hugs,

Dr. Mindy

APPENDIX A: OBESOGENS

Obesogens Found in Food

Acesulfame potassium (Sunett, Sweet One): This sweetener is commonly found in sugar-free and "diet" products, including soft drinks, fruit juices, ice creams, chewing gums, baked goods, and diabetic-friendly foods.

Aspartame (NutraSweet): Similar to acesulfame potassium, aspartame is used in many "diet" or sugar-free products, including diet sodas, sugar-free gum, low-calorie desserts, and yogurt, as well as a tabletop sweetener.

Polysorbate 80: It is often used as an emulsifier in foods like ice creams, whipped toppings, pickles, nondairy creamers, and some baked goods to improve texture and stability.

Benzoates (e.g., sodium benzoate): Found in acidic foods such as carbonated drinks, fruit juices, and pickles, as well as in condiments like ketchup and salad dressings, to inhibit microbial growth.

Propionate (e.g., calcium propionate): Used as a preservative in baked goods such as bread, cakes, and pastries to prevent mold and bacterial growth.

Butylated hydroxyanisole and butylated hydroxytoluene (BHA and BHT): These are found in a variety of foods, including cereals, snack foods, chewing gum, and preserved meats, to prevent oxidation and extend shelf life.

Saccharin: Like other artificial sweeteners, it's used in "diet" beverages, sugar-free candies, and chewing gums, and as a tabletop sweetener. It was once a common sweetener in "diet" soft drinks before being largely replaced by other sweeteners.

Carboxymethyl cellulose (CMC or cellulose gum): This thickener and stabilizer is found in ice creams, milk products, dressings, and sauces, and it is often used in gluten-free and reduced-fat food products.

Sucralose: Marketed under the brand name Splenda, it's used in a similar manner to aspartame and saccharin, and it is found in "diet" drinks and sugar-free desserts, and as a tabletop sweetener.

Sulfites (e.g., sodium sulfite): These are used as preservatives in dried fruits, wine, beer, and some packed seafood to prevent oxidation and preserve freshness.

Monosodium glutamate (MSG): Commonly added to savory snacks, soups, and stock cubes, and used in Asian cuisine to enhance flavor.

Perfluoroalkyl substances (PFAS): These chemicals are sometimes used in food packaging materials, such as grease-resistant paper and cardboard containers.

Polychlorinated biphenyls (PCBs): Although largely banned, PCBs can still be present in some fatty foods, especially those high in animal fats, due to their persistence in the environment.

Organophosphate pesticides: These are commonly used in agriculture and can be found as residues on fruits, vegetables, grains, and other food products.

Growth hormones: Some conventionally raised livestock may be treated with growth hormones, which can then be consumed through meat and dairy products.

High-fructose corn syrup (HFCS): Used as a sweetener in many processed foods and beverages, HFCS has been linked to obesity and metabolic disorders in some studies.

Heavy metals: Heavy metals, such as lead, mercury, arsenic, and cadmium, can be found in certain foods due to environmental contamination, agricultural practices, or processing methods. Common food sources of heavy metals are seafood, rice, certain fruit juices, water, processed foods, and inexpensive supplements.

HEALTHY KITCHEN UTENSIL ALTERNATIVES

To minimize exposure to obesogens, consider using these safer alternatives:

- Stainless-steel or cast-iron cookware instead of nonstick cookware.
- Silicone or wooden kitchen utensils instead of plastic ones.
- Glass or stainless-steel food storage containers instead of plastic ones.

Regularly inspect and replace kitchen items that show signs of wear or damage to prevent leaching of chemicals into food.

Choosing high-quality, durable kitchen items and avoiding products with questionable materials or coatings can help reduce exposure to obesogens in the kitchen.

30-DAY FASTING RESET / OMNIVORE

SUNDAY	MONDAY	TUESDAY	WEDNESDAY	THURSDAY	FRIDAY	SATURDAY
	DAY 1 | K	DAY 2 | K	DAY 3 | K	DAY 4 | K	DAY 5 | K	DAY 6 | K
	Day 1 of Cycle	**Power Phase 1**	**Power Phase 1**	**Power Phase 1**	**Power Phase 1**	**Power Phase 1**
	BEGINNER	BEGINNER	BEGINNER	BEGINNER	BEGINNER	BEGINNER
	IF: 13 hours	**IF:** 13 hours	**IF:** 13 hours	**IF:** 13 hours	**IF:** 15 hours	**IF:** 17 hours
	BF: Heal Your Body Smoothie	**BF:** Spinach, Kale, and Goat Cheese Frittata	**BF:** Fat-Bomb Smoothie	**BF:** Soft Scrambled Eggs with Za'atar and Feta	**BF:** Chocolate Almond Chia Pudding (no syrup)	**BF:** Coconut Oil Fudge (no sugar)
	L: Buddha Bowl (no syrup)	**L:** Avocado and Brazil Nut Salad (add protein)	**L:** Spanish Tomato and Tuna Salad (no sugar)	**L:** Cauliflower Rice Bowl (add protein)	**L:** Probiotic Bowl	**L:** Miso and Ginger Poke Bowl (no honey)
	D: Miso-Marinated Grilled Pork and Turmeric Sauerkraut	**D:** Salmon with Furikake (no sugar) and Korean Pickled Cucumbers	**D:** Lemongrass Chicken and Marinated Mushroom Salad	**D:** Chicken Cacciatore and Gazpacho	**D:** Kelp Noodle Pad Thai (no brown sugar; add protein)	**FS:** Fasting Herb Salad
	ADVANCED	ADVANCED	ADVANCED	ADVANCED	ADVANCED	ADVANCED
	IF: 15 hours (see menu above)	**IF:** 15 hours (see menu above)	**IF:** 15 hours (see menu above)	**IF:** 15 hours (see menu above)	**IF:** 15 hours (see menu above)	**F:** 24 hours
						***FS:** See menu above
						BF: Beef Bone Broth and ACV Turmeric Tea (no honey)
						***D:** Marinated Mushroom Salad (add protein)

LEGEND: BF = Break Fast, **FS** = Fasted Snack, **B** = Breakfast, **L** = Lunch, **D** = Dinner, **d** = Dessert,
K = Ketobiotic, HF = Hormone Feasting, **IF** = Intermittent Fasting, **A** = Autophagy, **F** = Fasting, ***** = Optional Meal

SUNDAY	MONDAY	TUESDAY	WEDNESDAY	THURSDAY	FRIDAY	SATURDAY
DAY 7 K	DAY 8 K	DAY 9 K	DAY 10 K	DAY 11 HF	DAY 12 HF	DAY 13 HF
Power Phase 1	**Power Phase 1**	**Power Phase 1**	**Power Phase 1**	**Manifestation**	**Manifestation**	**Manifestation**
BEGINNER AND ADVANCED	BEGINNER AND ADVANCED	BEGINNER AND ADVANCED	BEGINNER AND ADVANCED	BEGINNER	BEGINNER	BEGINNER
A: 17 hours	**A:** 17 hours	**A:** 17 hours	**A:** 17 hours	**IF:** 13 hours	**IF:** 13 hours	**IF:** 13 hours
BF: Nutty Granola Parfait (no syrup)	**BF:** Choco Maca Smoothie	**BF:** Chocolate Almond Chia Pudding (no syrup)	**BF:** Guacamole with Vegetable Chips	**BF:** Choco Maca Smoothie	**BF:** Purple Quinoa Porridge	**BF:** Japanese Savory Pancake
L: Turmeric Eggs with Smoked Salmon and Goat Cheese	**L:** Kimchi Edamame Bowl and Functional Mushroom Broth	**L:** Turkish Eggs with Yogurt and Chili Brown Butter	**L:** Probiotic Bowl	**L:** Buddha Bowl	**L:** Mediterranean Quinoa Salad (add protein)	**L:** Tortilla Española and Mexican-Style Pickled Jalapeños and Carrots
*FS: Lemon Basil Chia Seed Drink	***FS:** ACV Turmeric Tea (no honey)	***FS:** Fasting Herb Salad	***FS:** Lime Ginger Mint Mocktail	**D:** Socca Pizza (add protein topping)	**D:** Portuguese Pork, Kale, and Potato Stew	**D:** Spanish Garlic Shrimp and All the Greens Bowl
				*d: Maple Peanut Butter Fudge	***d:** Date Bark	***d:** Strawberry-and-Cream Protein Pops
				ADVANCED	ADVANCED	ADVANCED
				IF: 15 hours (see menu above)	**IF:** 15 hours (see menu above)	**IF:** 15 hours (see menu above)

30-DAY FASTING RESET / OMNIVORE   CONTINUED

SUNDAY	MONDAY	TUESDAY	WEDNESDAY	THURSDAY	FRIDAY	SATURDAY
DAY 14 HF	**DAY 15** HF	**DAY 16** K	**DAY 17** K	**DAY 18** K	**DAY 19** K	**DAY 20** HF
Manifestation	**Manifestation**	**Power Phase 2**	**Power Phase 2**	**Power Phase 2**	**Power Phase 2**	**Nurture**
BEGINNER	BEGINNER	BEGINNER	BEGINNER	BEGINNER	BEGINNER	BEGINNER
IF: 13 hours	**IF:** 13 hours	**IF:** 15 hours	**IF:** 15 hours	**IF:** 15 hours	**IF:** 15 hours	No fasting (See menu below)
BF: Nutty Granola Parfait	**BF:** Pumpkin Protein Pancakes	**BF:** Gazpacho	**BF:** Coconut Oil Fudge (no syrup)	**BF:** Fat-Bomb Smoothie	**BF:** Nutty Granola Parfait (no syrup)	
L: Height-of-Summer Veggie Salad (add protein)	**L:** Chana Masala (add protein) and Arugula Salad	**L:** Miso and Ginger Poke Bowl	**L:** Tahini Kale Salad (add protein)	**L:** Black-Eyed Pea Crunch Salad	**L:** Chana Masala (no sugar) and Gazpacho	
D: Lasagna (add protein) and Gazpacho	**D:** Greek Lamb T-Bones with Whipped Feta and Red, White, and Green Salad	**D:** Fettuccine "Alfredo" (add protein) and Marinated Mushroom Salad	**D:** Miso-Marinated Grilled Pork and Arugula Salad	**D:** Chicken Cacciatore and Pomegranate Grilled Asparagus with Cashew "Ricotta"	**D:** Spanish Garlic Shrimp and Turmeric Sauerkraut	
***d:** Date Bark	***d:** Chocolate Almond Chia Pudding					
ADVANCED	ADVANCED	ADVANCED	ADVANCED	ADVANCED	ADVANCED	ADVANCED
IF: 15 hours (see menu above)	**IF:** 15 hours (see menu above)	**F:** 24 hours	**A:** 17 hours	**A:** 17 hours	**A:** 17 hours	**IF:** 13 hours
		***FS:** Fat-Bomb Smoothie	**BF:** Beef Bone Broth	**BF:** Chicken Bone Broth	**BF:** Walnut Pâté and (5) Fasting Crackers	**B:** Purple Quinoa Porridge
		BF: Chicken Bone Broth	**L:** See menu above	**L:** See menu above	**L:** See menu above	**L:** Buddha Bowl
		***D:** See menu above	**FS:** Fasting Herb Salad	**FS:** Lime Ginger Mint Mocktail	**FS:** Coconut Oil Fudge (no syrup)	**D:** Beef Stew with Beer and Fasting Crackers or Guacamole with Vegetable Chips
						***d:** Date Bark

LEGEND: BF = Break Fast, **FS** = Fasted Snack, **B** = Breakfast, **L** = Lunch, **D** = Dinner, **d** = Dessert,
K = Ketobiotic, HF = Hormone Feasting, **IF** = Intermittent Fasting, **A** = Autophagy, **F** = Fasting, ***** = Optional Meal

SUNDAY	MONDAY	TUESDAY	WEDNESDAY	THURSDAY	FRIDAY	SATURDAY
DAY 21 (HF)	DAY 22 (HF)	DAY 23 (HF)	DAY 24 (HF)	DAY 25 (HF)	DAY 26 (HF)	DAY 27 (HF)
Nurture	**Nurture**	**Nurture**	**Nurture**	**Nurture**	**Nurture**	**Nurture**
BEGINNER	BEGINNER	BEGINNER	BEGINNER	BEGINNER	BEGINNER	BEGINNER
No fasting (See menu below)	No fasting (See menu below)	No fasting (See menu below)	No fasting (See menu below)	No fasting (See menu below)	No fasting (See menu below)	No fasting (See menu below)
ADVANCED	ADVANCED	ADVANCED	ADVANCED	ADVANCED	ADVANCED	ADVANCED
IF: 13 hours	**IF:** 13 hours	**IF:** 13 hours	**IF:** 13 hours	**IF:** 13 hours	**IF:** 13 hours	**IF:** 13 hours
B: Choco Maca Smoothie	**B:** Nutty Granola Parfait	**B:** Wild Blueberry Smoothie	**B:** Chia Protein Bars	**B:** Protein Banana Donut Holes	**B:** Purple Quinoa Porridge	**B:** Heal Your Body Smoothie
L: Spanish Tomato and Tuna Salad	**L:** Navy Bean Tuscan Kale Soup (add protein) and Fasting Crackers	**L:** Red, White, and Green Salad (add protein)	**L:** Buddha Bowl (add protein)	**L:** Lentil Soup (add protein) and Fasting Crackers	**L:** Kelp Noodle Pad Thai (add protein)	**L:** All the Greens Bowl (add protein)
D: Sardine Tostadas and Tahini Kale Salad	**D:** Chicken Cacciatore and Mediterranean Quinoa Salad	**D:** Red Thai Curry (add protein) and Gazpacho	**D:** Chili-Loaded Sweet Potato (add protein) and Avocado and Brazil Nut Salad	**D:** Socca Pizza (add protein topping) and Korean-Style Pickled Cucumbers	**D:** Lemongrass Chicken and Arugula Salad	**D:** Southwest Steak and Sweet Potato Hash and Pickled Red Onions
*d: Maple Peanut Butter Fudge	***d:** Chocolate Almond Chia Pudding	***d:** Coconut Oil Fudge	***d:** Coconut Oil Fudge	***d:** Date Bark	***d:** Keto Basque Cheesecake and Salted Caramel Sauce	***d:** Keto Basque Cheesecake and Salted Caramel Sauce

30-DAY FASTING RESET / OMNIVORE   CONTINUED

SUNDAY	MONDAY	TUESDAY	WEDNESDAY	THURSDAY	FRIDAY	SATURDAY
DAY 28 | HF **Nurture**	DAY 29 | HF **Nurture**	DAY 30 | HF **Nurture**				
BEGINNER	BEGINNER	BEGINNER				
No fasting (See menu below)	No fasting (See menu below)	No fasting (See menu below)				
ADVANCED	ADVANCED	ADVANCED				
IF: 13 hours	**IF:** 13 hours	**IF:** 13 hours				
B: Turmeric Eggs with Smoked Salmon and Goat Cheese and Orange Chia Seed Muffin	**B:** Turkish Eggs with Yogurt and Chili Brown Butter	**B:** Southwest Steak and Sweet Potato Hash				
L: Buddha Bowl (add protein)	**L:** Mediterra-nean Quinoa Salad (add protein)	**L:** Black-Eyed Pea Crunch Salad (add protein)				
D: Lasagna (add protein) and Red, White, and Green Salad	**D:** Red Thai Curry (add protein) and Gazpacho	**D:** Portuguese Pork, Kale, and Potato Stew and Fasting Crackers				
***d:** Flourless Chocolate Almond Torte	***d:** Flourless Chocolate Almond Torte and Salted Caramel Sauce	***d:** Strawberry-and-Cream Protein Pops				

LEGEND: BF = Break Fast, **FS** = Fasted Snack, **B** = Breakfast, **L** = Lunch, **D** = Dinner, **d** = Dessert,
K = Ketobiotic, **HF** = Hormone Feasting, **IF** = Intermittent Fasting, **A** = Autophagy, **F** = Fasting, ***** = Optional Meal

30-DAY FASTING RESET / PLANT-BASED

MONDAY	TUESDAY	WEDNESDAY	THURSDAY	FRIDAY	SATURDAY
DAY 1	Ⓚ	DAY 2	Ⓚ	DAY 3	Ⓚ	DAY 4	Ⓚ	DAY 5	Ⓚ	DAY 6	Ⓚ
Day 1 of Cycle	**Power Phase 1**	**Power Phase 1**	**Power Phase 1**	**Power Phase 1**	**Power Phase 1**
BEGINNER	BEGINNER	BEGINNER	BEGINNER	BEGINNER	BEGINNER
IF: 13 hours	**IF:** 13 hours	**IF:** 13 hours	**IF:** 13 hours	**IF:** 15 hours	**IF:** 17 hours
BF: Heal Your Body Smoothie	**BF:** Walnut Pâté and (5) Fasting Crackers	**BF:** Fat-Bomb Smoothie	**BF:** Gazpacho and (5) Fasting Crackers	**BF:** Tofu Scramble	**BF:** Chocolate Almond Chia Pudding (no syrup)
L: Buddha Bowl (no syrup)	**L:** Avocado and Brazil Nut Salad and Chia Protein Bar	**L:** Tahini Kale Salad and Pomegranate Grilled Asparagus with Cashew "Ricotta" and Roasted Garlic Dressing	**L:** Black-Eyed Pea Crunch Salad	**L:** Probiotic Bowl	**L:** Marinated Mushroom Salad and Turmeric Sauerkraut
D: Tempeh and Broccoli with Forbidden Rice and Keto Pickled Ginger	**D:** Kimchi Edamame Bowl and Korean-Style Pickled Cucumbers	**D:** Zucchini String Bean Soup and Fasting Crackers	**D:** Cauliflower Rice Bowl and Chia Protein Bar	**D:** Kelp Noodle Pad Thai (no sugar)	**FS:** Fasting Herb Salad
ADVANCED	ADVANCED	ADVANCED	ADVANCED	ADVANCED	ADVANCED
IF: 15 hours (see menu above)	**IF:** 15 hours (see menu above)	**IF:** 15 hours (see menu above)	**IF:** 15 hours (see menu above)	**IF:** 15 hours (see menu above)	**F:** 24 hours
					*FS: See menu above
					BF: Functional Mushroom Broth and ACV Turmeric Tea (no honey)
					*D: Kimchi Edamame Bowl

LEGEND: BF = Break Fast, **FS** = Fasted Snack, **B** = Breakfast, **L** = Lunch, **D** = Dinner, **d** = Dessert,
Ⓚ = Ketobiotic, Ⓗ = Hormone Feasting, **IF** = Intermittent Fasting, **A** = Autophagy, **F** = Fasting, ***** = Optional Meal

30-DAY FASTING RESET / PLANT-BASED CONTINUED

SUNDAY	MONDAY	TUESDAY	WEDNESDAY	THURSDAY	FRIDAY	SATURDAY
DAY 7 | K	DAY 8 | K	DAY 9 | K	DAY 10 | K	DAY 11 | HF	DAY 12 | HF	DAY 13 | HF
Power Phase 1	**Power Phase 1**	**Power Phase 1**	**Power Phase 1**	**Manifestation**	**Manifestation**	**Manifestation**
BEGINNER AND ADVANCED	BEGINNER AND ADVANCED	BEGINNER AND ADVANCED	BEGINNER AND ADVANCED	BEGINNER	BEGINNER	BEGINNER
A: 17 hours	**A:** 17 hours	**A:** 17 hours	**A:** 17 hours	**IF:** 13 hours	**IF:** 13 hours	**IF:** 13 hours
BF: Nutty Granola Parfait (no syrup)	**BF:** Olive Tapenade and (5) Fasting Crackers	**BF:** Fat-Bomb Smoothie	**BF:** Coconut Oil Fudge (no syrup)	**BF:** Chickpea "Omelet" and Orange Chia Seed Muffin	**BF:** Japanese Savory Pancake (use Dashi or water)	**BF:** Choco Maca Smoothie
L: Gazpacho and (5) Fasting Crackers	**L:** Cauliflower Rice Bowl	**L:** Kelp Noodle Pad Thai (no sugar)	**L:** Probiotic Bowl	**L:** Buddha Bowl	**L:** Mediterranean Quinoa Salad	**L:** Black-Eyed Pea Crunch Salad
*FS: Lemon Basil Chia Seed Drink	***FS:** Cherry-Mint Mocktail	***FS:** Fasting Herb Salad	***FS:** Lime Ginger Mint Mocktail	**D:** Fettuccine "Alfredo" and Pomegranate Grilled Asparagus with Cashew "Ricotta"	**D:** Quinoa Tabbouleh and Grilled Tofu	**D:** Lentil Mushroom Sweet Potato Shepherd's Pie and Arugula Salad
				*d: Chia Protein Bars	***d:** Date Bark	***d:** Strawberry-and-Cream Protein Pops
				ADVANCED	ADVANCED	ADVANCED
				IF: 15 hours (see menu above)	**IF:** 15 hours (see menu above)	**IF:** 15 hours (see menu above)

LEGEND: BF = Break Fast, **FS** = Fasted Snack, **B** = Breakfast, **L** = Lunch, **D** = Dinner, **d** = Dessert,
K = Ketobiotic, HF = Hormone Feasting, **IF** = Intermittent Fasting, **A** = Autophagy, **F** = Fasting, ***** = Optional Meal

SUNDAY	MONDAY	TUESDAY	WEDNESDAY	THURSDAY	FRIDAY	SATURDAY
DAY 14 (HF) **Manifestation**	**DAY 15** (HF) **Manifestation**	**DAY 16** (K) **Power Phase 2**	**DAY 17** (K) **Power Phase 2**	**DAY 18** (K) **Power Phase 2**	**DAY 19** (K) **Power Phase 2**	**DAY 20** (HF) **Nurture**
BEGINNER	BEGINNER	BEGINNER	BEGINNER	BEGINNER	BEGINNER	BEGINNER
IF: 13 hours	**IF:** 13 hours	**IF:** 15 hours	**IF:** 15 hours	**IF:** 15 hours	**IF:** 15 hours	No fasting (See menu below)
BF: Nutty Granola Parfait	**BF:** Pumpkin Protein Pancakes	**BF:** Functional Mushroom Broth	**BF:** Chia Protein Bars	**BF:** Fat-Bomb Smoothie	**BF:** Kimchi Edamame Bowl	
L: Height-of-Summer Veggie Salad	**L:** All the Greens Bowl	**L:** Black-Eyed Pea Crunch Salad	**L:** Tahini Kale Salad and Gazpacho	**L:** Marinated Mushroom Salad and Pumpkin Soup	**L:** Tofu Scramble and Turmeric Sauerkraut	
D: Lasagna and Pomegranate Grilled Asparagus with Cashew "Ricotta"	**D:** Chana Masala and Red, White, and Green Salad	**D:** Tempeh and Broccoli with Forbidden Rice and Keto Pickled Ginger	**D:** Kimchi Edamame Bowl	**D:** Mediterranean Quinoa Salad and Turmeric Sauerkraut	**D:** Kelp Noodle Pad Thai (no sugar)	
*d: Flourless Chocolate Almond Torte (V)	***d:** Flourless Chocolate Almond Torte (V)					
ADVANCED	ADVANCED	ADVANCED	ADVANCED	ADVANCED	ADVANCED	ADVANCED
IF: 15 hours (see menu above)	**IF:** 15 hours (see menu above)	**F:** 24 hours	**A:** 17 hours	**A:** 17 hours	**A:** 17 hours	**IF:** 13 hours
		*FS: ACV Turmeric Tea (no honey)	**BF:** Functional Mushroom Broth	**BF:** Functional Mushroom Broth	**BF:** See menu above	**B:** Purple Quinoa Porridge
		BF: See menu above	**L:** See menu above	**L:** See menu above	**L:** See menu above	**L:** Buddha Bowl
		*D: Probiotic Bowl	**FS:** Fasting Herb Salad	**FS:** Lime Ginger Mint Mocktail	**FS:** Coconut Oil Fudge (no syrup)	**D:** Black Bean Soup and Guacamole with Vegetable Chips
						*d: Date Bark

30-DAY FASTING RESET / PLANT-BASED CONTINUED

SUNDAY	MONDAY	TUESDAY	WEDNESDAY	THURSDAY	FRIDAY	SATURDAY
DAY 21 (HF) **Nurture**	**DAY 22** (HF) **Nurture**	**DAY 23** (HF) **Nurture**	**DAY 24** (HF) **Nurture**	**DAY 25** (HF) **Nurture**	**DAY 26** (HF) **Nurture**	**DAY 27** (HF) **Nurture**
BEGINNER	BEGINNER	BEGINNER	BEGINNER	BEGINNER	BEGINNER	BEGINNER
No fasting (See menu below)	No fasting (See menu below)	No fasting (See menu below)	No fasting (See menu below)	No fasting (See menu below)	No fasting (See menu below)	No fasting (See menu below)
ADVANCED	ADVANCED	ADVANCED	ADVANCED	ADVANCED	ADVANCED	ADVANCED
IF: 13 hours	**IF:** 13 hours	**IF:** 13 hours	**IF:** 13 hours	**IF:** 13 hours	**IF:** 13 hours	**IF:** 13 hours
B: Chocolate Almond Chia Pudding	**B:** Your Best Workout Smoothie	**B:** Wild Blueberry Smoothie	**B:** Choco Maca Smoothie	**B:** Protein Banana Donut Holes	**B:** Heal Your Body Smoothie	**B:** Pumpkin Protein Pancake
L: Navy Bean Tuscan Kale Soup and Fasting Crackers	**L:** Buddha Bowl	**L:** Black Bean Soup and Red, White, and Green Salad	**L:** Spaghetti Lentil Bolognese and Gazpacho	**L:** Lentil Soup and Fasting Crackers	**L:** Kelp Noodle Pad Thai	**L:** All the Greens Bowl and Fasting Crackers
D: Sweet Potato and Tempeh Tacos and Arugula Salad	**D:** Red Thai Curry (with forbidden rice)	**D:** Lasagna and Fasting Herb Salad	**D:** Chili-Loaded Sweet Potato and Pomegranate Grilled Asparagus with Cashew "Ricotta"	**D:** Socca Pizza and Arugula Salad	**D:** Chana Masala and Arugula Salad	**D:** Split Pea Soup with Chickpea Crunchies
***d:** Maple Peanut Butter Fudge (V)	***d:** Strawberry and Cream Protein Pops	***d:** Date Bark	***d:** Coconut Oil Fudge	***d:** Date Bark	***d:** Maple Peanut Butter Fudge (V)	***d:** Maple Peanut Butter Fudge (V)

LEGEND: BF = Break Fast, **FS** = Fasted Snack, **B** = Breakfast, **L** = Lunch, **D** = Dinner, **d** = Dessert,
(K) = Ketobiotic, (HF) = Hormone Feasting, **IF** = Intermittent Fasting, **A** = Autophagy, **F** = Fasting, * = Optional Meal

SUNDAY	MONDAY	TUESDAY
DAY 28	HF	DAY 29	HF	DAY 30	HF
Nurture	**Nurture**	**Nurture**
BEGINNER	BEGINNER	BEGINNER
No fasting (See menu below)	No fasting (See menu below)	No fasting (See menu below)
ADVANCED	ADVANCED	ADVANCED
IF: 13 hours	**IF:** 13 hours	**IF:** 13 hours
B: Tofu Scramble and Orange Chia Seed Muffin	**B:** Purple Quinoa Porridge	**B:** Choco Maca Smoothie
L: Chili-Loaded Sweet Potato and Arugula Salad	**L:** Mediterranean Quinoa Salad	**L:** Black-Eyed Pea Crunch Salad
D: Lentil Mushroom Sweet Potato Shepherd's Pie and Gazpacho	**D:** Sweet Potato and Tempeh Tacos and Avocado and Brazil Nut Salad	**D:** Quinoa Tabbouleh and Grilled Tofu
*d: Flourless Chocolate Almond Torte (V)	***d:** Flourless Chocolate Almond Torte (V)	***d:** Strawberry-and-Cream Protein Pops

METRIC CONVERSION CHART

STANDARD CUP	FINE POWDER (E.G., FLOUR)	GRAIN (E.G., RICE)	GRANULAR (E.G., SUGAR)	LIQUID SOLIDS (E.G., BUTTER)	LIQUID (E.G., MILK)
1	140 g	150 g	190 g	200 g	240 ml
¾	105 g	113 g	143 g	150 g	180 ml
⅔	93 g	100 g	125 g	133 g	160 ml
½	70 g	75 g	95 g	100 g	120 ml
⅓	47 g	50 g	63 g	67 g	80 ml
¼	35 g	38 g	48 g	50 g	60 ml
⅛	18 g	19 g	24 g	25 g	30 ml

USEFUL EQUIVALENTS FOR COOKING/OVEN TEMPERATURES

Process	Fahrenheit	Celsius	Gas Mark
Freeze Water	32°F	0°C	
Room Temperature	68°F	20°C	
Boil Water	212°F	100°C	
Bake	325°F	160°C	3
	350°F	180°C	4
	375°F	190°C	5
	400°F	200°C	6
	425°F	220°C	7
	450°F	230°C	8
Broil			Grill

USEFUL EQUIVALENTS FOR LIQUID INGREDIENTS BY VOLUME

¼ tsp				1 ml
½ tsp				2 ml
1 tsp				5 ml
3 tsp	1 tbsp		½ fl oz	15 ml
	2 tbsp	⅛ cup	1 fl oz	30 ml
	4 tbsp	¼ cup	2 fl oz	60 ml
	5⅓ tbsp	⅓ cup	3 fl oz	80 ml
	8 tbsp	½ cup	4 fl oz	120 ml
	10⅔ tbsp	⅔ cup	5 fl oz	160 ml
	12 tbsp	¾ cup	6 fl oz	180 ml
	16 tbsp	1 cup	8 fl oz	240 ml
	1 pt	2 cups	16 fl oz	480 ml
	1 qt	4 cups	32 fl oz	960 ml

USEFUL EQUIVALENTS FOR DRY INGREDIENTS BY WEIGHT

(To convert ounces to grams, multiply the number of ounces by 30.)

1 oz	¹⁄₁₆ lb	30 g
4 oz	¼ lb	120 g
8 oz	½ lb	240 g
12 oz	¾ lb	360 g
16 oz	1 lb	480 g

USEFUL EQUIVALENTS FOR LENGTH

(To convert inches to centimeters, multiply the number of inches by 2.5.)

1 in			2.5 cm	
6 in	½ ft		15 cm	
12 in	1 ft		30 cm	
36 in	3 ft	1 yd	90 cm	
40 in			100 cm	1 m

DR. MINDY'S
FAVORITE RESOURCES

If you're interested in exploring some of my favorite products, simply scan the QR code below to access my resource page. There, you'll find products that I've carefully researched and personally use for both myself and my patients. These items are provided by some truly wonderful, heart-centered people who specialize in unique, toxin-free solutions to enhance your health journey. Be sure to check for special discounts exclusive to readers of this book.

Cheers to healthy living!

ENDNOTES

Chapter 1: How to Eat for Your Hormones

1. Helena Bottemiller Evich, "The FDA's Food Failure," *Politico*, April 8, 2022, https://www.politico.com/interactives/2022/fda-fails-regulate-food-health-safety-hazards/.

2. Angela Amico et al., "The Demise of Artificial Trans Fat: A History of a Public Health Achievement," *The Milbank Quarterly* 99, no. 3 (September 2021): 746–70, https://doi.org/10.1111%2F1468-0009.12515.

3. Lisa Lefferts, *Obesogens: Assessing the Evidence Linking Chemicals in Food to Obesity*, Washington, D.C.: Center for Science in the Public Interest, January 2023, https://www.cspinet.org/sites/default/files/2023-02/CSPI_Obesogens_Report_2-2023.pdf.

4. World Health Organization, *Obesity and Overweight Fact Sheet*, accessed April 14, 2024, https://www.who.int/news-room/fact-sheets/detail/obesity-and-overweight.

5. Lisa Lefferts, *Obesogens: Assessing the Evidence Linking Chemicals in Food to Obesity*.

6. Jiongxing Fu et al., "Dietary Fiber Intake and Gut Microbiota in Human Health," *Microorganisms* 10, no. 12 (December 2022): 2507, http://dx.doi.org/10.3390/microorganisms10122507.

7. Jacqueline A. Barnett, Maya L. Bandy, and Deanna L. Gibson, "Is the Use of Glyphosate in Modern Agriculture Resulting in Increased Neuropsychiatric Conditions through Modulation of the Gut-Brain-Microbiome Axis?," *Frontiers in Nutrition* 9 (March 8, 2022): 827384, https://doi.org/10.3389%2Ffnut.2022.827384.

8. Rie Matsuzaki et al., "Pesticide Exposure and the Microbiota-Gut-Brain Axis," *The ISME Journal* 17 (August 2023): 1153–66, https://doi.org/10.1038/s41396-023-01450-9.

9. Joint FAO/WHO/UNU Expert Consultation, *Protein and Amino Acid Requirements in Human Nutrition*, WHO Technical Report Series, 935 (Geneva, Switzerland: World Health Organization, 2007), 138, https://iris.who.int/bitstream/handle/10665/43411/WHO?sequence=1.

Chapter 3: The Eat Like a Girl Philosophy

1. Maura Palmery et al., "Oral Contraceptives and Changes in Nutritional Requirements," *European Review for Medical and Pharmacological Sciences* 17, no. 13 (July 2013): 1804–13, https://pubmed.ncbi.nlm.nih.gov/23852908/.

Chapter 4: Creating Fasting and Eating Windows

1. Pamela M. Peeke et al., "Effect of Time Restricted Eating on Body Weight and Fasting Glucose in Participants with Obesity: Results of a Randomized, Controlled, Virtual Clinical Trial," *Nutrition & Diabetes*, January 15, 2021, https://doi.org/10.1038/s41387-021-00149-0.

Chapter 5: Your First Meal Matters: The Art of Breaking Your Fast

1. Jessie Inchauspé, "Improving Health through Glucose Control," interview by Dr. Mindy Pelz, *The Resetter Podcast*, February 26, 2024, podcast, 38:17, https://drmindypelz.com/ep224/.

2. Hamed Mirzaei, Jorge A. Suarez, and Valter D. Longo, "Protein and Amino Acid Restriction, Aging and Disease: From Yeast to Humans," *Trends in Endocrinology and*

Metabolism 25, no. 11 (November 2014): 558–66, https://doi.org/10.1016/j.tem.2014.07.002.

3. Yan Zhao et al., *Frontiers in Cell and Developmental Biology* 9 (April 2021): 646482, https://doi.org/10.3389%2Ffcell.2021.646482.

4. Meerza Abdul Razak et al., "Multifarious Beneficial Effect of Nonessential Amino Acid, Glycine: A Review," *Oxidative Medicine and Cellular Longevity*, 1716701 (March 2017): 1–8, http://dx.doi.org/10.1155/2017/1716701.

Chapter 6: Your Power Phases

1. Christopher R. Cederroth and Serge Nef, "Soy, Phytoestrogens and Metabolism: A Review," *Molecular and Cellular Endocrinology* 304, no. 1–2 (May 25, 2009): 30–42, https://doi.org/10.1016/j.mce.2009.02.027.

2. I. J. Rowe and Rodney J. Baber, "The Effects of Phytoestrogens on Postmenopausal Health," *Climacteric* 24, no. 1 (February 2021): 57–63, https://doi.org/10.1080/13697137.2020.1863356.

3. T. Y. Tai et al., "The Effect of Soy Isoflavone on Bone Mineral Density in Postmenopausal Taiwanese Women with Bone Loss: A 2-Year Randomized Double-Blind Placebo-Controlled Study," *Osteoporosis International* 23, no. 5 (September 2011): 1571–80, https://doi.org/10.1007/s00198-011-1750-7; De-Fu Ma et al., "Soy Isoflavone Intake Increases Bone Mineral Density in the Spine of Menopausal Women: Meta-Analysis of Randomized Controlled Trials," *Clinical Nutrition* 27, no. 1 (February 2008): 57–64, https://doi.org/10.1016/j.clnu.2007.10.012.

4. Shiho Nakai, Mariko Fujita, and Yasutomi Kamei, "Health Promotion Effects of Soy Isoflavones," *Journal of Nutritional Science and Vitaminology* 66, no. 6 (December 2020): 502–7, https://doi.org/10.3177/jnsv.66.502.

5. Heyi Yang et al., "Proteomic Analysis of Menstrual Blood," *Molecular & Cellular Proteomics* 11, no. 10 (July 2012): 1024–35, http://dx.doi.org/10.1074/mcp.M112.018390.

6. Emily L. Silva et al., "Untargeted Metabolomics Reveals That Multiple Reproductive Toxicants Are Present at the Endometrium," *The Science of the Total Environment* 843, no. 6 (June 2022): 157005, http://dx.doi.org/10.1016/j.scitotenv.2022.157005.

Chapter 7: The Manifestation Phase

1. Nobuhiro Kawai et al., "The Sleep-Promoting and Hypothermic Effects of Glycine Are Mediated by NMDA Receptors in the Suprachiasmatic Nucleus," *Neuropsychopharmacology* 40, no. 6 (May 2015): 1405–16, http://dx.doi.org/10.1038/npp.2014.326.

Chapter 9: What to Do If You Have No Cycle

1. A. Janet Tomiyama et al., "Low Calorie Dieting Increases Cortisol," *Psychosomatic Medicine* 72, no. 4 (May 2010): 357–64, https://doi.org/10.1097%2FPSY.0b013e3181d9523c.

2. Maria M. Mihaylova et al., "Fasting Activates Fatty Acid Oxidation to Enhance Intestinal Stem Cell Function during Homeostasis and Aging," *Cell Stem Cell* 22, no. 5 (May 2019): 769–78, https://doi.org/10.1016%2Fj.stem.2018.04.001.

3. Rachel T. Buxton et al., "A Synthesis of Health Benefits of Natural Sounds and Their Distribution in National Parks," *Proceedings of the National Academy of Sciences* 118, no. 14 (April 2021): e2013097118, https://doi.org/10.1073/pnas.2013097118.

Chapter 10: The 30-Day Fasting Reset

1. Salk Institute for Biological Studies, "A Matter of Time: Living in Circadian Rhythm," *Inside Salk*, Winter 2018, https://inside.salk.edu/winter-2018/a-matter-of-time/.

BIBLIOGRAPHY

Amico, Angela, Margo G. Wootan, Michael F. Jacobson, Cindy Leung, and Walter Willett. "The Demise of Artificial Trans Fat: A History of a Public Health Achievement." *The Milbank Quarterly* 99, no. 3 (September 2021): 746–7. https://doi.org/10.1111%2F1468-0009.12515.

Barnett, Jacqueline A., Maya L. Bandy, and Deanna L. Gibson. "Is the Use of Glyphosate in Modern Agriculture Resulting in Increased Neuropsychiatric Conditions through Modulation of the Gut-Brain-Microbiome Axis?" *Frontiers in Nutrition* 9 (March 8, 2022): 827384. https://doi.org/10.3389%2Ffnut.2022.827384.

Buxton, Rachel T., Amber L. Pearson, Claudia Allou, and George Wittemyer. "A Synthesis of Health Benefits of Natural Sounds and Their Distribution in National Parks." *Proceedings of the National Academy of Sciences* 118, no. 14 (April 2021): e2013097118. https://doi.org/10.1073/pnas.2013097118.

Cederroth, Christopher R., and Serge Nef. "Soy, Phytoestrogens and Metabolism: A Review." *Molecular and Cellular Endocrinology* 304, no. 1–2 (May 25, 2009): 30–42. https://doi.org/10.1016/j.mce.2009.02.027.

Evich, Helena Bottemiller. "The FDA's Food Failure." *Politico*, April 8, 2022. https://www.politico.com/interactives/2022/fda-fails-regulate-food-health-safety-hazards/.

Fu, Jiongxing, Yan Zheng, Ying Gao, and Wanghong Xu. "Dietary Fiber Intake and Gut Microbiota in Human Health." *Microorganisms* 10, no. 12 (December 2022): 2507. http://dx.doi.org/10.3390/microorganisms10122507.

Inchauspé, Jesse. "Improving Health through Glucose Control." Interview by Dr. Mindy Pelz. *The Resetter Podcast*, February 26, 2024. Podcast, 38:17. https://drmindypelz.com/ep224/.

Joint FAO/WHO/UNU Expert Consultation. *Protein and Amino Acid Requirements in Human Nutrition*. WHO Technical Report Series, 935. Geneva, Switzerland: World Health Organization, 2007. https://iris.who.int/bitstream/handle/10665/43411/WHO?sequence=1.

Kawai, Nobuhiro, Noriaki Sakai, Masashi Okuro, Sachie Karakawa, Yosuke Tsuneyoshi, Noriko Kawasaki, Tomoko Takeda, Makoto Bannai, and Seiji Nishino. "The Sleep-Promoting and Hypothermic Effects of Glycine Are Mediated by NMDA Receptors in the Suprachiasmatic Nucleus." *Neuropsychopharmacology* 40, no. 6 (May 2015): 1405–16. http://dx.doi.org/10.1038/npp.2014.326.

Lefferts, Lisa. *Obesogens: Assessing the Evidence Linking Chemicals in Food to Obesity*. Washington, D.C.: Center for Science in the Public Interest, January 2023. https://www.cspinet.org/sites/default/files/2023-02/CSPI_Obesogens_Report_2-2023.pdf.

Ma, De-Fu, Li-Qiang Qin, Pei-Yu Wang, and Ryohei Katoh. "Soy Isoflavone Intake Increases Bone Mineral Density in the Spine of Menopausal Women: Meta-Analysis of Randomized Controlled Trials." *Clinical Nutrition* 27, no. 1 (February 2008): 57–64. https://doi.org/10.1016/j.clnu.2007.10.012.

Matsuzaki, Rie, Eoin Gunnigle, Violette Geissen, Gerard Clarke, Jatin Nagpal, and John F. Cryan. "Pesticide Exposure and the Microbiota-Gut-Brain Axis." *The ISME Journal* 17 (August 2023): 1153–66. https://doi.org/10.1038/s41396-023-01450-9.

Mihaylova, Maria M., Chia-Wei Cheng, Amanda Q. Cao, Surya Tripathi, Miyeko D. Mana, Khristian E. Bauer-Rowe, Monther Abu-Remaileh et al. "Fasting Activates Fatty Acid Oxidation to Enhance Intestinal Stem Cell Function during Homeostasis and Aging." *Cell Stem Cell* 22, no. 5 (May 2019): 769–78. https://doi.org/10.1016%2Fj.stem.2018.04.001.

Mirzaei, Hamed, Jorge A. Suarez, and Valter D. Longo. "Protein and Amino Acid Restriction, Aging and Disease: From Yeast to Humans." *Trends in Endocrinology and Metabolism* 25, no. 11 (November 2014): 558–66. https://doi.org/10.1016/j.tem.2014.07.002.

Nakai, Shiho, Mariko Fujita, and Yasutomi Kamei. "Health Promotion Effects of Soy Isoflavones." *Journal of Nutritional Science and Vitaminology* 66, no. 6 (December 2020): 502–7. https://doi.org/10.3177/jnsv.66.502.

Palmery, Maura, A. Saraceno. Alberto Vaiarelli, and Gianfranco Carlomagno. "Oral Contraceptives and Changes in Nutritional Requirements." *European Review for Medical and Pharmacological Sciences* 17, no. 13 (July 2013): 1804–13. https://pubmed.ncbi.nlm.nih.gov/23852908/.

Peeke, Pamela M., Frank L. Greenway, Sonja K. Billes, Dachuan Zhang, and Ken Fujioka. "Effect of Time Restricted Eating on Body Weight and Fasting Glucose in Participants with Obesity: Results of a Randomized, Controlled, Virtual Clinical Trial." *Nutrition & Diabetes*, January 15, 2021. https://doi.org/10.1038/s41387-021-00149-0.

Razak, Meerza Abdul, Pathan Shajahan Begum, Buddolla Viswanath, and Senthilkumar Rajagopal. "Multifarious Beneficial Effect of Nonessential Amino Acid, Glycine: A Review," *Oxidative Medicine and Cellular Longevity*, 1716701 (March 2017): 1–8. http://dx.doi.org/10.1155/2017/1716701.

Rowe, I. J., and Rodney J. Baber. "The Effects of Phytoestrogens on Postmenopausal Health." *Climacteric* 24, no. 1 (February 2021): 57–63. https://doi.org/10.1080/13697137.2020.1863356.

Salk Institute for Biological Studies. "A Matter of Time: Living in Circadian Rhythm." *Inside Salk*, Winter 2018. https://inside.salk.edu/winter-2018/a-matter-of-time/.

Silva, Emily L., Douglas I. Walker, Zoe Coates Fuentes, Brismar Pinto-Pacheco, Christine N. Metz, Peter K. Gregersen, and Shruthi Mahalingaiah. "Untargeted Metabolomics Reveals That Multiple Reproductive Toxicants Are Present at the Endometrium." *The Science of the Total Environment* 843, no. 6 (June 2022): 157005. http://dx.doi.org/10.1016/J.scitotenv.2022.157005.

Tai, T. Y., Keh Sung Tsai, S. T. Tu, J. S. Wu, Chingi Chang, C. L. Chen, N. S. Shaw, H. Y. Peng, S. Y. Wang, and Chih-Hsing Wu. "The Effect of Soy Isoflavone on Bone Mineral Density in Postmenopausal Taiwanese Women with Bone Loss: A 2-Year Randomized Double-Blind Placebo-Controlled Study." *Osteoporosis International* 23, no. 5 (September 2011): 1571–80. https://doi.org/10.1007/s00198-011-1750-7.

Tomiyama, A. Janet, Traci Mann, Danielle Vinas, Jeffrey M. Hunger, Jill DeJager, and Shelley E. Taylor. "Low Calorie Dieting Increases Cortisol." *Psychosomatic Medicine* 72, no. 4 (May 2010): 357–64. https://doi.org/10.1097%2FPSY.0b013e3181d9523c.

World Health Organization. *Obesity and Overweight Fact Sheet*. Accessed April 14, 2024. https://www.who.int/news-room/fact-sheets/detail/obesity-and-overweight.

Yang, Heyi, Bo Zhou, Mechthild Prinz, and Donald Siegel. "Proteomic Analysis of Menstrual Blood." *Molecular & Cellular Proteomics* 11, no. 10 (July 2012): 1024–35. http://dx.doi.org/10.1074/mcp.M112.018390.

Zhao, Yan, Jason Cholewa, Huayu Shang, Yueqin Yang, Xiaomin Ding, Qianjin Wang, Quansheng Su, Nelo Eidy Zanchi, and Zhi Xia. *Frontiers in Cell and Developmental Biology* 9 (April 2021): 646482. https://doi.org/10.3389%2Ffcell.2021.646482.

INDEX

RECIPES BY EATING STYLE

Ketobiotic Recipes

VEGAN, VEGETARIAN, AND OMNIVORE RECIPES

Vegan Recipes

Vegetarian Recipes

Omnivore Recipes

ACKNOWLEDGMENTS

MY FIRST WORDS of gratitude go to you. In a world where we have been taught to outsource our health to trendy diets, popular health influencers, expensive supplements, or expert doctors, your decision to learn how to take amazing care of your feminine body is the first step to taking your health power back. Recently, a cultural conversation has emerged around the health struggles that so many women are experiencing as they try and keep up with the demands of a patriarchal society. A definition of *patriarch* that rings true for me is any structure that has power over you. And to date, our healthcare system has acted in a patriarchal manner. Contrast that with a matriarchal approach, which encourages us to source our power from within ourselves. My deepest desire for you is that you keep turning within and start trusting the natural rhythms of your beautiful feminine body.

I have been blessed to have been guided by many incredible health practitioners along my own health journey. One practitioner, Dr. Luc De Schepper, literally saved my life. Dr. Luc guided me out of the ashes of a healing fire that was brewing inside me at 19 years old, when I was diagnosed with severe chronic fatigue syndrome. When other doctors gave up on me, Dr. Luc taught me how to use food to heal myself. At a tender young age, when I felt like my world was crashing in on me, Dr. Luc lifted me up and walked the path of healing with me. He showed me which foods were

destroying my body and which foods I needed to lean into to restore my health. Dr. Luc, if you are out there somewhere, know I have taken your passion for using food as medicine and am now sharing it with the world. I am forever grateful for your guidance, care, and support at an extremely dark moment in my life.

Putting together a book of this magnitude requires a team of incredibly dedicated people. What an impressive team rallied around this project! A massive thank-you goes to my amazing agent, Stephanie Tade, who wore many hats while I wrote this book—therapist, career advisor, plant-based enthusiast, chef curator, recipe tester, mindfulness expert, and patient listener. I am eternally grateful for your wisdom, support, and friendship. To Colleen Martell, my amazing collaborative writer and editor—thank you, thank you, thank you! Holy cow, girl! Without you, I could not have pulled this book together as fast as we did. I am so grateful for your willingness to walk the neuronal pathways of my mind, exploring all the wonderful ways we could arm women with empowering knowledge. I love writing books with you!

To the One+One Books packaging team— Kristin, Leah, Leslie, Mi Ae, Erin, Phyllis, Kay, Frances, and David—thank you for your persistence and vision to get this project out in what felt like the quickest timeline ever created for a book. Thank you as well to Erin, the brilliant photographer who put up with my exuberant family and made a day of posing for photos a whole lot of fun.

To my beautiful Hay House family—Reid, Mags, Patty, Melody, and Shannon—thank you for always believing in me, supporting my mission to empower women, and collaborating with me on projects we know will help change the direction of women's healthcare. I love that our universes are united!

To my amazing team, who shows up every day to support our massively growing audience. Thank you for caring as deeply as I do about the beautiful women who continue to reach out to us for support. I love serving health with all of you!

To my dedicated chefs, Leslie and Jeff, thank you for listening so intently to my vision to take your culinary magic and turn it into hormonal medicine. You both were such a joy to work with. I can't wait for the world to taste your culinary greatness! Having your masterful recipes live here in my book is an incredible honor.

Lastly, to my mom. Your vision for teaching Molly and me about the importance of healthy food set us up for lifelong health. Thank you for caring about the quality of the food we ate. My younger self may have grumbled a few thousand times as you said no to bringing sugary treats or trendy commercial food products into our home, but my adult self now stands in awe of your commitment to our health. Thank you for making my childhood home a health sanctuary. I feel so blessed to have been born into your arms.

ABOUT THE AUTHOR

DR. MINDY PELZ, DC, is a renowned advocate for women's health and is passionately committed to empowering women to embrace and trust their body's natural healing processes. With an extensive background in women's health, Dr. Mindy has developed groundbreaking approaches that help women navigate the complexities of hormonal fluctuations throughout different life stages and the specific needs of women as they age.

Throughout her career, Dr. Mindy has advised a diverse group of clients, ranging from celebrities and Olympic athletes to corporate and cultural leaders, helping them achieve their health goals. Her dedication to accessible health education is evident in her writing, speaking engagements, and podcast, *The Resetter Podcast*, which is a favored source for the latest health-science and wellness discussions.

Dr. Mindy is the author of several influential books, including international bestsellers *Fast Like a Girl* and *The Menopause Reset*. Her work has been featured on many top global podcasts, like *The Diary of a CEO*; *Feel Better, Live More*; *The Mel Robbins Podcast*; *Women of Impact*; and *Impact Theory*. Her YouTube channel, with over 80 million lifetime views, continues to be the go-to resource for fasting and women's health.

Dr. Mindy's educational journey began at the University of Kansas, where her studies focused on exercise physiology and nutritional sciences. She took her passion for studying the human body and went on to receive a Doctor of Chiropractic degree, graduating with clinical honors. She founded one of the largest lifestyle clinics in the San Francisco Bay Area, where her clinical practice focused largely on nutrition, detox, hormone education, and helping women and families customize a lifestyle to keep all family members healthy. She also serves as a faculty member at the American Academy of Anti-Aging Medicine.

Currently residing in California, Dr. Mindy continues to inspire and educate women worldwide, advocating for a holistic approach that integrates comprehensive dietary strategies, an understanding of hormonal health, the transformative power of fasting, and now, "eating like a girl."

HAY HOUSE TITLES OF RELATED INTEREST

YOU CAN HEAL YOUR LIFE, *the movie,*
starring Louise Hay & Friends
(available as an online streaming video)
www.hayhouse.com/louise-movie

THE SHIFT, *the movie,*
starring Dr. Wayne W. Dyer
(available as an online streaming video)
www.hayhouse.com/the-shift-movie

* * *

THE BONE BROTH SECRET:
A Culinary Adventure in Health, Beauty, and Longevity
by Louise Hay and Heather Dane

FAST LIKE A GIRL:
*A Woman's Guide to Using the Healing Power of Fasting
to Burn Fat, Boost Energy, and Balance Hormones*
by Dr. Mindy Pelz

FUEL UP:
*Harness the Power of Your Blender and
"Cheat" Your Way to Good Health*
by Dana Cohen MD and Colin Sapire

THE OFFICIAL FAST LIKE A GIRL JOURNAL:
*A 60-Day Guided Journey to Healing, Self-Trust,
and Inner Wisdom Through Fasting*
by Dr. Mindy Pelz

REAL SUPERFOODS:
Everyday Ingredients to Elevate Your Health
by Ocean Robbins and Nichole Dandrea-Russert, MS, RDN

All of the above are available at your local bookstore,
or may be ordered by contacting Hay House (see next page).

We hope you enjoyed this Hay House book. If you'd like to receive our online catalog featuring additional information on Hay House books and products, or if you'd like to find out more about the Hay Foundation, please contact:

Hay House LLC, P.O. Box 5100, Carlsbad, CA 92018-5100
(760) 431-7695 or (800) 654-5126
www.hayhouse.com® • www.hayfoundation.org

———

Published in Australia by:
Hay House Australia Publishing Pty Ltd
18/36 Ralph St., Alexandria NSW 2015
Phone: +61 (02) 9669 4299
www.hayhouse.com.au

Published in the United Kingdom by:
Hay House UK Ltd
The Sixth Floor, Watson House,
54 Baker Street, London W1U 7BU
Phone: +44 (0) 203 927 7290
www.hayhouse.co.uk

Published in India by:
Hay House Publishers (India) Pvt Ltd
Muskaan Complex, Plot No. 3,
B-2, Vasant Kunj, New Delhi 110 070
Phone: +91 11 41761620
www.hayhouse.co.in

———

Let Your Soul Grow

Experience life-changing transformation—one video
at a time—with guidance from the world's leading experts.

www.healyourlifeplus.com

GET READY TO TRANSFORM YOUR HEALTH WITH THESE POWERFUL BOOKS BY DR. MINDY PELZ

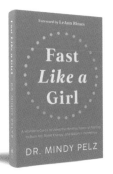

An INTERNATIONAL BESTSELLER, *WALL STREET JOURNAL* BESTSELLER, and *PUBLISHER'S WEEKLY* BESTSELLER!

Are you among the many women who feel unheard and unseen by their doctors and health professionals? Have you become exhausted by the promise of quick-fix diets that only leave you disappointed? Well in *Fast Like a Girl*, Dr. Mindy helps you to take back control of your health by using the quickest path back to better health—fasting.

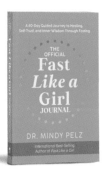

Join Dr. Mindy Pelz as she makes fasting easy to do and easy to understand in this 60-day fasting journal!

Never before has keeping track of your fasting been this simple! Dr. Mindy Pelz's new 60-day fasting journal is designed to make sure that you feel supported, encouraged, and inspired as you work your way through your fasting journey.

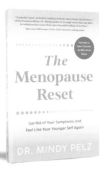

Are you struggling through your menopausal years?

As if from out of nowhere, you experience symptoms such as sleepless nights, irritable moods, unexplained anxiety, trouble retrieving words, and hot flashes. Your weight won't budge, no matter how hard you try. How great would it feel to wake up feeling rested; have a brain that is calm, joyful, and clear; and to finally lose weight in an easy and sustainable way? The good news is that there is a way for you to do all of this and more.

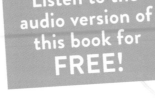

NOTES

NOTES

NOTES

NOTES